Hydrogen Sulfide in Kidney Diseases

George J. Dugbartey • Alp Sener

Hydrogen Sulfide in Kidney Diseases

A Novel Pharmacotherapy

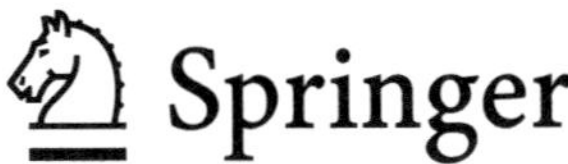 Springer

George J. Dugbartey
Department of Pharmacology
and Toxicology
School of Pharmacy, College of Health
Sciences, University of Ghana
Legon, Accra, Ghana

Alp Sener
Departments of Surgery and Microbiology
and Immunology
Schulich School of Medicine & Dentistry
Western University
London, ON, Canada

ISBN 978-3-031-44043-4   ISBN 978-3-031-44041-0   (eBook)
https://doi.org/10.1007/978-3-031-44041-0

This Springer imprint is published by the registered company Springer Nature Switzerland AG
The registered company address is: Gewerbestrasse 11, 6330 Cham, Switzerland

Paper in this product is recyclable.

This book is a product of my long walk from a difficult African background to the highest global stage of academia, and experimental and clinical medicine. I dedicate this book to my beloved mother, Hannah Akondo of blessed memory, and all my teachers at the various stages of my education, who went above and beyond the call of duty in my academic journey to success. I would like to make a special mention of my PhD project supervisor, Prof. Dr. Robert H. Henning, who mentored and introduced me into the promising scientific world of hydrogen sulfide research.
- George J. Dugbartey
It has been a tremendous journey to carry out the research that has enabled us to better understand the impact of hydrogen sulfide and its role in renal injury. None of this would have been possible without the dedication and effort of all students who have contributed to the body of research that has made this book possible—it has been an honor to be involved in their training. I dedicate this book to my dear wife (Melanie), my children (Ella and Brenden), and my parents (Isik and Ilhan) who have all been endless sources of inspiration, support, and encouragement.
- Alp Sener

Foreword

The quest for innovative therapies to combat kidney diseases is having its moment. However, existing clinically approved drugs offer limited efficacy, highlighting the need for a better understanding of the underlying pathological mechanisms. This understanding is crucial in developing more effective therapeutic strategies. In this context, it gives me great pleasure to introduce the book, "Hydrogen Sulfide in Kidney Diseases: A Novel Pharmacotherapy," authored by George J. Dugbartey and Alp Sener.

Within the pages of this enlightening volume, the authors present a collection of ten meticulously crafted chapters, each exploring a distinct aspect of therapeutic applications of hydrogen sulfide (H_2S) in nephrology. These chapters go beyond providing a mere enumeration of findings and observations; they guide the readers to examine the intricacies of the role of H_2S in renal health and disease. For example, it even delves into the potential of H_2S as a therapy for COVID-19-associated nephropathy, showcasing its relevance in addressing current health challenges.

Alp Sener's team is among the pioneers in the world who explored the role of H_2S in kidney transplantation. Their groundbreaking works, along with the works of many other research teams, shed light and offered promise on the therapeutic role of H_2S against a host of kidney diseases. With this insightful book, George J. Dugbartey and Alp Sener have bestowed upon us a gift—a comprehensive assimilation of the latest advancements in the field, which draws upon a wealth of preclinical studies that showcases the therapeutic potential of H_2S—that has the power to revolutionize the way we approach kidney diseases and, indeed, the broader field of medicine.

This timely book serves as an indispensable reference for those seeking to explore novel treatment modalities in nephrology. It is also a valuable resource for individuals engaged in the fundamental learning and research of H_2S biology and medicine. My heartiest congratulations to the authors on this laudable initiative.

I invite you to immerse yourself in the captivating world of hydrogen sulfide and its potential as a therapeutic marvel. This book stands as a testament to the indomitable spirit of scientific inquiry and human ingenuity, reminding us of the importance of being creative and imaginative in everything we do. Enjoy your reading experience.

Faculty of Science   Rui Wang, MD, PhD, FRSC, FCAHS, FAHA
York University
Toronto, ON, Canada

Preface

For over three centuries, hydrogen sulfide (H_2S) has been known as a toxic and deadly gas at high concentrations, with a distinctive smell of rotten eggs. However, studies over the past two decades have shown that H_2S has risen above its historically notorious label and has now received significant scientific attention as an endogenously produced gaseous signaling molecule that participates in cellular homeostasis and influences a myriad of physiological and pathological processes at low concentrations. Its production is enzymatically regulated, and when dysregulated, it contributes to pathogenesis of renal diseases. Several recent preclinical studies have demonstrated that at low micromolar concentrations, H_2S exhibits important therapeutic characteristics that target multiple molecular pathways and thereby prevent the development and progression of several pathologies. In the face of limited efficacy of available clinically approved drugs, the beneficial effect of exogenous H_2S administration as a potential alternative and/or a supplemental therapeutic agent targeted against common renal pathologies in which reduced levels of renal and plasma H_2S were observed should not be ignored. From preclinical and clinical perspectives, this book is topical and timely and seeks to lay the foundation for future clinical applications of H_2S in nephrology. The book serves as a good resource for both educational and didactic purposes towards novel alternative and/ or additional treatments of kidney diseases and other aspects of clinical medicine.

<table>
<tr><td>London, ON, Canada</td><td>George J. Dugbartey</td></tr>
<tr><td>London, ON, Canada</td><td>Alp Sener</td></tr>
</table>

Contents

1 Hydrogen Sulfide and the Renal System 1
George J. Dugbartey

2 Hydrogen Sulfide for Cisplatin- and Gentamicin-Induced Acute Kidney Injury 23
George J. Dugbartey

3 Hydrogen Sulfide as a Potential Future Therapy for Chronic Kidney Disease, Hyperhomocysteinemia, and Management of Polycystic Kidney Disease 39
George J. Dugbartey

4 Hydrogen Sulfide for Diabetic Kidney Disease and Focal Segmental Glomerulosclerosis 69
George J. Dugbartey

5 Hydrogen Sulfide for the Treatment of Hypertensive Nephropathy and Calcium-Based Nephrolithiasis 93
George J. Dugbartey

6 Hydrogen Sulfide as a Potential Therapy for COVID-19-Associated Nephropathy 119
George J. Dugbartey, Karl K. Alornyo, Vincent Boima,
Sampson Antwi, and Alp Sener

7 Hydrogen Sulfide for Prevention of Obstructive Nephropathy 143
Shouzhe Lin, Smriti Juriasingani, George J. Dugbartey,
and Alp Sener

8 Hydrogen Sulfide Therapy as the Future of Renal Graft Preservation 159
George J. Dugbartey, Hjalmar R. Bouma, Manujendra N. Saha,
Ian Lobb, Robert H. Henning, and Alp Sener

9 Hydrogen Sulfide Against Ischemia-Reperfusion Injury in Transplantation of Kidney and Other Transplantable Solid Organs 181
George J. Dugbartey and Alp Sener

10 FDA-Approved Hydrogen Sulfide Donor Drug and Its Clinical Applications in Nephrology 203
George J. Dugbartey, Max Y. Zhang, and Alp Sener

Index... 223

Authors and Contributors

About the Authors

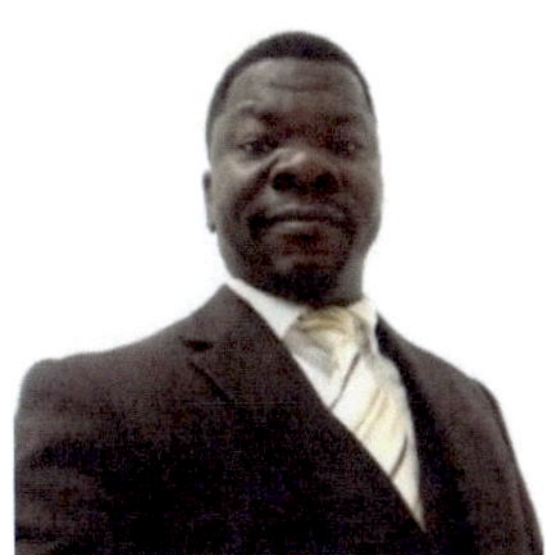

George J. Dugbartey BSc, MSc, PhD, is a faculty member of the University of Ghana and Accra College of Medicine, Ghana, where he teaches Clinical and Experimental Pharmacology, Medical Physiology and Scientific Writing at undergraduate and postgraduate levels. He is also a Medical Scientist in kidney transplant surgery at London Health Sciences Centre, University of Western Ontario, Canada, where his research focuses on hydrogen sulfide in kidney transplantation. In addition, his research areas also include hydrogen sulfide therapy for diabetic kidney disease, hypertensive nephropathy, and drug-induced acute kidney injury. He has over 10 years of research experience in the field of hydrogen sulfide. Dr. Dugbartey is a well-traveled scholar, educator, and a versatile scientist and has presented his research findings at a lot of scientific conferences worldwide. He is also the recipient of several conference awards and research awards, including the prestigious Canadian Institutes of Health Research Award. He is an author, Academic Editor and Reviewer for a lot of respectable scientific journals worldwide. Dr. Dugbartey has over 50 publications in internationally reputable peer-reviewed journals, for most of which he is the first or senior responsible author.

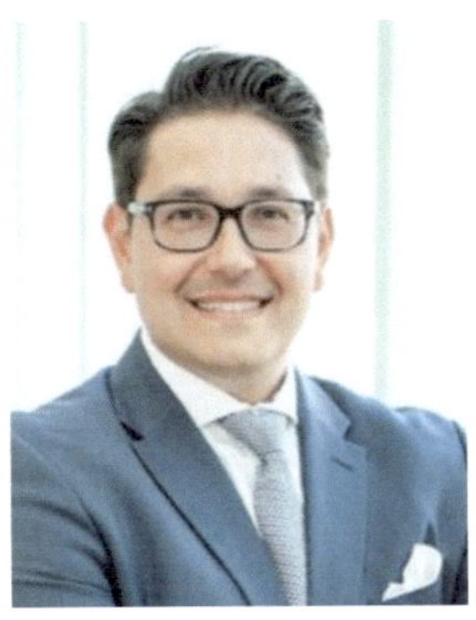

Alp Sener MD, PhD, FRCSC, is the Chief and Chair of Urology and Director of Kidney and Pancreas Transplant Fellowship Program at Schulich School of Medicine and Dentistry, London Health Sciences Centre, and St. Joseph's Hospital, London, Canada. He is an accomplished researcher, with over 20 years of research experience in the areas of kidney/pancreas transplantation and hydrogen sulfide as a novel pharmacological approach for improved organ graft preservation. Dr. Sener is also a urologist whose research areas also include bladder cancer, with interest in hydrogen sulfide involvement. He is an internationally recognized kidney transplant surgeon, educator, and researcher, with over 350 publications. He has been an invited speaker at numerous national and international conferences. He is also a recipient of several prestigious local, national, and international research contribution awards, including the Canadian Society of Transplantation Research Excellence Award, Western University Dean's Award of Excellence, and Vanguard Award from the American Society of Transplant Surgeons.

Contributors

Karl K. Alornyo Department of Pharmacology and Toxicology, School of Pharmacy, College of Health Sciences, University of Ghana, Accra, Ghana

Sampson Antwi Department of Child Health, School of Medical Sciences, Kwame Nkrumah University of Science and Technology and Komfo Anokye Teaching Hospital, Kumasi, Ghana

Vincent Boima Department of Medicine and Therapeutics, University of Ghana Medical School, College of Health Sciences, University of Ghana, Accra, Ghana

Hjalmar R. Bouma Department of Clinical Pharmacy and Pharmacology, University of Groningen, University Medical Center Groningen, Groningen, The Netherlands

George J. Dugbartey Division of Urology, Department of Surgery, London Health Sciences Center, Western University, London, ON, Canada

Multi-Organ Transplant Program, London Health Sciences Center, Western University, London, ON, Canada

Matthew Mailing Center for Translational Transplant Studies, London Health Sciences Center, Western University, London, ON, Canada

Department of Pharmacology and Toxicology, School of Pharmacy, College of Health Sciences, University of Ghana, Accra, Ghana

Department of Physiology and Pharmacology, Accra College of Medicine, Accra, Ghana

Matthew Mailing Centre for Translational Transplant Studies, University Hospital, London Health Sciences Centre, London, ON, Canada

Department of Surgery, Schulich School of Medicine and Dentistry, St. Joseph's Health Care London, London, ON, Canada

Robert H. Henning Department of Clinical Pharmacy and Pharmacology, University of Groningen, University Medical Center Groningen, Groningen, The Netherlands

Smriti Juriasingani Department of Microbiology and Immunology, Schulich School of Medicine and Dentistry, University of Western Ontario, London, ON, Canada

Matthew Mailing Centre for Translational Transplant Studies, University Hospital, London Health Sciences Centre, London, ON, Canada

Shouzhe Lin Department of Microbiology and Immunology, Schulich School of Medicine and Dentistry, University of Western Ontario, London, ON, Canada

Matthew Mailing Centre for Translational Transplant Studies, University Hospital, London Health Sciences Centre, London, ON, Canada

Ian Lobb Matthew Mailing Center for Translational Transplant Studies, London Health Sciences Center, Western University, London, ON, Canada

Department of Microbiology and Immunology, London Health Sciences Center, Western University, London, ON, Canada

Manujendra N. Saha Division of Urology, Department of Surgery, London Health Sciences Center, Western University, London, ON, Canada

Matthew Mailing Center for Translational Transplant Studies, London Health Sciences Center, Western University, London, ON, Canada

Alp Sener Division of Urology, Department of Surgery, London Health Sciences Center, Western University, London, ON, Canada

Multi-Organ Transplant Program, London Health Sciences Center, Western University, London, ON, Canada

Matthew Mailing Center for Translational Transplant Studies, London Health Sciences Center, Western University, London, ON, Canada

Department of Microbiology and Immunology, London Health Sciences Center, Western University, London, ON, Canada

Department of Microbiology and Immunology, Schulich School of Medicine and Dentistry, University of Western Ontario, London, ON, Canada

Matthew Mailing Centre for Translational Transplant Studies, University Hospital, London Health Sciences Centre, London, ON, Canada

Department of Surgery, Schulich School of Medicine and Dentistry, St. Joseph's Health Care London, London, ON, Canada

Max Y. Zhang Matthew Mailing Center for Translational Transplant Studies, London Health Sciences Center, Western University, London, ON, Canada

Department of Microbiology and Immunology, Schulich School of Medicine and Dentistry, University of Western Ontario, London, ON, Canada

Chapter 1
Hydrogen Sulfide and the Renal System

George J. Dugbartey

Historical Account of Hydrogen Sulfide as an Environmental Toxin

Hydrogen sulfide (H_2S) is commonly known as a *"sewer gas"* with a pungent smell of rotten eggs, whose history dates back to the beginning of the eighteenth century as an environmental toxin. It is a colorless, flammable, water- and lipid-soluble, and membrane-permeable gas [1]. This obnoxious gas gained notoriety for centuries for its toxicity and death especially among industrial workers. H_2S was first described in 1713 by the Italian physician Bernardino Ramazzini, who was known as the Father of Occupational Medicine. He published a book titled *De Morbis Artificum*, or *Diseases of Workers*, in which he described in Chap. 14 (titled "Diseases of

---

This chapter is an expanded version by the same author in the publication titled Physiological role of hydrogen sulfide in the kidney and its therapeutic implications for kidney diseases. Biomed Pharmacother. 2023; 116:115396.

G. J. Dugbartey (✉)
Division of Urology, Department of Surgery, London Health Sciences Center, Western University, London, ON, Canada

Multi-Organ Transplant Program, London Health Sciences Center, Western University, London, ON, Canada

Matthew Mailing Center for Translational Transplant Studies, London Health Sciences Center, Western University, London, ON, Canada

Department of Pharmacology and Toxicology, School of Pharmacy, College of Health Sciences, University of Ghana, Accra, Ghana

Department of Physiology and Pharmacology, Accra College of Medicine, Accra, Ghana
e-mail: gdugbart@uwo.ca

G. J. Dugbartey, A. Sener, *Hydrogen Sulfide in Kidney Diseases*,
https://doi.org/10.1007/978-3-031-44041-0_1

Cleaners of Privies and Cesspits") an ocular inflammation among sewer workers, which could lead to total blindness from secondary bacterial invasion. He then postulated that an unknown volatile acid was produced when these workers disturbed the excrement while working, which irritated their eyes and could be responsible for the pungent odor of the excrement. He also hypothesized that the same acid could be responsible for turning the surfaces of copper and silver coins black in the pockets of these workers [1]. In 1777, a series of accidents occurred in Paris, some of which resulted in death, due to inhalation of a gas emanating from the ancient Parisian sewer system. An investigative report from this accident indicated a mild ocular inflammation, as previously described by Ramazzini, and severe asphyxia. Subsequent reports and a series of chemical tests associated the sewer gas with H_2S and implicated it as the cause of the Parisian accidents, leading to the birth of H_2S as an environmental toxin [2–5].

The first biological investigation on the lethal effect of H_2S gas in animals was reported by the French anatomist Francois Chaussier in 1803, in which he described dermal absorption of the gas in horses when they were exposed to fresh air. He also reported the toxic effect of this gas in the animals following intragastric and intrarectal administration of H_2S-saturated solutions [6]. Subsequently, intravenous administration of the same solutions produced hyperpnea (deep breathing) and seizures and resulted in asphyxia and death at high doses. Other scientists of the day who labored in that vineyard observed the presence of H_2S in expired air from animals and a change in blood color after intravenous administration of H_2S-containing solutions in these animals, which was attributed to the formation of sulfhemoglobin, a dangerous oxidation product from hemoglobin reaction with H_2S. Mitchell and Davenport published an excellent review of the findings from these studies and in addition provided informative further reading on the subject [5]. It is worth reiterating that the clinical manifestations of H_2S toxicity are concentration dependent. For example, H_2S has been reported to cause mucosal irritation, headache, dizziness, nausea, vomiting, coughing, breathing difficulty, keratoconjunctivitis, and corneal ulceration at 50–100 ppm [7]. Olfactory paralysis was observed at 100–150 ppm, while bronchitis and pulmonary edema occurred at a concentration approaching 300 ppm. Also, cardiopulmonary arrest usually occurs at concentrations higher than 700 ppm, and sudden syncope and death occur following acute exposure at concentrations higher than 1000 ppm [7]. Using ex vivo tissues following H_2S exposure in animals, investigations on the mechanism(s) underlying H_2S toxicity began from the late twentieth century to early years of the twenty-first century. From these studies, it is now established that H_2S toxicity at the molecular level is primarily due to its ability to inhibit cytochrome *c* oxidase, a terminal enzyme of the mitochondrial respiratory chain, thereby blocking oxygen consumption and adenosine triphosphate (ATP) production, resulting in *"oxygen hunger"* in cells and tissues [8–12]. This suggests that H_2S poisoning shares close similarities with suffocation. In addition to antagonizing the activity of cytochrome *c* oxidase, H_2S can also interact with and inhibit intra- and extracellular proteins such as monoamine oxidase and Na^+/K^+-ATPase via a host of reactions including sulfhydration (a posttranslational modification of proteins by H_2S) to drive its toxicological action [8–11]. Altogether, the pioneering work of Bernardino Ramazzini laid the foundation for three centuries of research on H_2S as an environmental toxin.

From an Environmental Toxin to an Endogenous Biological Signaling Molecule

Ever since Bernardino Ramazzini first described H_2S as a toxic gas in 1713, subsequent studies on this foul-smelling gas have focused on its toxicological profile. Considering that patients recovering from acute H_2S poisoning exhibit cognitive decline, and the fact that animals exposed to H_2S also show a change in the levels of neurotransmitters in their brains [13], the brain could therefore be considered as one of the target primary organs in H_2S toxicity. Inspired by this report, Warenycia and colleagues [14] demonstrated in 1989 the existence of endogenous H_2S in the brains of normal healthy rats even without H_2S exposure. Their discovery suggests a possible physiological role of H_2S. Following this discovery, Abe and Kimura [15] also demonstrated in 1996 that H_2S is a potential biological signaling molecule that is enzymatically produced in the hippocampus at low physiological and nontoxic concentrations using the sulfur-containing amino acid, L-cysteine, as a substrate and that the cytosolic H_2S-producing enzyme, cystathionine beta-synthase (CBS), can be activated and inhibited pharmacologically. They suggested that endogenous H_2S could be a neuromodulator as well as a neuroprotectant that regulates neuronal function. In a subsequent study in 1997, Kimura's group again discovered a second cytosolic enzyme, cystathionine gamma-lyase (CSE), that produced H_2S also from L-cysteine in vascular smooth muscles [16]. They observed that the H_2S produced by CSE relaxed vascular smooth muscles either alone or in synergy with nitric oxide [16]. Interestingly, the findings of Kimura's group became the starting point for several recent studies including those from our own group, testing the involvement of endogenous H_2S in regulation of several signaling pathways in various organ systems including the renal system. From 2001 to 2011, a group led by Rui Wang also demonstrated that H_2S exhibits vasodilatory effect by regulating vascular tone and blood pressure via activation and opening of ATP-sensitive potassium (K_{ATP}) channels [17–21]. This informed him to propose the term *"gasotransmitters"* in 2002 to characterize a class of small endogenously produced gaseous signaling molecules that play important roles in cellular homeostasis and impact physiological and pathological processes. Nitric oxide (NO) was the first identified member of the family of gasotransmitters, followed by carbon monoxide (CO), while H_2S is now established as the third member [22–24]. Using brain homogenates of CBS-knockout and wild-type mice, Kimura's team identified the mitochondrial enzyme, 3-mercaptopyruvate sulfurtransferase (3-MST) in 2009 as another H_2S-generating enzyme, which together with cysteine aminotransferase (CAT) produced H_2S from L-cysteine [25]. Interestingly, the level of H_2S produced from 3-MST was not different in both experimental groups [25]. Four years later, they also identified a fourth pathway in the cerebellum and kidneys of mice, which produced H_2S from D-cysteine, a naturally occurring enantiomer of L-cysteine. This pathway involved the peroxisomal enzyme, D-amino acid oxidase (DAO), coupled with 3-MST [26].

Over the last three decades, it became increasingly evident from a substantial body of experimental studies that there is a rapid paradigm shift in the H_2S field in which low physiological concentrations of H_2S produce pharmacological effects, thus overcoming its negative public image in the toxicological literature. For example, several studies have shown that H_2S exhibits antioxidant and anti-inflammatory effects at low concentrations as opposed to prooxidant and pro-inflammatory effects at high concentrations [27–30]. Also, H_2S protects against DNA damage and preserves its integrity at low concentrations while high concentrations were previously known to damage DNA [31, 32]. In addition, low H_2S concentrations stimulate cellular respiration, whereas the inhibitory effect on cytochrome c oxidase at high concentrations has been well documented [33–36]. Thus, H_2S exerts cytoprotection at low concentrations in contrast to cytotoxicity at high concentrations. In line with this, researchers are employing various H_2S donor compounds and inhibitors as well as creation of mice lacking H_2S-synthesizing enzymes to alter the physiological levels of endogenous H_2S and its synthesizing enzymes in an attempt to further understand the signaling cascades in the physiological and pathophysiological roles of H_2S, which could serve as a therapeutic target in the treatment or prevention of certain diseases. In summary, it can be inferred from recent experimental results that H_2S has been promoted from an environmental toxin to an endogenous biological signaling molecule with physiological relevance and therapeutic potential.

Effects of Hydrogen Sulfide on Renal Physiology

Functional Anatomy of the Kidney

The kidney is a complex organ and crucial to survival. As a pair, they are highly vascularized, receiving about 25% of the total cardiac output. They filter about 150–200 L of fluid daily from renal blood flow (RBF). This allows for toxins, metabolic waste products, and excess electrolytes to be excreted while preserving important substances in the blood that are needed by the body. In addition, the kidneys are actively involved in water regulation, a role which is supported by high expression of aquaporins (AQPs), integral membrane proteins that serve as water channels. By regulating body fluids and maintaining electrolyte and acid-base balance, the kidneys regulate blood pressure and ensure normal function of other organs [37–39]. The anatomical and functional unit of the kidney is the nephron, which is divided into two portions, namely, the glomerulus (a network of capillary filtration unit) and the tubular system that is responsible for selective reabsorption and secretion in the process of urine production. The tubular system is subdivided into proximal tubule, descending and ascending limbs of loop of Henle, distal tubule, connecting tubule, and collecting duct [37–39]. Following filtration by the glomeruli, the filtrate is transported along the regions of the tubular system, where the proximal tubule selectively reabsorbs about two-thirds of the filtered sodium from the filtrate, a process that is regulated by transmembranal sodium-proton (Na^+/H^+) antiporter and sodium-potassium-ATPase (Na^+/K^+-ATPase). Sodium reabsorption also occurs in the ascending limb of the loop of Henle via the action of sodium-potassium-chloride (Na^+-K^+-$2Cl^-$) cotransporter, while sodium transport in distal tubule is by the actions of sodium-chloride (Na-Cl) cotransporter, and transport in the connecting tubule and collecting duct is under the control of epithelial sodium channel (ENaC) [37]. It is important to note that the descending limb of the loop of Henle reabsorbs water from the glomerular filtrate as well as in other regions of the tubular system through AQP, except for the thick ascending limb of the loop of Henle and the early distal tubule, which are water impermeable. Hence, these two regions are known as the diluting segments of the nephron, producing free water (or solute-free water) [37]. It is of interest to note that nine AQPs, 1, 2, 3, 4, 5, 6, 7, 8 and 11, are localized in the kidneys, participating in short- and long-term regulation of water balance as well as involving in water balance disorders [37]. Surrounding the renal tubules are peritubular capillaries, which originate from efferent arteriole and return the bulk of the solutes and water reabsorbed by the tubular system into systemic circulation (i.e., the venous system) and conserved for the body's use. The tubular system is also equipped with secretory pathways that dispose of drugs and metabolites and other unwanted substances such as creatinine, ammonia, urea, and uric acid from the peritubular capillaries into the glomerular filtrate and excreted in urine [37]. Thus, the elaborate reabsorption and secretory pathways modify the composition of the glomerular filtrate such that the kidneys produce about 1–2 L of urine per day.

Renal Production of Hydrogen Sulfide

Following the discoveries by Kimura's group, it later became increasingly evident that all four H_2S-producing enzymes are also abundantly localized in the kidney, with CBS and CSE being the most dominant. Using marker enzymes of known localization in a study to characterize the renal involvement in homocysteine metabolism, both CBS and CSE were reported to be localized in the proximal tubules of rat kidneys. While CBS was expressed by proximal tubular cells in the outer cortex, CSE was localized in the inner cortex and outer medulla [40]. Subsequent studies corroborated this finding using different methods in mouse and rat kidneys [41–43]. Specifically, both enzymes are expressed in the brush border and cytoplasm of epithelial cells of the renal proximal tubules, distal tubules, and peritubular capillaries [26, 44–48]. In addition to the tubular localization of CBS and CSE, we also found both enzymes in the glomeruli of rats subjected to hypothermic injury and diabetic nephropathy [49, 50]. However, CSE is the main H_2S-producing enzyme in the glomeruli, which is expressed by endothelial cells, mesangial cells, and podocytes [46–48]. Besides animal kidneys, CSE was also found to be expressed in the glomerular and tubulointerstitial compartments of human kidneys [48]. Unlike CBS and CSE, which are the main H_2S-synthesizing enzymes in the kidney, 3-MST and DAO have been less studied and their significance in mediating H_2S-generating pathways has so far received little scientific attention. Nevertheless, they are also expressed in the kidney [26, 51, 52], with 3-MST specifically found in epithelial cells of the proximal tubule [52]. In total, about 75% of all renal cells and 87% of endothelial cells express H_2S-producing enzymes [46, 48], making the kidney a rich source of endogenous H_2S production and with important roles in renal function. This explains why all the known pathways of H_2S production have been described in the kidney. Interestingly, deficiency in H_2S-synthesizing enzymes and significantly reduced plasma H_2S levels have recently been reported in human patients and experimental animals, which correlated with the severity of kidney diseases [53–56]. These findings imply that H_2S restoration could be a therapeutic target in human kidney diseases. Figure 1.1 is a simplified illustration of endogenous H_2S production in the kidney. It is important to note that besides its endogenous production, H_2S can also be administered exogenously via H_2S donor compounds to augment

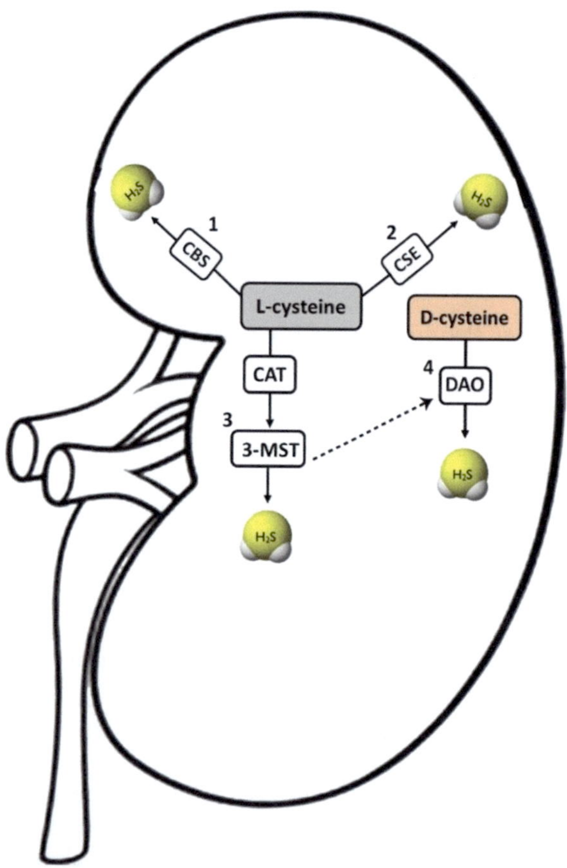

Fig. 1.1 Simplified view of hydrogen sulfide production in the kidney. (1) H_2S production by CBS using L-cysteine as a substrate; (2) H_2S production by CSE using L-cysteine as a substrate; (3) H_2S production by 3-MST using L-cysteine as a substrate; (4) H_2S production by DAO using D-cysteine as a substrate. *H_2S* Hydrogen sulfide, *CBS* Cystathionine beta-synthase, *CSE* Cystathionine gamma-lyase, *CAT* Cysteine aminotransferase, *3-MST* 3-mercaptopyruvate sulfurtransferase, *DAO* D-amino acid oxidase

endogenous H_2S level. These H_2S donor compounds include sodium hydrosulfide (NaHS), sodium sulfide (Na_2S), sodium thiosulfate, GYY4137, AP39, AP123, SG1002, S-propargyl cysteine (SPRC, also known as ZYZ-802), sulfurous mineral water, and garlic-derived polysulfide [57–62].

Hydrogen Sulfide Involvement in Renal Function

Several lines of empirical evidence have established the involvement of H_2S in the regulation of cellular physiology via a wide array of mechanisms such as regulation of kinases, ion channels, and transcription factors through posttranslational S-sulfhydration of cysteine residues. H_2S also binds to heme in heme-containing proteins, as well as functions as a free radical scavenger and a donor of electrons to the mitochondrial electron transport chain to increase mitochondrial ATP production and regulate bioenergetics [33, 63–65]. In the kidney, H_2S functions to regulate many physiological processes including renal blood flow, glomerular filtration rate, diuresis, natriuresis, kaliuresis, and blood pressure. In addition, H_2S also functions as an oxygen sensor in the renal medulla to ensure oxygen balance and improve medullary blood flow.

Effect of Hydrogen Sulfide on Renal Excretory Function

In the kidney, H_2S has been shown to alter cellular function in a variety of ways, which result in diverse downstream effects. In a porcine model of kidney transplantation, for example, infusion of Na_2S (an H_2S donor) 10 min before and 20 min after reperfusion of cold-stored porcine kidneys reversed cyclosporine-induced vasoconstriction and other pathological changes through increased renal blood flow (RBF) and glomerular filtration rate (GFR, an index of renal clearance function) [66]. Similarly, in a genetic model of hyperhomocysteinemia (a risk factor in chronic kidney disease progression), heterozygous CBS mice ($CBS^{+/-}$) showed a reduced GFR, which was associated with elevated systolic blood pressure and renal dysfunction, while GFR was restored and renal protection observed in $CBS^{+/-}$ mice which received H_2S-supplemented drinking water (30 μM NaHS for 8 weeks) [67]. Also, in a study to determine the effect of H_2S on renal hemodynamics and function in rats, intrarenal arterial infusion of NaHS (another H_2S donor) at a rate of 50 $\mu L/min$ increased RBF and GFR and also promoted natriuresis and kaliuresis, which correlated positively with increased plasma H_2S level and renal CBS and CSE expression [45]. In addition, pharmacological inhibition of endogenous H_2S with aminooxyacetic acid (AOAA; CBS inhibitor) and propargylglycine (PAG; CSE inhibitor) together reduced RBF and GFR, resulting in increased Na^+ and K^+ reabsorption [45, 68, 69]. It is worth noting that failure of the kidney to remove excess Na^+, for example, is associated with detrimental pathological effects, due to its role in regulating blood volume, fluid balance, and blood pressure. In a recent clinical study involving 157 non-dialysis patients with chronic kidney disease (CKD), Kung and colleagues [70] reported that plasma H_2S and mRNA levels of CBS and CSE in blood mononuclear cells of these patients were significantly lower compared to healthy controls, which corresponded with reduced GFR and severity of the disease. However, mRNA level of 3-MST was markedly increased in the CKD patients [70], suggesting a compensatory effect between the H_2S-producing enzymes.

Mechanistically, the increased RBF and GFR by H_2S suggests a vasodilatory effect on afferent arterioles by reducing renal vascular resistance possibly via activation of K_{ATP} channels (the main vascular target of H_2S), as pharmacological blockade of K_{ATP} channels with 10 μM glibenclamide during renal ischemia-reperfusion injury potentiated further injury on renal epithelial integrity in a rat model of isolated perfused kidney [71]. Also, H_2S activates NO/cGMP/sGC/PKG pathway [72, 73], one of the most extensively studied vasodilatory pathways, which altogether could account for the increased RBF and GFR in the above studies. This also suggests that H_2S interacts with other members of the gasotransmitter family to induce vasodilation. In the case of increased natriuresis and kaliuresis, H_2S administration through NaHS inhibited the activities of Na^+/K^+-ATPase and Na^+-K^+-$2Cl^-$ cotransporter in the renal tubules [45, 69], thereby preventing the reabsorption of these ions and potentiating their excretion (Fig. 1.2). In a greater detail, the inhibitory effect of

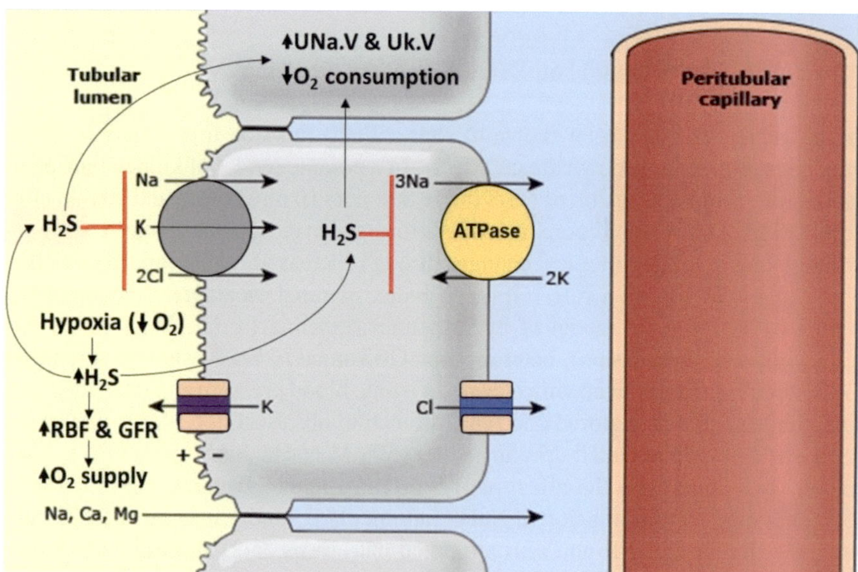

Fig. 1.2 Effects of H_2S on renal function. H_2S induces vasodilation and also blocks renal tubular transport by inhibiting the activities of Na^+/K^+-ATPase and Na^+-K^+-$2Cl^-$ cotransporter, thereby increasing RBF and GFR and promoting natriuresis (UNa.V) and kaliuresis (Uk.V). H_2S also functions as an oxygen sensor under hypoxic condition in the renal medulla in which its production increases, leading to oxygen restoration and further enhancing RBF and GFR as well as suppressing tubular transport. *H_2S* hydrogen sulfide, *RBF* renal blood flow, *GFR* glomerular filtration rate, *UNa.V* urinary sodium, *Uk.V* urinary potassium

H$_2$S on Na$^+$/K$^+$-ATPase has been shown to be due to its ability to directly target H$_2$S-sensitive disulfide bonds in epidermal growth factor receptor (EGFR) in the proximal tubule, resulting in endocytosis and inhibition of Na$^+$/K$^+$-ATPase via EGFR/GAB1/PI3K/Akt signaling pathway [69]. In addition, exogenous H$_2$S administration prevents hydrogen peroxide-induced activation and opening of ENaC in the distal tubule via phosphatidylinositol 3,4,5-trisphosphate (PI(3,4,5)P3) pathway [74], thereby reducing Na$^+$ reabsorption and increasing its excretion. Furthermore, pharmacological inhibition of CBS and CSE with AOAA (10 mg/kg/day) and PAG (30 mg/kg/day), respectively, is associated with decreased AQP-2 protein expression in the inner medullary collecting duct, resulting in decreased urine osmolality and urinary concentration defects in mice [75]. However, intraperitoneal administration of the H$_2$S donor, GYY4137 (50 mg/kg/day), upregulated renal AQP-2 expression and significantly promoted urine concentration via cAMP-dependent protein kinase signaling pathway [75]. There are studies also showing increased activity of Cl$^-$/HCO$_3^-$ exchanger in aortic tissues of rats as well as in vascular smooth muscle cells [76, 77]. Although this has not been studied in the kidney, it is possible that H$_2$S exhibits the same effect in renal tissues considering the crucial role of Cl$^-$/HCO$_3^-$ exchanger in regulating ion excretion and maintaining physiological pH. Taken together, H$_2$S increases RBF, GFR, and excretory function of the kidney by inhibiting the activities of transporters such as Na$^+$-K$^+$-2Cl$^-$ and Na$^+$/K$^+$-ATPase.

Role of Hydrogen Sulfide as an Oxygen Sensor in Renal Function

As mentioned in section "Functional Anatomy of the Kidney" above, the kidney receives about 25% of the total cardiac output. However, the medullary compartment receives only about 10% of the total renal perfusion in functionally normal kidney due to intrarenal arteriovenous oxygen shunt [78]. This makes the renal medulla highly vulnerable to pathological conditions. Available evidence indicates that H$_2$S is an oxygen sensor and mediates tubulovascular cross talk in the renal medulla [79–84]. While the production of H$_2$S is independent of oxygen, its oxidative metabolism in mitochondria is oxygen dependent. Thus, the low oxygen partial pressure in the renal medulla creates a hypoxic environment that leads to H$_2$S accumulation, which increases the activity of H$_2$S including electron donation for ATP production in the mitochondria and restoration of oxygen balance by increasing medullary flow and decreasing tubular Na$^+$ transport, which accounts for 60% of renal oxygen consumption [45, 79–84] (Fig. 1.2). Considering that the majority of Na$^+$-K$^+$-2Cl$^-$ channels are found in thick ascending limb of the loop of Henle, which also expresses CBS and requires a balance between oxygen supply and hyperosmolality for urine concentration [42], the finding that H$_2$S functions as an oxygen sensor in the renal medulla is very important. The oxygen-sensing ability of H$_2$S is also supported by the fact that CBS and CSE translocate into mitochondria under hypoxic conditions to increase endogenous H$_2$S production along with 3-MST [33, 85]. Besides the kidney, H$_2$S-mediating oxygen sensing has also been reported in the heart, lungs, and gastrointestinal tract, thus affecting blood flow and regulating oxygen balance in these tissues [86–88]. However, the specific mechanisms and downstream signaling events require further investigations. In summary, H_2S functions as an oxygen sensor under hypoxic conditions, thereby increasing medullary flow, inhibiting tubular transport, and restoring oxygen balance.

Effect of Hydrogen Sulfide on Renal Renin Release

The renal-angiotensin-aldosterone system (RAAS) is a critical renovascular humoral regulatory system in the body that is composed of hormones, enzymes, proteins, and a series of reactions that regulate blood volume, blood pressure, renal hemodynamics, and systemic vascular resistance by regulating water, plasma sodium (salt) excretion, and vascular tone on a long-term basis through coordinated effects on the heart, blood vessels, and kidneys. As a compensatory protective mechanism, the RAAS is activated by a pressure transducer mechanism involving mechanoreceptors in afferent arterioles in response to conditions such as renal hypoperfusion and hypotension (such as during hemorrhage or dehydration) in the early stages of cardiovascular and renal diseases [37, 89, 90]. The RAAS is also activated by abnormally low concentration of sodium chloride, which is sensed by macula densa cells in the distal convoluted tubule and generates paracrine signals in the juxtaglomerular cells present within the walls of the afferent arterioles of the kidney to release renin [37, 91, 92]. However, chronic activation of RAAS is pathological, as it produces adverse effects such as syndromes of congestive heart failure, systemic hypertension, and chronic kidney disease [93, 94]. Thus, RAAS activity is determined and regulated by the release of renin, a process which has been well documented to be mediated by intracellular cyclic adenosine monophosphate (cAMP, a second messenger in signal transduction) [95–98].

Administration of H_2S has been found to modulate renin release when RAAS is overactivated. In a two-kidney-one-clip (2K1C) model of renovascular hypertension in rats, daily intraperitoneal administration of 5.6 mg/kg NaHS resulted in significant reduction in renin activity and levels of angiotensin II (a potent vasoconstrictor in the RAAS), which positively correlated with downregulation of renal renin mRNA and protein expressions as well as blood pressure in 2K1C rats compared to vehicle control rats [99]. Using primary cultures of renin-rich kidney cells in a separate study, the same authors also reported that treatment with 100 μmol/L of NaHS also significantly suppressed renin activity along with reduction in intracellular cAMP level [99]. This observation was supported by results from later studies in which NaHS (0.1–10 μM) strongly suppressed cAMP production in As4.1 cells (renin-expressing cell line) treated with isoproterenol (a β-adrenoceptor agonist), forskolin (an adenylyl cyclase activator), or 3-isobutyl-1-methylxanthine (a phosphodiesterase inhibitor) by inhibiting the activity of adenylyl cyclase (an enzyme that catalyzes the production of cAMP from ATP), thus regulating renin activity and blood pressure [100, 101]. In a model of high-salt-induced hypertension in Dahl salt-sensitive rats, feeding on high-salt diet containing 8% NaCl for 8 weeks inhibited RAAS activation in the rat kidney, reversed pathological remodeling, and prevented salt-sensitive hypertension, which corresponded with upregulation in renal CBS mRNA and protein expression, and 3-MST mRNA expression, and significantly increased renal and serum H_2S levels to near-normal levels compared to rats fed with high-salt diet without NaHS supplementation [102]. Interestingly, H_2S had no effect on renin activity in normal rats [99], which suggests that H_2S only inhibits renin release when RAAS is overactivated. Using human umbilical vein endothelial cells (a model system for studying endothelial cell function), Laggner et al. [103] also demonstrated that H_2S directly inhibits the activity of angiotensin-converting enzyme (ACE, a zinc-containing vasoconstricting enzyme in the RAAS) in a dose-dependent manner by interfering with zinc in the active center of ACE. Collectively, these empirical findings accentuate the vasodilatory effect of H_2S in addition to suppressing angiotensin II production under conditions in which RAAS is overactivated (Fig. 1.3).

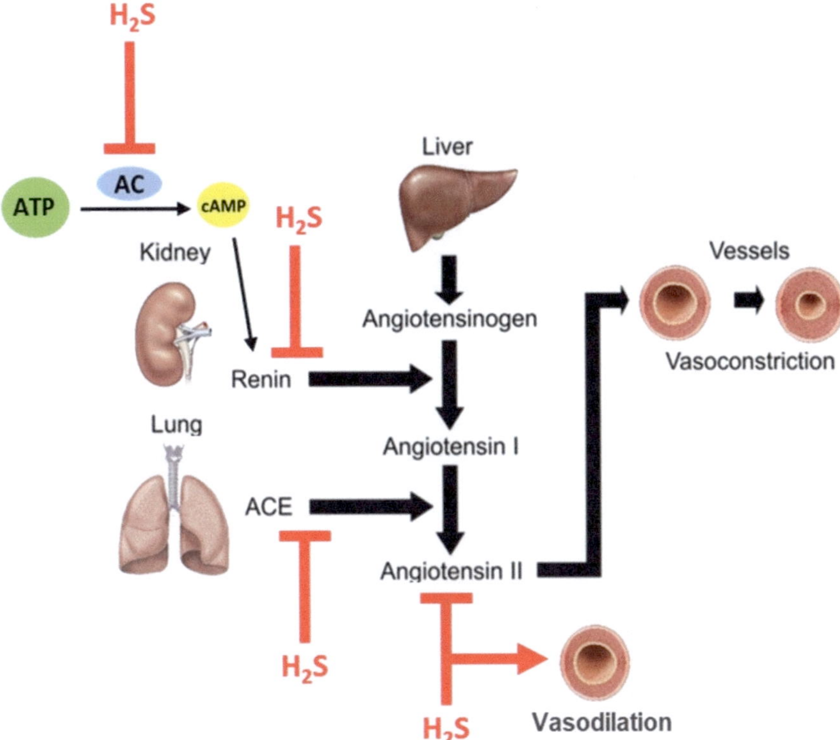

Fig. 1.3 H_2S modulates renin-angiotensin-aldosterone system (RAAS). Under conditions in which RAAS is overactivated, administration of H_2S inhibits the activities of renin and angiotensin-converting enzyme (ACE) as well as reduces angiotensin II level by suppressing intracellular cyclic adenosine monophosphate (cAMP) production via inhibition of adenylyl cyclase (AC)

Role of Hydrogen Sulfide in Renal Water Handling

As mentioned in section "Functional Anatomy of the Kidney", aquaporins (AQPs), also known as water channels, are a family of transmembrane proteins that regulate intracellular and intercellular water flow by mediating bidirectional flow of water and small uncharged solutes such as glycerol, urea, ammonia, and hydrogen peroxide down an osmotic gradient, thus influencing the overall process of urine concentration [104]. AQPs are widely expressed in specific cell types in various tissues. In the kidney, there are nine AQPs distributed at various regions of the nephron. They are AQP1–8 and AQP11 [104]. AQP1 is a highly selective water-permeable channel localized in the apical and basolateral membranes of the epithelial cells of the proximal tubules, thin descending limb of loop of Henle, and descending vasa recta [105], while AQP2 is highly concentrated in the apical membrane of collecting duct principal cells (epithelial cells) and involved in regulating urine concentration [106]. AQP3 and AQP4 are found in the basolateral cell membrane of principal collecting duct cells, exporting water in the cytoplasm [107, 108]. AQP5 and AQP6 are localized in intercalated cells of the collecting duct. However, their functions are not completely understood [109, 110]. AQP7 is localized in the brush border of the S3 segment (straight portion) of the proximal tubule and regulates glycerol transport [111], whereas AQP8 is found in the epithelial cells of proximal tubule, principal cells of collecting duct, and mitochondrial membrane, where it regulates ammonia transport [112]. AQP11 is expressed in the endoplasmic reticulum of epithelial cells of the proximal tubules and plays a crucial role in water and glucose reabsorption [113]. Among the renal AQPs, AQP2 is the major regulator of urine concentration, whose function is regulated by arginine vasopressin via activation of intracellular cyclic adenosine monophosphate (cAMP)/protein kinase A (PKA) signaling pathway [114, 115]. In addition, cAMP response element-binding protein (CREB), a ubiquitously expressed nuclear transcription factor, has been reported to enhance transcription from AQP2 promoter through cAMP response element [116, 117]. It is important to mention that PKA phosphorylates AQP2 in addition to other kinases that regulate localization of AQP2, thereby facilitating AQP2 accumulation on the plasma membrane [118]. Interestingly, alteration in AQP2 protein expression is associated with water balance disorders such as nephrogenic diabetes insipidus, nephrogenic syndrome of inappropriate antidiuresis, syndrome of inappropriate antidiuretic hormone secretion, and autosomal dominant polycystic kidney disease [75, 119, 120]. This finding suggests that vasopressin-AQP2 pathway could be a therapeutic target in the treatment and/or pharmacological management of water balance disorders and that urinary AQP2 could serve as a useful biomarker for diagnosis of these disorders.

Burgeoning preclinical evidence shows that H_2S upregulates renal AQP2 expression via cAMP/PKA signaling pathway, thereby improving urine concentration in water balance disorders (Fig. 1.4). In a mouse model of lithium-induced nephrogenic diabetes insipidus (NDI), a rare water balance disorder characterized by polyuria and polydipsia, Luo et al. [75] reported that coadministration of the endogenous

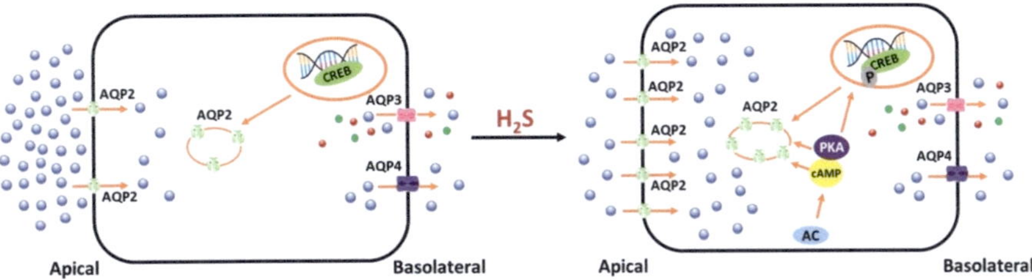

Fig. 1.4 Role of H_2S in renal water handling. H_2S activates intracellular cyclic adenosine monophosphate (cAMP)/protein kinase A (PKA) signaling pathway, thereby upregulating renal aquaporin 2 (AQP2) expression. This decreases urine osmolality and improves urine concentration in water balance disorders such as nephrogenic diabetes insipidus

H_2S inhibitors, AOAA (10 mg/kg/day; against CBS) and PAG (30 mg/kg/day; against CSE) for 5 days, was associated with a 40% decrease in AQP2 protein expression in the inner medullary collecting duct, along with significant downregulation in the expression of renal phosphorylated CREB (p-CREB) protein compared to control mice. This observation aligned with marked downregulation of renal AQP2 mRNA expression and a 70% reduction in endogenous H_2S production in the renal inner medulla. Similar results were obtained in the renal cortex. In a separate experiment by the same authors, AOAA and PAG coadministration in dehydrated mice exhibited a 20% decrease in urine osmolality and 25% increase in urine production compared to dehydrated control mice. This corresponded with significant downregulation in AQP2 and p-CREB protein expression in the renal inner medulla [75] and suggests a urine concentration defect following inhibition of endogenous H_2S production. However, daily intraperitoneal administration of the H_2S donor, GYY4137 (50 mg/kg), for 7 days markedly upregulated AQP2 protein expression in the renal inner medulla of lithium-induced NDI mice compared to control mice. As expected, this was consistent with increased urine osmolality and significantly improved urine concentration [75]. Using an in vitro model, treatment of primary cultured inner medullary collecting duct cells of rats with NaHS and GYY4137 resulted in increased AQP2 protein expression after 5 min of treatment and was associated with increased cAMP level in the cell lysate. However, this effect was significantly abrogated with the PKA inhibitor, H89 or adenylyl cyclase, in rat inner medullary collecting duct suspensions [75]. This result further affirms the observation that increased renal AQP2 expression and improvement in urine concentration by H_2S are via cAMP/PKA signaling pathway (Fig. 1.4). As H_2S is an activator cAMP/PKA pathway under NDI condition, it is important to note that H_2S also activates cAMP/PKA signaling pathway in different cell types under different conditions [18].

Apart from the study by Luo and colleagues [75] on the effect of H_2S on renal AQPs, there is no other study in the literature on this subject. However, alpha-lipoic acid (ALA), an endogenous source of H_2S, has been reported to exhibit similar effects on AQP1–3. Using a rat model of lipopolysaccharide (LPS)-induced acute kidney injury, intraperitoneal administration of 50 mg/kg of ALA preserved renal expression of AQP2 and Na^+/H^+ exchanger, which were significantly downregulated by LPS and partly contributed to attenuating LPS-induced renal damage [121]. Similarly, administration of the same dose of ALA via the same route on days 2 and 1, and 8 h prior to 6 mg/kg cisplatin administration, followed by injection on days 1, 2, and 3 after cisplatin administration resulted in increased renal expression of AQP1–3, improved urine concentration, and tubular sodium reabsorption, with increased renal expression of adenylyl cyclase VI and vasopressin-induced cAMP production. These effects were reversed in cisplatin-treated rats without ALA administration [122, 123]. Specifically, the increased expression of AQP1–3 by ALA was localized in the cortical and medullary regions of the kidney as revealed by semiquantitative immunoblotting and immunohistochemical staining [122, 123]. These results corroborate the result of Bae et al. [124] who also observed that intraperitoneal injection of 80 mg/kg of ALA before and after 40 min of ischemia (renal pedicle clamping) attenuated the downregulation of renal AQP1–3 by activating local protective systems such as arginine-vasopressin/cAMP and nitric oxide/cGMP [130]. Overall, these promising experimental findings suggest that H_2S treatment could represent a novel therapy that targets vasopressin-AQP pathway in water balance disorders such as NDI. However, considering that this research area has not been extensively studied, the findings from these few studies make clinical translation difficult. Therefore, more studies with other H_2S donors and at different doses are required to corroborate these interesting results.

Conclusion

Hydrogen sulfide (H_2S), a foul-smelling gas with historic notoriety as an environmental toxin, has recently emerged as an endogenous gaseous signaling molecule that plays important roles in cellular homeostasis. The kidney is considered one of the major sources of endogenous H_2S production due to the abundant expression of H_2S-producing enzymes in the glomerular and tubular compartments, thereby influencing normal renal function such as regulation of renal blood flow, glomerular filtration rate, tubular transport, blood pressure, and renal bioenergetics. Thus, the role of H_2S in renal function implies that it could be considered as a novel targeted therapeutic agent or biomarker for common renal pathologies, which are discussed in the subsequent chapters of this book.

Conflict of Interest None.

References

1. Ramazzini B. The Latin text of 1713, rev. with translation and notes by W. C. Wright. Chicago: University of Chicago Press. 1940; De Morbis Anificum Diatriba. pp. 151–157.
2. Dupuyturen M. Rapport sur une espece de mephitisme des fosses d'aisance, produite par le gas azote. J Med. 1806;IX:187–213.
3. Hugo V. Les Miserables. Translated by L. Wraxall, illustrations by L. Ward. New York: The Heritage Press. 1938.
4. Nichollas P, Kim JK. Oxidation of sulphide by cytochrome aa3. Biochim Biophys Acta. 1981;637:312–20.
5. Mitchell CW, Davenport SJ. Hydrogen sulphide literature. Public Health Rep. 1924;39:1–13.
6. Chaussier F. Precis d'experiences faites sur les animaux avec le gaz hydrogene sulfure. J Gen de Med, Chir et Pharm Paris. 1908;15:19–39.
7. Gabbay DS, De Roos F, Perrone J. Twenty-foot fall averts fatality from massive hydrogen sulfide exposure. J Emerg Med. 2001;20(2):141–4.
8. Beauchamp RO Jr, Bus JS, Popp JA, Boreiko CJ, Andjelkovich DA. A critical review of the literature on hydrogen sulfide toxicity. Crit Rev Toxicol. 1984;13(1):25–97.
9. Khan AA, Schuler MM, Prior MG, Yong S, Coppock RW, Florence LZ, et al. Effects of hydrogen sulfide exposure on lung mitochondrial respiratory chain enzymes in rats. Toxicol Appl Pharmacol. 1990;103:482–90.
10. Nicholson RA, Roth SH, Jian Zheng AZ. Inhibition of respiratory and bioenergetic mechanisms by hydrogen sulfide in mammalian brain. J Toxicol Environ Health. 1998;54:491–507.
11. Dorman DC, Moulin FJM, McManus BE, Mahle KC, James RA, Struve MF. Cytochrome oxidase inhibition induced by acute hydrogen sulfide inhalation: correlation with tissue sulfide concentrations in the rat brain, liver, lung, and nasal epithelium. Toxicol Sci. 2002;65:18–25.
12. Blackstone E, Morrison M, Roth MB. H_2S induces a suspended animation-like state in mice. Science. 2005;308(5721):518.
13. Reiffenstein RJ, Hulbert WC, Roth SH. Toxicology of hydrogen sulfide. Annu Rev Pharmacol Toxic. 1992;32:109–34.
14. Warenycia MW, Goodwin LR, Benishin CG, Reiffenstein RJ, Francom DM, Taylor JD, et al. Acute hydrogen sulfide poisoning. Demonstration of selective uptake of sulfide by the brainstem by measurement of brain sulfide levels. Biochem Pharmacol. 1989;38:973–81.
15. Abe K, Kimura H. The possible role of hydrogen sulfide as an endogenous neuromodulator. J Neurosci. 1996;16:1066–71.
16. Hosoki R, Matsuki N, Kimura H. The possible role of hydrogen sulfide as an endogenous smooth muscle relaxant in synergy with nitric oxide. Biochem Biophys Res Commun. 1997;237:527–31.
17. Zhao W, Zhang J, Lu Y, Wang R. The vasorelaxant effect of H_2S as a novel endogenous gaseous KATP channel opener. EMBO J. 2001;20:6008–16.
18. Zhao W, Wang R. H2S-induced vasorelaxation and underlying cellular and molecular mechanisms. Am J Physiol Heart Circ Physiol. 2002;283:H474–80.
19. Tang G, Wu L, Liang W, Wang R. Direct stimulation of K_{ATP} channels by exogenous and endogenous hydrogen sulfide in vascular smooth muscle cells. Mol Pharmacol. 2005;68:1757–64.
20. Yang G, Wu L, Jiang B, Yang W, Qi J, Cao K, et al. H_2S as a physiologic vasorelaxant: hypertension in mice with deletion of cystathionine gamma-lyase. Science. 2008;322:587–90.
21. Mustafa AK, Sikka G, Gazi SK, Steppan J, Jung SM, Bhunia AK, et al. Hydrogen sulfide as endothelium-derived hyperpolarizing factor sulfhydrates potassium channels. Circ Res. 2011;109:1259–68.
22. SoRelle R. Nobel prize awarded to scientists for nitric oxide discoveries. Circulation. 1998;98(22):2365–6.

23. Untereiner AA, Wu L, Wang R. The role of carbon monoxide as a gasotransmitter in cardiovascular and metabolic regulation. In: Hermann A, Sitdikova G, Weiger T, editors. Gasotransmitters: physiology and pathophysiology. Berlin: Springer; 2012. p. 37–70.

24. Wang R. Hydrogen sulfide: the third gasotransmitter in biology and medicine. Antioxid Redox Signal. 2010;12(9):1061–4.

25. Shibuya N, Tanaka M, Yoshida M, Ogasawara Y, Togawa T, Ishii K, Kimura H. 3-Mercaptopyruvate sulfurtransferase produces hydrogen sulfide and bound sulfane sulfur in the brain. Antioxid Redox Signal. 2009;11:703–14.

26. Shibuya N, Koike S, Tanaka M, Ishigami-Yuasa M, Kimura Y, Ogasawara Y, Fukui K, Nagahara N, Kimura H. A novel pathway for the production of hydrogen sulfide from D-cysteine in mammalian cells. Nat Commun. 2013;4:1366.

27. Kimura Y, Kimura H. Hydrogen sulfide protects neurons from oxidative stress. FASEB J. 2004;18:1165–7.

28. Whiteman M, Armstrong JS, Chu SH, Jia-Ling S, Wong BS, Cheung NS, et al. The novel neuromodulator hydrogen sulfide: an endogenous peroxynitrite 'scavenger'? J Neurochem. 2004;90:765–8.

29. Kimura Y, Goto Y, Kimura H. Hydrogen sulfide increases glutathione production and suppresses oxidative stress in mitochondria. Antioxid Redox Signal. 2010;12:1–13.

30. Li L, Bhatia M, Zhu YZ, Zhu YC, Ramnath RD, Wang ZJ, et al. Hydrogen sulfide is a novel mediator of lipopolysaccharide-induced inflammation in the mouse. FASEB J. 2005;19:1196–8.

31. Szczesny B, Módis K, Yanagi K, Coletta C, Le Trionnaire S, Perry A, et al. AP39, a novel mitochondria-targeted hydrogen sulfide donor, stimulates cellular bioenergetics, exerts cytoprotective effects and protects against the loss of mitochondrial DNA integrity in oxidatively stressed endothelial cells in vitro. Nitric Oxide. 2014;41:120–30.

32. Szczesny B, Marcatti M, Zatarain JR, Druzhyna N, Wiktorowicz JE, Nagy P, et al. Inhibition of hydrogen sulfide biosynthesis sensitizes lung adenocarcinoma to chemotherapeutic drugs by inhibiting mitochondrial DNA repair and suppressing cellular bioenergetics. Sci Rep. 2016;6:36125.

33. Fu M, Zhang W, Wu L, Yang G, Li H, Wang R. Hydrogen sulfide (H2S) metabolism in mitochondria and its regulatory role in energy production. Proc Natl Acad Sci U S A. 2012;109:2943–8.

34. Goubern M, Andriamihaja M, Nübel T, Blachier F, Bouillaud F. Sulfide, the first inorganic substrate for human cells. FASEB J. 2007;21:1699–706.

35. Szabo C, Coletta C, Chao C, Módis K, Szczesny B, Papapetropoulos A, et al. Tumor-derived hydrogen sulfide, produced by cystathionine-β-synthase, stimulates bioenergetics, cell proliferation, and angiogenesis in colon cancer. Proc Natl Acad Sci U S A. 2013;110:12474–9.

36. Módis K, Coletta C, Erdélyi K, Papapetropoulos A, Szabo C. Intramitochondrial H_2S production by 3-mercaptopyruvate sulfurtransferase maintains mitochondrial electron flow and supports cellular bioenergetics. FASEB J. 2013;27:601–11.

37. Eaton DC, Pooler JP. Vanders renal physiology. 9th ed. New York: McGraw Hill Publisher; 2018.

38. Giebisch G, Windhanger E. Glomerular filtration and renal blood flow. In: Boron WF, Boulpaep EL, editors. Medical physiology: a cellular and molecular approach. Philadelphia: Saunders; 2009. p. 767–81.

39. Bhaskar A, Oommen V. A simple model for demonstrating the factors affecting glomerular filtration rate. Adv Physiol Educ. 2018;42(2):380–2.

40. House JD, Brosnan ME, Brosnan JT. Characterization of homocysteine metabolism in the rat kidney. Biochem J. 1997;328(Pt 1):287–92.

41. Ishii I, Akahoshi N, Yu XN, Kobayashi Y, Namekata K, Komaki G, Kimura H. Murine cystathionine gamma-lyase: complete cDNA and genomic sequences, promoter activity, tissue distribution and developmental expression. Biochem J. 2004;381(Pt 1):113–23.

42. Li N, Chen L, Muh RW, Li PL. Hyperhomocysteinemia associated with decreased renal transsulfuration activity in Dahl S rats. Hypertension. 2006;47:1094–100.
43. Tripatara P, Patel NS, Brancaleone V, Renshaw D, Rocha J, Sepodes B, Mota-Filipe H, Perretti M, Thiemermann C. Characterisation of cystathionine gamma-lyase/hydrogen sulphide pathway in ischaemia/reperfusion injury of the mouse kidney: an in vivo study. Eur J Pharmacol. 2009;606(1–3):205–9.
44. Yamamoto J, Sato W, Kosugi T, Yamamoto T, Kimura T, Taniguchi S, et al. Distribution of hydrogen sulfide (H2S)-producing enzymes and the roles of the H2S donor sodium hydrosulfide in diabetic nephropathy. Clin Exp Nephrol. 2013;17(1):32–40.
45. Xia M, Chen L, Muh RW, Li PL, Li N. Production and actions of hydrogen sulfide, a novel gaseous bioactive substance, in the kidneys. J Pharmacol Exp Ther. 2009;329(3):1056–62.
46. Lee HJ, Mariappan MM, Feliers D, Cavaglieri RC, Sataranatarajan K, Abboud HE, et al. Hydrogen sulfide inhibits high glucose-induced matrix protein synthesis by activating AMP-activated protein kinase in renal epithelial cells. J Biol Chem. 2012;387(7):4451–61.
47. Bos EM, Leuvinink HG, Snijder PM, et al. Hydrogen sulfide-induced hypometabolism prevents renal ischemia/reperfusion injury. J Am Soc Nephrol. 2009;20(9):1901–5.
48. Bos EM, Wang R, Snijder PM, et al. Cystathionine γ-lyase protects against renal ischemia/reperfusion by modulating oxidative stress. J Am Soc Nephrol. 2013;24(5):759–70.
49. Dugbartey GJ, Talaei F, Houwertjes MC, Goris M, Epema AH, Bouma HR, Henning RH. Dopamine treatment attenuates acute kidney injury in a rat model of deep hypothermia and rewarming—the role of renal H$_2$S-producing enzymes. Eur J Pharmacol. 2015;769:225–33.
50. Dugbartey GJ, Alornyo KK, Diaba DE, Adams I. Activation of renal CSE/H$_2$S pathway by alpha-lipoic acid protects against histological and functional changes in the diabetic kidney. Biomed Pharmacother. 2022;153:113386.
51. Aminzadeh MA, Vaziri ND. Downregulation of the renal and hepatic hydrogen sulfide (H2S)-producing enzymes and capacity in chronic kidney disease. Nephrol Dial Transplant. 2012;27(2):498–504.
52. Nagahara N, Ito T, Kitamura H, Nishino T. Tissue and subcellular distribution of mercaptopyruvate sulfurtransferase in the rat: confocal laser fluorescence and immunoelectron microscopic studies combined with biochemical analysis. Histochem Cell Biol. 1998;110(3):243–50.
53. Brancaleone V, Roviezzo F, Vellecco V, De Gruttola L, Bucci M, Cirino G. Biosynthesis of H2S is impaired in non-obese diabetic (NOD) mice. Br J Pharmacol. 2008;155(5):673–80.
54. Jain SK, Bull R, Rains JL, Bass PF, Levine SN, Reddy S, McVie R, Bocchini JA. Low levels of hydrogen sulfide in the blood of diabetes patients and streptozotocin-treated rats causes vascular inflammation? Antioxid Redox Signal. 2010;12(11):1333–7.
55. Dutta M, Biswas UK, Chakraborty R, Banerjee P, Raychaudhuri U, Kumar A. Evaluation of plasma H$_2$S levels and H$_2$S synthesis in streptozotocin induced type-2 diabetes-an experimental study based on Swietenia macrophylla seeds. Asian Pac J Trop Biomed. 2014;4(1):S483–7.
56. Yuan X, Zhang J, Xie F, Tan W, Wang S, Huang L, Tao L, Xing Q, Yuan Q. Loss of the protein cystathionine β-synthase during kidney injury promotes renal tubulointerstitial fibrosis. Kidney Blood Press Res. 2017;42(3):428–43.
57. Ginter E, Simko V. Garlic (Allium sativum L.) and cardiovascular diseases. Bratisl Lek Listy. 2010;111(8):452–6.
58. Kashfi K, Olson KR. Biology and therapeutic potential of hydrogen sulfide and hydrogen sulfide-releasing chimeras. Biochem Pharmacol. 2013;85(5):689–703.
59. Safar MM, Abdelsalam RM. H2S donors attenuate diabetic nephropathy in rats: modulation of oxidant status and polyol pathway. Pharmacol Rep. 2015;67(1):17–23.
60. Gerő D, Torregrossa R, Perry A, Waters A, Le-Trionnaire S, Whatmore JL, Wood M, Whiteman M. The novel mitochondria-targeted hydrogen sulfide (H2S) donors AP123 and AP39 protect against hyperglycemic injury in microvascular endothelial cells in vitro. Pharmacol Res. 2016;113(Pt A):186–98.

61. Polhemus DJ, Li Z, Pattillo CB, Gojon G Sr, Gojon G Jr, Giordano T, Krum H. A novel hydrogen sulfide prodrug, SG1002, promotes hydrogen sulfide and nitric oxide bioavailability in heart failure patients. Cardiovasc Ther. 2015;33(4):216–26.
62. Zhang MY, Dugbartey GJ, Juriasingani S, Akbari M, Liu W, Haig A, McLeod P, Arp J, Sener A. Sodium thiosulfate-supplemented UW solution protects renal grafts against prolonged cold ischemia-reperfusion injury in a murine model of syngeneic kidney transplantation. Biomed Pharmacother. 2022;145:112435.
63. Mustafa AK, Gadalla MM, Sen N, Kim S, Mu W, Gazi SK, Barrow RK, Yang G, Wang R, Snyder SH. H_2S signals through protein S-sulfhydration. Sci Signal. 2009;2(96):ra72.
64. Kabil O, Banerjee R. Redox biochemistry of hydrogen sulfide. J Biol Chem. 2010;285(29):21903–7.
65. Liu YH, Yan CD, Bian JS. Hydrogen sulfide: a novel signaling molecule in the vascular system. J Cardiovasc Pharmacol. 2011;58(6):560–9.
66. Lee G, Hosgood SA, Patel MS, Nicholson ML. Hydrogen sulphide as a novel therapy to ameliorate cyclosporine nephrotoxicity. J Surg Res. 2015;197:419–26.
67. Pushpakumar S, Kundu S, Sen U. Hydrogen sulfide protects hyperhomocysteinemia-induced renal damage by modulation of Caveolin and eNOS interaction. Sci Rep. 2019;9(1):2223.
68. Roy A, Khan AH, Islam MT, Prieto MC, Majid DS. Interdependency of cystathione γ-lyase and cystathione β-synthase in hydrogen sulfide-induced blood pressure regulation in rats. Am J Hypertens. 2012;25(1):74–81.
69. Ge SN, Zhao MM, Wu DD, Chen Y, Wang Y, Zhu JH, Cai WJ, Zhu YZ, Zhu YC. Hydrogen sulfide targets EGFR Cys797/Cys798 residues to induce Na(+)/K(+)-ATPase endocytosis and inhibition in renal tubular epithelial cells and increase sodium excretion in chronic salt-loaded rats. Antioxid Redox Signal. 2014;21(15):2061–82.
70. Kuang Q, Xue N, Chen J, Shen Z, Cui X, Fang Y, Ding X. Low plasma hydrogen sulfide is associated with impaired renal function and cardiac dysfunction. Am J Nephrol. 2018;47(5):361–71.
71. Rahgozar M, Willgoss DA, Gobé GC, Endre ZH. ATP-dependent K+ channels in renal ischemia reperfusion injury. Ren Fail. 2003;25(6):885–96.
72. Wang R. Signaling pathways for the vascular effects of hydrogen sulfide. Curr Opin Nephrol Hypertens. 2011;20:107–12.
73. Wang R, Szabo C, Ichinose F, Ahmed A, Whiteman M, Papapetropoulos A. The role of H_2S bioavailability in endothelial dysfunction. Trends Pharmacol Sci. 2015;36:568–78.
74. Zhang J, Chen S, Liu H, Zhang B, Zhao Y, Ma K, Zhao D, Wang Q, Ma H, Zhang Z. Hydrogen sulfide prevents hydrogen peroxide-induced activation of epithelial sodium channel through a PTEN/PI(3,4,5)P3 dependent pathway. PLoS One. 2013;8(5):e64304.
75. Luo R, Hu S, Liu Q, Han M, Wang F, Qiu M, Li S, Li X, Yang T, Fu X, Wang W, Li C. Hydrogen sulfide upregulates renal AQP-2 protein expression and promotes urine concentration. FASEB J. 2019;33(1):469–83.
76. Liu YH, Bian JS. Bicarbonate-dependent effect of hydrogen sulfide on vascular contractility in rat aortic rings. Am J Physiol Cell Physiol. 2010;299(4):C866–72.
77. Lee SW, Cheng Y, Moore PK, Bian JS. Hydrogen sulphide regulates intracellular pH in vascular smooth muscle cells. Biochem Biophys Res Commun. 2007;358(4):1142–7.
78. Maruno M, Kiyosue H, Tanoue S, Hongo N, Matsumoto S, Mori H, et al. Renal arteriovenous shunts: clinical features, imaging appearance, and transcatheter embolization based on angio-architecture. Radiographics. 2016;36(2):580–95.
79. Olson KR, Dombkowski RA, Russell MJ, Doellman MM, Head SK, Whitfield NL, Madden JA. Hydrogen sulfide as an oxygen sensor/transducer in vertebrate hypoxic vasoconstriction and hypoxic vasodilation. J Exp Biol. 2006;209(Pt 20):4011–23.
80. Koning AM, Frenay AR, Leuvenink HG, van Goor H. Hydrogen sulfide in renal physiology, disease and transplantation—the smell of renal protection. Nitric Oxide. 2015;46:37–49.

81. Bełtowski J. Hypoxia in the renal medulla: implications for hydrogen sulfide signaling. J Pharmacol Exp Ther. 2010;334(2):358–63.
82. Olson KR. Hydrogen sulfide as an oxygen sensor. Antioxid Redox Signal. 2015;22(5):377–97.
83. Olson KR. Hydrogen sulfide as an oxygen sensor. Clin Chem Lab Med. 2013;51(3):623–32.
84. Prieto-Lloret J, Aaronson PI. Hydrogen sulfide as an O2 sensor: a critical analysis. Adv Exp Med Biol. 2017;967:261–76.
85. Teng H, Wu B, Zhao K, Yang G, Wu L, Wang R. Oxygen-sensitive mitochondrial accumulation of cystathionine β-synthase mediated by Lon protease. Proc Natl Acad Sci U S A. 2013;110(31):12679–84.
86. Olson KR, Whitfield NL. Hydrogen sulfide and oxygen sensing in the cardiovascular system. Antioxid Redox Signal. 2010;12(10):1219–34.
87. Hu H, Shi Y, Chen Q, Yang W, Zhou H, Chen L, Tang Y, Zheng Y. Endogenous hydrogen sulfide is involved in regulation of respiration in medullary slice of neonatal rats. Neuroscience. 2008;156(4):1074–82.
88. Dombkowski RA, Naylor MG, Shoemaker E, Smith M, DeLeon ER, Stoy GF, Gao Y, Olson KR. Hydrogen sulfide (H2S) and hypoxia inhibit salmonid gastrointestinal motility: evidence for H2S as an oxygen sensor. J Exp Biol. 2011;214(Pt 23):4030–40.
89. Yang T, Xu C. Physiology and pathophysiology of the intrarenal renin-angiotensin system: an update. J Am Soc Nephrol. 2017;28(4):1040–9.
90. Fountain JH, Kaur J, Lappin SL. Physiology, renin angiotensin system. In: StatPearls [Internet]. Treasure Island: StatPearls Publishing; 2023.
91. Vargas SL, Toma I, Kang JJ, Meer EJ, Peti-Peterdi J. Activation of the succinate receptor GPR91 in macula densa cells causes renin release. J Am Soc Nephrol. 2009;20(5):1002–11.
92. Peti-Peterdi J, Harris RC. Macula densa sensing and signaling mechanisms of renin release. J Am Soc Nephrol. 2010;21(7):1093–6.
93. Remuzzi G, Perico N, Macia M, Ruggenenti P. The role of renin-angiotensin-aldosterone system in the progression of chronic kidney disease. Kidney Int Suppl. 2005;99:S57–65.
94. Ames MK, Atkins CE, Pitt B. The renin-angiotensin-aldosterone system and its suppression. J Vet Intern Med. 2019;33(2):363–82.
95. Peters J, Münter K, Bader M, Hackenthal E, Mullins JJ, Ganten D. Increased adrenal renin in transgenic hypertensive rats, TGR(mREN2)27, and its regulation by cAMP, angiotensin II, and calcium. J Clin Invest. 1993;91(3):742–7.
96. Gambaryan S, Wagner C, Smolenski A, Walter U, Poller W, Haase W, Kurtz A, Lohmann SM. Endogenous or overexpressed cGMP-dependent protein kinases inhibit cAMP-dependent renin release from rat isolated perfused kidney, microdissected glomeruli, and isolated juxtaglomerular cells. Proc Natl Acad Sci U S A. 1998;95(15):9003–8.
97. Friis UG, Jensen BL, Sethi S, Andreasen D, Hansen PB, Skott O. Control of renin secretion from rat juxtaglomerular cells by cAMP-specific phosphodiesterases. Circ Res. 2002;90:996–1003.
98. Friis UG, Stubbe J, Uhrenholt TR, Svenningsen P, Nusing RM, Skøtt O, Jensen BL. Prostaglandin E2 EP2 and EP4 receptor activation mediates cAMP-dependent hyperpolarization and exocytosis of renin in juxtaglomerular cells. Am J Physiol Renal Physiol. 2005;289:F989–97.
99. Lu M, Liu YH, Goh HS, Wang JJ, Yong QC, Wang R, Bian JS. Hydrogen sulfide inhibits plasma renin activity. J Am Soc Nephrol. 2010;21(6):993–1002.
100. Lu M, Liu YH, Ho CY, Tiong CX, Bian JS. Hydrogen sulfide regulates cAMP homeostasis and renin degranulation in As4.1 and rat renin-rich kidney cells. Am J Physiol Cell Physiol. 2012;302(1):C59–66.
101. Liu YH, Lu M, Xie ZZ, Hua F, Xie L, Gao JH, Koh YH, Bian JS. Hydrogen sulfide prevents heart failure development via inhibition of renin release from mast cells in isoproterenol-treated rats. Antioxid Redox Signal. 2014;20(5):759–69.

102. Huang P, Chen S, Wang Y, Liu J, Yao Q, Huang Y, Li H, Zhu M, Wang S, Li L, Tang C, Tao Y, Yang G, Du J, Jin H. Down-regulated CBS/H2S pathway is involved in high-salt-induced hypertension in Dahl rats. Nitric Oxide. 2015;46:192–203.

103. Laggner H, Hermann M, Esterbauer H, Muellner MK, Exner M, Gmeiner BM, Kapiotis S. The novel gaseous vasorelaxant hydrogen sulfide inhibits angiotensin-converting enzyme activity of endothelial cells. J Hypertens. 2007;25(10):2100–4.

104. Li Y, Wang W, Jiang T, Yang B. Aquaporins in urinary system. Adv Exp Med Biol. 2017;969:131–48.

105. Chou CL, Knepper MA, Hoek AN, Brown D, Yang B, Ma T, Verkman AS. Reduced water permeability and altered ultrastructure in thin descending limb of Henle in aquaporin-1 null mice. J Clin Invest. 1999;103(4):491–6.

106. Ren H, Yang B, Molina PA, Sands JM, Klein JD. NSAIDs alter phosphorylated forms of AQP2 in the inner medullary tip. PLoS One. 2015;10(10):e0141714.

107. Ma T, Song Y, Yang B, Gillespie A, Carlson EJ, Epstein CJ, Verkman AS. Nephrogenic diabetes insipidus in mice lacking aquaporin-3 water channels. Proc Natl Acad Sci U S A. 2000;97(8):4386–91.

108. Kim YH, Earm JH, Ma T, Verkman AS, Knepper MA, Madsen KM, Kim J. Aquaporin-4 expression in adult and developing mouse and rat kidney. J Am Soc Nephrol. 2001;12(9):1795–804.

109. Procino G, Mastrofrancesco L, Sallustio F, Costantino V, Barbieri C, Pisani F, Schena FP, Svelto M, Valenti G. AQP5 is expressed in type-B intercalated cells in the collecting duct system of the rat, mouse and human kidney. Cell Physiol Biochem. 2011;28(4):683–92.

110. Promeneur D, Kwon TH, Yasui M, Kim GH, Frøkiaer J, Knepper MA, Agre P, Nielsen S. Regulation of AQP6 mRNA and protein expression in rats in response to altered acid-base or water balance. Am J Physiol Renal Physiol. 2000;279(6):F1014–26.

111. Ishibashi K, Imai M, Sasaki S. Cellular localization of aquaporin 7 in the rat kidney. Exp Nephrol. 2000;8(4–5):252–7.

112. Su W, Cao R, Zhang XY, Guan Y. Aquaporins in the kidney: physiology and pathophysiology. Am J Physiol Renal Physiol. 2020;318(1):F193–203.

113. Atochina-Vasserman EN, Biktasova A, Abramova E, Cheng DS, Polosukhin VV, et al. Aquaporin 11 insufficiency modulates kidney susceptibility to oxidative stress. Am J Physiol Renal Physiol. 2013;304(10):F1295–307.

114. Ren H, Yang B, Ruiz JA, Efe O, Ilori TO, Sands JM, Klein JD. Phosphatase inhibition increases AQP2 accumulation in the rat IMCD apical plasma membrane. Am J Physiol Renal Physiol. 2016;311(6):F1189–97.

115. Lei L, Huang M, Su L, Xie D, Mamuya FA, Ham O, Tsuji K, Păunescu TG, Yang B, Lu HAJ. Manganese promotes intracellular accumulation of AQP2 via modulating F-actin polymerization and reduces urinary concentration in mice. Am J Physiol Renal Physiol. 2018;314(2):F306–16.

116. Matsumura Y, Uchida S, Rai T, Sasaki S, Marumo F. Transcriptional regulation of aquaporin-2 water channel gene by cAMP. J Am Soc Nephrol. 1997;8(6):861–7.

117. Jung HJ, Raghuram V, Lee JW, Knepper MA. Genome-wide mapping of DNA accessibility and binding sites for CREB and C/EBPβ in vasopressin-sensitive collecting duct cells. J Am Soc Nephrol. 2018;29(5):1490–500.

118. Kharin A, Klussmann E. Many kinases for controlling the water channel aquaporin-2. J Physiol. 2023. https://doi.org/10.1113/JP284100.

119. Ranieri M, Di Mise A, Tamma G, Valenti G. Vasopressin-aquaporin-2 pathway: recent advances in understanding water balance disorders. F1000Res. 2019;8:F1000 Faculty Rev-149.

120. Valenti G, Tamma G. The vasopressin-aquaporin-2 pathway syndromes. Handb Clin Neurol. 2021;181:249–59.

121. Suh SH, Lee KE, Kim IJ, Kim O, Kim CS, Choi JS, Choi HI, Bae EH, Ma SK, Lee JU, Kim SW. Alpha-lipoic acid attenuates lipopolysaccharide-induced kidney injury. Clin Exp Nephrol. 2015;19(1):82–91.
122. Bae EH, Lee J, Ma SK, Kim IJ, Frøkiaer J, Nielsen S, Kim SY, Kim SW. Alpha-lipoic acid prevents cisplatin-induced acute kidney injury in rats. Nephrol Dial Transplant. 2009;24(9):2692–700.
123. Bae EH, Lee J, Kim SW. Effects of antioxidant drugs in rats with acute renal injury. Electrolyte Blood Press. 2007;5(1):23–7.
124. Bae EH, Lee KS, Lee J, Ma SK, Kim NH, Choi KC, Frøkiaer J, Nielsen S, Kim SY, Kim SZ, Kim SH, Kim SW. Effects of alpha-lipoic acid on ischemia-reperfusion-induced renal dysfunction in rats. Am J Physiol Renal Physiol. 2008;294(1):F272–80.

Chapter 2
Hydrogen Sulfide for Cisplatin- and Gentamicin-Induced Acute Kidney Injury

George J. Dugbartey

Cisplatin-Induced Acute Kidney Injury

Cisplatin (*cis*-diamminedichloroplatinum (II), CDDP) is one of the most commonly used chemotherapeutic agents for the treatment of several solid-organ cancers. These include head and neck cancer, penile cancer, endometrial cancer, esophageal cancer, carcinoids, mesothelioma, non-small cell lung cancer, malignant melanoma, adrenocortical carcinoma, testicular cancer, ovarian cancer, breast cancer, as well as cervical and bladder cancer [1, 2]. In testicular cancer, for example, cisplatin is a very potent antineoplastic agent, with cure rates of over 90% [3]. Historic evidence reveals that cisplatin was accidentally discovered to

This chapter is an expanded version by the same author in the publication titled Hydrogen sulfide: a novel nephroprotectant against cisplatin-induced renal toxicity. Nitric Oxide. 2016;57:15–20.

G. J. Dugbartey (✉)
Department of Pharmacology and Toxicology, School of Pharmacy, College of Health Sciences, University of Ghana, Accra, Ghana

Department of Physiology and Pharmacology, Accra College of Medicine, Accra, Ghana

Division of Urology, Department of Surgery, London Health Sciences Center, Western University, London, ON, Canada

Multi-Organ Transplant Program, London Health Sciences Center, Western University, London, ON, Canada

Matthew Mailing Center for Translational Transplant Studies, London Health Sciences Center, Western University, London, ON, Canada
e-mail: gdugbart@uwo.ca

G. J. Dugbartey, A. Sener, *Hydrogen Sulfide in Kidney Diseases*,
https://doi.org/10.1007/978-3-031-44041-0_2

inhibit cell division in 1965 by the American biophysicist and chemist Barnett Rosenberg [4]. By 1969, the antineoplastic property of cisplatin was demonstrated in animal models [5]. This anticancer property of cisplatin is, however, not completely clear, although increasing evidence suggests that cisplatin binds to DNA, resulting in the formation of inter- and intrastrand cross-links, which disrupt DNA synthesis and replication [6]. As cancer cells are rapidly dividing cells, the cisplatin-DNA adduct inhibits their replication, and they are destroyed by the cross-links.

Although cisplatin is currently the drug of choice in many platinum-based therapy regimens, acute kidney injury (AKI) has been reported to be a major side effect of high-dose cisplatin therapy that occurs in 20–30% of patients receiving high-dose cisplatin [7]. Cisplatin was first reported to induce AKI in animal studies [8], in which the authors observed tubular necrosis and high serum creatinine, as well as elevated levels of urea and other nitrogen-rich compounds in the blood. Cisplatin-induced AKI was reported in the initial clinical trials of cisplatin chemotherapy, showing acute renal failure in 14–100% of patients in cumulative dose [9]. Clinical reports indicate that cisplatin-induced AKI is often seen following 10 days of cisplatin treatment and is characterized by renal vasoconstriction leading to reduced renal blood flow (RBF) and consequently a reduced glomerular filtration rate (GFR) and elevated serum levels of creatinine, particularly after repeated doses of cisplatin [10, 11]. Quiescent proximal tubular cells are most vulnerable to cisplatin-induced AKI, as this is where the formation of DNA adducts cannot account for the dose-limiting toxicity [12]. Also, the presence of organic cation transporters and high-affinity copper transporters in the inner cortex and the outer medulla of proximal tubules contributes to disproportionate accumulation of cisplatin in kidney tissue, leading to cisplatin-induced AKI [13, 14]. Although the molecular pathway of cisplatin-induced AKI is not completely understood, results from several experimental studies suggest a sequential tubular injury pathway, which includes (1) uptake and bioconversion of cisplatin to a nephrotoxin, (2) induction of oxidative stress and mitochondrial DNA damage, (3) induction of inflammation, and (4) activation of apoptotic machinery (Fig. 2.1). Thus, these important mechanisms of injury (as well as other less important mechanisms) are potential therapeutic targets for reducing the nephrotoxic effects associated with cisplatin treatment.

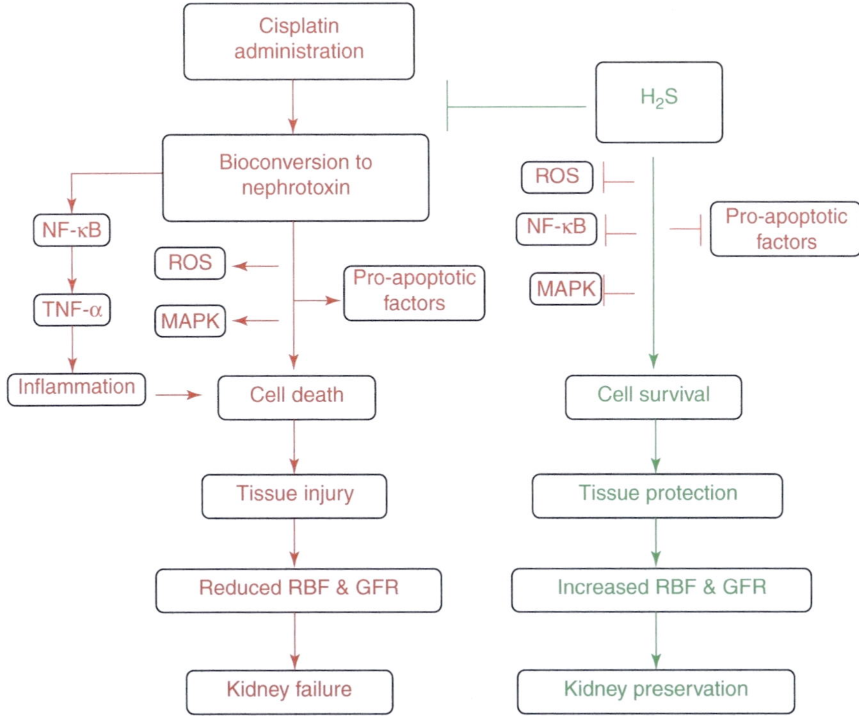

Fig. 2.1 Effects of H$_2$S on cisplatin-induced acute kidney injury. Cisplatin is bioconverted into a nephrotoxic metabolite upon uptake into proximal tubular epithelial cells. The nephrotoxic metabolite induces activation of nuclear factor kappa B (NF-κB) and consequently tumor necrosis factor alpha (TNF-α) production, which triggers inflammation and further potentiates cell injury and cell death. This culminates in decreased renal blood flow (RBF) and glomerular filtration rate (GFR) and ultimately renal failure. H$_2$S treatment disrupts the bioconversion pathway of cisplatin into a nephrotoxin and inhibits NF-κB activation as well as ROS production and pro-apoptotic stimuli. The disruption of the bioconversion of cisplatin into a nephrotoxin by H$_2$S leads to cell and tissue protection, increased (and maintenance of) RBF and GFR, and ultimately kidney preservation

Hydrogen Sulfide Ameliorates Cisplatin-Induced AKI

For several centuries, hydrogen sulfide (H$_2$S) was perceived to be a highly toxic gas and an environmental hazard, with the smell of rotten eggs. However, extensive research in the last two decades has shown that H$_2$S, produced endogenously at low micromolar concentrations, functions as an important physiological signaling molecule with potentially beneficial therapeutic properties [15, 16]. It has emerged as a third gasotransmitter, exhibiting similar properties to nitric oxide (NO) and carbon monoxide (CO), and is produced in all mammalian species studied thus far, including humans [15, 16]. Endogenous H$_2$S is synthesized by two cytosolic enzymes, cystathionine-β-synthase (CBS) and cystathionine-γ-lyase (CSE), a mitochondrial enzyme, 3-mercaptopyruvate sulfurtransferase (3-MST), and a peroxisomal enzyme, D-amino acid oxidase (DAO) [17–19]. In the kidney, these H_2S-producing enzymes are mainly localized in the brush border and cytoplasm of the proximal tubules [17–20], the same region of the nephron in which cisplatin accumulates and exerts its nephrotoxic action. The therapeutic potential of both endogenous and exogenous H_2S has been identified through its cyto- and organo-protective properties in a diverse array of in vitro and in vivo experimental models such as renal ischemia/reperfusion injury and whole-body hypothermia and rewarming [21–23]. Interestingly, H_2S has recently been identified to possess several renal protective properties that could disrupt the molecular pathways that lead to cisplatin-induced AKI and may thereby ameliorate renal injury in cancer patients undergoing cisplatin therapy (Fig. 2.1).

H₂S Disrupts the Bioconversion of Cisplatin into Nephrotoxic Metabolites

The bioconversion of cisplatin into a nephrotoxic metabolite is initially catalyzed by the enzyme glutathione-*S*-transferase (GST), which facilitates the binding of cisplatin to glutathione (GSH), a naturally occurring antioxidant in renal tubular cells, causing the formation of glutathione conjugates [24, 25]. The glutathione conjugate, which is not toxic by itself, is cleaved into a potent nephrotoxic metabolite by the enzymes gamma-glutamyl transpeptidase (GGT) and aminopeptidase N (APN), which are abundantly expressed on the surface of plasma membranes of proximal tubular cells. This metabolite can be further converted into highly reactive cysteine thiols by the enzyme cysteine-*S*-conjugate beta-lyase (CCBL), causing cytotoxicity [24, 25]. Dwivedi et al. [26] reported a significant decrease in GSH and GST activity in rat kidney following cisplatin treatment, suggesting an important role for these enzymes in the pathogenesis of cisplatin-induced AKI. Interestingly, treatment of rats with garlic-derived diallyl disulfide (DADS) and diallyl sulfide (DAS) (natural sources of H_2S) has been shown to enhance GSH and GST activities in the presence of cisplatin and reduce cisplatin-induced AKI [26, 27]. This increase in GSH and GST activity and subsequent mitigation of cisplatin-induced AKI suggest that H_2S increases natural antioxidant activity (Fig. 2.1). While this phenomenon requires further investigation, it is possible that modulation of GSH and GST by H_2S could disrupt the enzymatic conversion of glutathione conjugates into nephrotoxic metabolites, thereby limiting cisplatin-induced AKI.

H₂S Exerts Antioxidant Action that Limits Cisplatin-Induced AKI

A plethora of evidence indicates that cisplatin metabolites accumulate in the mitochondrial matrix where they inhibit complexes I–IV of the mitochondrial respiratory chain, decrease intracellular ATP, significantly reduce mitochondrial GSH activity, and consequently increase production of reactive oxygen species (ROS) [28, 29]. This increased ROS production overwhelms and impairs cellular antioxidant defense systems, leading to oxidative stress and subsequent cell dysfunction and apoptotic cell death [28, 29]. Moreover, the formation of cisplatin-DNA crosslinks in mitochondria leads to mitochondrial DNA damage [6]. Interestingly, H_2S has been shown to exhibit antioxidant effects that may reduce cisplatin-induced AKI. In a rat model of cisplatin-induced AKI, Fard et al. [30] showed a significant increase in the activity of renal antioxidant enzymes and reduced oxidative stress, as well as a marked decrease in renal injury and preservation of renal function following treatment with the sulfide salt, sodium hydrosulfide (NaHS) [31, 32]. Recent in vitro studies reported that treatment with AP39, a mitochondrially targeted H_2S donor, decreased mitochondrial ROS production, preserved mitochondrial function and integrity, and improved cellular viability during oxidative stress in both endothelial and renal epithelial cells [33, 34]. Treatment of rats with AP39 also resulted in decreased renal injury and oxidative stress as well as improved renal function following in vivo renal ischemia/reperfusion injury [34]. While the potential of H_2S to preserve mitochondrial DNA integrity and function during cisplatin-induced AKI remains to be revealed, these previous findings suggest that targeting of H_2S release to mitochondria may result in more potent antioxidant effects and hence may offer promising potential therapeutic avenue in ameliorating renal injury and failure due to cisplatin-induced AKI (Fig. 2.1).

Anti-inflammatory Property of H_2S Ameliorates Cisplatin-Induced AKI

Inflammatory response is an inevitable event that leads to cytotoxicity. The presence of cisplatin metabolites in renal tubular cells induces translocation of transcription factor nuclear factor *kappa* B (NF-κB) from the cytosol to the nucleus and activation of mitogen-activated protein kinases (MAPKs) [35]. Downstream gene expression induced by MAPK and NF-κB includes tumor necrosis factor alpha (TNF-α), a prototypical inflammatory cytokine which plays a key role in cisplatin-induced inflammation [36, 37]. Cisplatin accumulation in the renal tubular cells promotes the binding of TNF-α to its receptors (TNFR1 and TNFR2) expressed on the cell surface, triggering induction of inflammatory factors and recruitment of immune cells such as macrophages and neutrophilic granulocytes [38]. These immune cells produce (chemotactic) cytokines and ROS, which together enhance the nephrotoxic effect of cisplatin and may eventually progress into loss of kidney function [38–40]. Recent evidence has suggested that H_2S may exhibit beneficial anti-inflammatory properties in the context of drug-induced AKI [30]. In a rat model of cisplatin-induced AKI, intraperitoneal administration of NaHS suppressed TNF-α production, reduced inflammation, and ameliorated cisplatin nephrotoxicity [30]. In addition, treatment of rats with DAS during gentamicin-induced AKI has previously been shown to limit the activation of NF-κB and expression of TNF-α production [41], although this is yet to be tested in cisplatin-induced AKI model.

The first slow-release H$_2$S donor, GYY4137, has also been shown to exhibit anti-inflammatory effects in alternate models of inflammation. Treatment of rats with GYY4137 was shown to reduce production of pro-inflammatory cytokines and mediators (e.g., TNF-α, IL-6, IL-1ß, iNOS) and also inhibited NF-κB activation and MAPK signaling pathway in a model of endotoxic shock in rat lung and liver as well as LPS-challenged RAW 264.7 cells—macrophage cell line [42]. Similarly, in a rat model of myocardial ischemia/reperfusion injury, GYY3147 was reported to inhibit inflammation in cardiomyocytes by inhibiting activation of NF-κB and MAPK signaling pathway [43]. Considering the substantial anti-inflammatory properties of H$_2$S, mitigation of the inflammatory response following cisplatin injury is another potential mechanism by which H$_2$S ameliorates cisplatin-induced AKI (Fig. 2.1).

H$_2$S Disrupts the Apoptotic Machinery and Protects Proximal Tubular Cells Against Cisplatin-Induced AKI

Apoptosis of renal tubular cells has been demonstrated as a major mechanism that leads to early tubular cell death in several in vivo and in vitro models of cisplatin-induced AKI [44, 45]. Multiple pathways of apoptosis have been implicated in cisplatin-induced AKI of which the most critical involves opening of mitochondrial permeability transition pore (MPTP) of proximal tubular cells due to accumulation of ROS and influx of cytosolic calcium ions (Ca^{2+}) into the mitochondria. This leads to the release of pro-apoptotic factors such as cytochrome *c*, endonuclease G, and apoptosis-inducing factor from the mitochondria into the cytosol and nucleus [44–46]. In turn, this activates several events downstream, which results in caspase-dependent and caspase-independent apoptotic cell death [47, 48]. Interestingly, H$_2$S has also been recently shown to exhibit anti-apoptotic properties in response to cisplatin-induced AKI. Administration of NaHS to rats was reported to protect proximal tubular epithelial cells from apoptotic cell death and reverse cisplatin-induced mesangial matrix changes, attenuating the progression of cisplatin-induced toxicity [30–32]. Although the authors did not report the effect of H$_2$S on MPTP, it is possible that H$_2$S reduces apoptosis during cisplatin-induced AKI by inhibiting the opening of MPTP as has been previously demonstrated in spontaneously hypertensive rat model [49]. It should also be noted that other mechanisms of mitochondrial protection by H$_2$S have been previously reported to include electron donation and stimulation of mitochondrial electron transport flow [50, 51] and attenuation of homocysteine-induced mitochondrial toxicity [52]. Thus, apoptosis is a major factor in the pathogenesis of cisplatin-induced renal injury, which may be reduced through the specific anti-apoptotic effects of H$_2$S (Fig. 2.1).

H$_2$S Increases RBF and GFR and Might Improve Renal Function During Cisplatin Therapy

As illustrated in Fig. 2.1, another unique property of H$_2$S is its ability to increase RBF and GFR, a property which may help improve renal function in cancer patients undergoing cisplatin therapy. H$_2$S participates in several homeostatic functions including the control of vascular function and electrolyte balance [53–55], which are associated with the control of renal vascular and tubular functions. This implies that H$_2$S may participate in the regulation of renal function. In an experimental model to determine the effects of H$_2$S on renal function, Xia et al. [17] observed that intrarenal arterial infusion of NaHS increased RBF and GFR in rats by increasing vasodilation in pre- and post-glomerular arterioles. These effects were obliterated following administration of H$_2$S inhibitors. As declines in RBF and GFR are common clinical characteristics of cisplatin-induced AKI, it is possible that H$_2$S administration could improve RBF and GFR, thereby maintaining renal function during cisplatin treatment. Although this sounds promising, it is yet to be put forward in other studies. Thus, the ability of H$_2$S to increase and maintain RBF and GFR may allow maintenance of normal renal perfusion and consequently preserve renal function during cisplatin treatment.

Gentamicin-Induced AKI

Gentamicin belongs to the class of aminoglycoside antibiotics that has long been used against a broad range of Gram-negative bacteria and is still commonly used in clinical practice today. It is also used together with β-lactam antibiotics against *Staphylococcus* and *Enterococcus* spp. It remains the antibiotic of choice for many dangerous and life-threatening bacterial infections such as endocarditis, meningitis, pneumonia, urinary tract infections, bone infections, sepsis, and pelvic inflammatory disease [56]. However, just like cisplatin, AKI is a major complication of gentamicin administration, which has often been reported in about 20% of patients receiving gentamicin therapy and in 55–58% of patients in intensive care units [57–59]. Interestingly, single doses of gentamicin have also been reported to cause AKI [60]. The clinical manifestations of gentamicin-induced AKI include elevated levels of serum creatinine and blood urea nitrogen, proteinuria, reduced urine carnitine level, RBF, and GFR [61–65]. Histologically, gentamicin therapy has been associated with glomerular atrophy and hypertrophy, glomerular congestion, tubular necrosis and fibrosis with loss of brush border, tubular and perivascular edema, and infiltration of neutrophils and macrophages in the interstitium, which exacerbates the renal injury [66–70].

Mechanisms Underlying Gentamicin-Induced AKI

Burgeoning experimental evidence shows that the pathological mechanism underlying gentamicin-induced AKI is multifactorial. Like cisplatin, the primary route of gentamicin excretion is by the kidney. Following administration, gentamicin, a cationic drug, selectively accumulates in the renal proximal tubular cells, where it binds to phosphoinositides (negatively charged lipids of the brush border membrane) and forms a complex. This complex is then internalized by pinocytosis followed by reversible lysosomal phospholipidosis that negatively impacts several intracellular processes in the kidney [71, 72]. This includes activation of pro-apoptotic pathway in the proximal tubular epithelial cells; increased expression of the fibrotic protein, transforming growth factor-beta 1 (TGF-β1), and endothelin-1 (ET-1, a potent vasoconstrictor); activation of pro-inflammatory pathways involving NF-κB, p38MAPK, and TNF-α; recruitment of intercellular adhesion molecule-1 (ICAM-1) and monocyte chemoattractant protein-1 (MCP-1) to the site of injury; as well as increased influx of neutrophils and macrophages into the renal cortex and medulla, all of which contribute significantly to the pathogenesis and progression of renal injury along with reduced RBF and GFR [67, 73–77] (Fig. 2.2). In addition to this and as illustrated in Fig. 2.2, gentamicin also increases production of ROS such as superoxide anions, hydrogen peroxide, and hydroxyl radicals, as well as increases generation of reactive nitrogen species (RNS) in the renal cortex including the cortical mitochondria, leading to induction of oxidative and nitrosative stress and culminating in necrosis and apoptosis of tubular epithelial cells [78–81]. In summary, the pathophysiology of gentamicin-induced AKI is similar to that of cisplatin-AKI and involves activation of several pathological pathways including fibrotic, inflammatory, apoptotic, and oxidant pathways.

Hydrogen Sulfide Attenuates Gentamicin-Induced AKI

As with cisplatin-induced AKI, similar protective effects of H_2S have been reported in gentamicin-induced AKI although in only a few studies. In a rat model of gentamicin-induced AKI, Pedraza-Chaverrí et al. [61] observed that administration of DADS (50 mg/kg/24 h/4 days) attenuated renal injury induced by gentamicin. The renal protection was characterized by increased activities of manganese superoxide dismutase, glutathione peroxidase, and glutathione reductase, suggesting that H_2S attenuates gentamicin-induced AKI partly by activating renal antioxidant pathway and inhibiting induction of oxidative stress. The same authors later reported in another study the same salutary effect following administration of DAS at the same dose and duration as DADS, with preservation of renal structure and function evidenced by inhibition of proximal tubular epithelial cell necrosis and reduced proteinuria, serum creatinine, and blood urea nitrogen compared to gentamicin-induced AKI rats [82]. In addition to activating renal antioxidant pathway and thereby

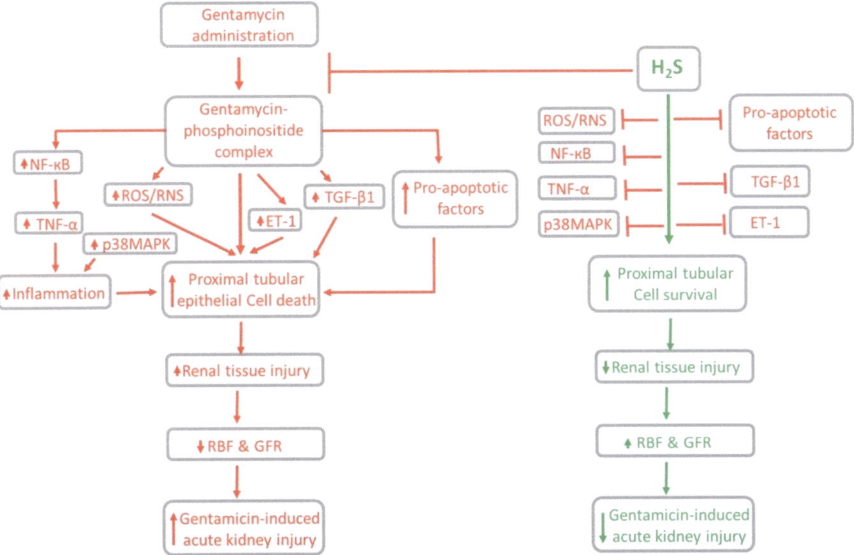

Fig. 2.2 Effects of H$_2$S on gentamicin-induced acute kidney injury. Gentamicin forms a complex with phosphoinositide upon uptake into proximal tubular epithelial cells. The complex induces activation of p38 mitogen-activated protein kinase (p38MAPK) and nuclear factor kappa B (NF-κB) and consequently tumor necrosis factor alpha (TNF-α) production, which triggers inflammation and further potentiates proximal tubular injury and cell death. Also, increased expression of transforming growth factor-beta 1 (TGF-β1) leads to renal fibrosis, while induction of oxidative and nitrosative stress through increased production of reactive oxygen species (ROS) and reactive nitrogen species (RNS), respectively, contributes to renal injury. The gentamicin-phosphoinositide complex also activates pro-apoptotic pathway, leading to death of proximal tubular epithelial cells. Increased expression of endothelin-1 (ET-1) by the complex also induces renal vasoconstriction, which culminates in reduced renal blood flow (RBF) and glomerular filtration rate (GFR) and exacerbates renal injury. H$_2$S inhibits all these pathological mechanisms, leading to cell survival and tissue protection along with increased (and maintenance of) RBF and GFR

contributing to protection against gentamicin-induced AKI, DAS was also reported by another research group to inhibit pro-inflammatory pathway by suppressing the activation of NF-κB and reducing the levels of pro-inflammatory mediators such as TNF-α, iNOS, and myeloperoxidase (MPO), which were significantly higher in the kidneys of control rats treated with gentamicin alone [83]. Besides DADS and DAS, administration of rats with NaHS also protected against gentamicin-induced AKI by reducing renal tubular necrosis and interstitial fibrosis and preserved glomerular and tubular integrity. Additionally, NaHS treatment also markedly reduced levels of renal cortical nitric oxide and malondialdehyde (MDA, a by-product of lipid peroxidation and an indication of ROS production) and significantly increased renal glutathione level relative to rats that received gentamicin alone [84]. It is important to note that these H$_2$S donors did not negatively influence the antibiotic action of gentamicin, as individual treatment with DADS and DAS was reported to even exhibit bacteriostatic effect against *Escherichia coli* and further enhanced the antibiotic effect of gentamicin in vitro [85]. This exciting finding suggests that H_2S donor compounds could be used as antibacterial agents that could be administered along with gentamicin to treat bacterial infections and at the same time prevent the occurrence of clinical gentamicin-induced AKI. However, considering that this finding is from only one study, more studies including in vivo models are required to corroborate this result. Overall, the antioxidant, anti-inflammatory, anti-apoptotic, anti-fibrotic, and vasodilatory properties of H_2S are beneficial in attenuating AKI associated with gentamicin administration.

Limitations and Future Perspectives

Despite the promising effects of H_2S on cisplatin- and gentamicin-induced AKI, studies demonstrating a direct protective role of H_2S are scarce. As well, data on the renal protective effect of H_2S during cisplatin- and gentamicin-induced AKI is limited to administration of garlic-derived sulfur compounds DAS and DADS, and the sulfide salt, NaHS, which are less effective and/or physiologically accurate H_2S producers compared to newer generations of synthetic H_2S donors such as GYY4137 and AP39 [26, 27, 30–32]. Moreover, the dose of sulfide administered in these studies (i.e., NaHS, >100 micromolar/kg intravenous or intraperitoneal) is extremely higher compared to endogenous levels of sulfide (i.e., H_2S, <2 micromolar in plasma and tissue). Furthermore, intracellular levels of H_2S were not measured following administration of NaHS, cisplatin, or gentamicin [30–32]. Despite these shortcomings, H_2S derived from DAS, DADS, and NaHS does appear to reduce oxidative stress, inflammation, apoptosis, and renal injury associated with cisplatin- and gentamicin-induced AKI [26, 27, 30–32]. More recently, sodium thiosulfate (a clinically used H_2S donor drug) protected the kidneys of cancer patients under cisplatin chemotherapy against cisplatin-induced AKI [86]. In contrast to these findings, inhibition of endogenous H_2S formation by DL-propargylglycine (PAG, a specific inhibitor of CSE) has been shown in different studies to improve renal function and reduce the expression of TNF-α and the influx of macrophages, neutrophils, and T lymphocytes into the kidney following administration of cisplatin and gentamicin [87–89]. The findings that inhibition of endogenous H_2S production also mitigates renal injury and inflammation associated with cisplatin and gentamicin treatments stand in direct contradiction of the previous studies showing the protective effects of exogenous H_2S against cisplatin- and gentamicin-induced AKI. This discrepancy may be because PAG could negatively affect the functions of a number of other enzymes that may play a role in the cellular response to cisplatin and gentamicin toxicity. This explanation is supported by the fact that incubation of renal tubular epithelial cells with increasing concentrations of NaHS did not decrease cell survival by itself, casting doubt on whether PAG is only inhibiting H_2S production in this case [87]. Also, since sulfide is a chelator of heavy metals and can readily react with platinum to form a platinum sulfide (PtS) complex, it is possible that the protective effects of exogenous H_2S administration shown in these cisplatin studies are not due to a direct modulation of oxidative stress, inflammation, or apoptotic pathways, but rather a direct detoxification and/or removal of cisplatin itself. Furthermore, the studies reporting the renal protective effect of H_2S inhibition on gentamicin-induced AKI used exclusively female rats with a greater risk of developing gentamicin-induced AKI [88] compared to male animals that are often used in such studies. This also suggests a possible hormonal role in renal protection against gentamicin-induced AKI. Future studies involving measurement of cellular sulfide levels during cisplatin- and gentamicin-induced AKI, as well as potential detoxification of both drugs by H_2S alone, should help to shed light on these contradicting findings. As new and more targeted H_2S donor molecules and inhibitors are being synthesized, we will gain a closer understanding of its roles as a renal protective molecule. In addition, the role of the other H_2S-producing enzymes (CBS, 3-MST, and DAO) should be studied in the context of cisplatin- and gentamicin-induced AKI.

Conclusion

Among other side effects of cisplatin therapy, AKI is the chief limiting factor. The observed AKI during cisplatin treatment is the net result of several molecular pathways including uptake and bioconversion of cisplatin to nephrotoxic metabolites, dysfunction of mitochondrial DNA, induction of inflammation, and activation of apoptotic pathways by cisplatin metabolites. Despite several clinical and experimental interventions to ameliorate this problem including prophylactic intensive hydration and forced diuresis, there is still incomplete protection against cisplatin-induced AKI in cancer patients receiving cisplatin therapy. Gentamicin treatment against Gram-negative bacterial infections induces AKI in a similar pathophysiological fashion as cisplatin. H_2S seems to be a promising nephroprotective agent, as it possesses combinatorial molecular properties which target multiple molecular mechanisms underlying cisplatin- and gentamicin-induced AKI. While administration of exogenous sources of H_2S protects against renal injury following cisplatin and gentamicin treatments, production of endogenous H_2S seems to have the opposite effect. Thus, the precise effects of H_2S on the molecular pathways affected by cisplatin and gentamicin that may lead to renal injury remain to be unraveled. Pharmacological modulation of levels of H_2S together with involvement of other H_2S-synthesizing enzymes may represent an important therapeutic alternative for limiting cisplatin- and gentamicin-induced AKI and could open new avenues to enhance cisplatin- and gentamicin-based therapies.

Conflict of Interest None.

References

1. Cohen SM, Lippard SJ. Cisplatin: from DNA damage to cancer chemotherapy. Prog Nucleic Acid Res Mol Biol. 2001;67:93–130.
2. Siddik ZH. Cisplatin: mode of cytotoxic action and molecular basis of resistance. Oncogene. 2003;22:7265–79.
3. Loehrer PJ, Gonin R, Nichols CR, Weathers T, Einhorn LH. Vinblastine plus ifosphamide plus cisplatin as initial salvage therapy in recurrent germ cell tumor. J Clin Oncol. 1998;16:2500–4.
4. Rosenberg B, Vancamp L, Krigas T. Inhibition of cell division in Escherichia coli by electrolysis products from a platinum electrode. Nature. 1965;205:698–9.
5. Rosenberg B, VanCamp L, Trosko JE, Mansour VH. Platinum compounds: a new class of potent antitumour agents. Nature. 1969;222:385–6.
6. Dzagnidze A, Katsarava Z, Makhalova J, Liedert B, et al. Repair capacity for platinum-DNA adducts determines the severity of cisplatin-induced peripheral neuropathy. J Neurosci. 2007;27:9451–7.
7. Yao X, Panichpisal K, Kurtzman N, Nugent K. Cisplatin nephrotoxicity: a review. Am J Med Sci. 2007;334:115–24.
8. Kociba RJ, Sleight SD. Acute toxicologic and pathologic effects of *cis*- diamminedichloroplatinum (NSC-119875) in the male rat. Cancer Chemother Rep. 1971;55:1–8.
9. Goldstein RS, Mayor GH. Minireview. The nephrotoxicity of cisplatin. Life Sci. 1983;32:685–90.
10. Winston JA, Safirstein R. Reduced renal blood flow in early cisplatin-induced acute renal failure in the rat. Am J Physiol. 1985;249:F490–6.
11. Miura K, Goldstein RS, Pasino DA, Hook J. Cisplatin nephrotoxicity: role of filtration and tubular transport of cisplatin in isolated perfused kidneys. Toxicology. 1987;44:147–58.
12. Townsend DM, Tew KD, Lin H, King JB, Hanigan MH. Role of glutathione-S- transferase Pi in cisplatin-induced nephrotoxicity. Biomed Pharmacother. 2009;63:79–85.
13. Ciarimboli G, Ludwig T, Lang D, et al. Cisplatin nephrotoxicity is critically mediated via human organ cation transporter 2. Am J Pathol. 2005;167:1477–84.
14. Pabla N, Murphy RF, Liu K, Dong Z. The copper transporter Ctrl contributes to cisplatin uptake by renal tubular cells during cisplatin-induced nephrotoxicity. Am J Physiol Renal Physiol. 2009;296:F505–11.
15. Abe K, Kimura H. The possible role of hydrogen sulfide as an endogenous neuromodulator. J Neurosci. 1996;16(3):1066–71.
16. Wang R. Two's company, three's a crowd: can H_2S be the third endogenous gaseous transmitter? FASEB J. 2002;16:1792–8.
17. Xia M, Chen L, Muh RW, Li PL, Li N. Production and action of hydrogen sulfide, a novel gaseous bioactive substance in the kidneys. J Pharmacol Exp Ther. 2009;329:1056–62.
18. Mikami Y, Shinuya N, Kimura Y, Nagahara N, Ogasawara Y, Kimura H. Thioredoxin and dihydrolipoic acid are required for 3-mercaptopyruvate sulfurtransferase to produce hydrogen sulfide. Biochem J. 2011;439(3):479–85.
19. Shibuya N, Koike S, Tanaka M, et al. A novel pathway for the production of hydrogen sulfide from D-cysteine in mammalian cells. Nat Commun. 2013;4:1366.
20. Yamamoto J, Sato W, Kosugi T, et al. Distribution of hydrogen sulfide (H2S)-producing enzymes and the roles of the H2S donor sodium hydrosulfide in diabetic nephropathy. Clin Exp Nephrol. 2013;17:32–40.
21. Talaei F, Bouma HR, van der Graaf AC, et al. Serotonin and dopamine protect from hypothermia/rewarming damage through the CBS/H_2S pathway. PLoS One. 2011;6(7):e22568.
22. Lobb I, Zhu J, Liu W, Haig A, Lan Z, Sener A. Hydrogen sulfide treatment ameliorates long-term renal dysfunction resulting from prolonged warm renal ischemia-reperfusion injury. Can Urol Assoc J. 2014;8(5–6):E413–8.
23. Dugbartey GJ, Talaei F, Houwertjes MC, Goris M, Epema AH, Bouma HR, Henning RH. Dopamine treatment attenuates acute kidney injury in a rat model of deep hypo-

thermia and rewarming—the role of renal H_2S-producing enzymes. Eur J Pharmacol. 2015;2999(15):30361–7.

24. Nishimura T, Newkirk K, Sessions RB, et al. Association between expression of glutathione-associated enzymes and response to platinum-based chemotherapy in head and neck cancer. Chem Biol Interact. 1998;111–112:187–98.

25. Paolicchi A, Sotiropuolou M, Perego P, et al. γ-Glutamyl transpeptidase catalyses the extracellular detoxification of cisplatin in a human cell line derived from the proximal convoluted tubule of the kidney. Eur J Cancer. 2002;39:996–1003.

26. Dwivedi C, Abu-Ghazaleh A, Guenther J. Effects of diallyl sulfide and diallyl disulfide on cisplatin-induced changes in glutathione and glutathione-S-transferase activity. Anticancer Drugs. 1996;7(7):792–4.

27. Chiarandini Fiore JP, Fanelli SL, de Ferreyra EC, Castro JA. Diallyl disulfide prevention of cis-Diamminedichloroplatinum-induced nephrotoxicity and leukopenia in rats: potential adjuvant effects. Nutr Cancer. 2008;60(6):784–91.

28. Davis CA, Nick HS, Agarwal A. Manganese superoxide dismutase attenuates cisplatin-induced renal injury: importance of superoxide. J Am Soc Nephrol. 2001;12:2683–90.

29. Kruidering M, van der Water B, de Heer E, et al. Cisplatin-induced nephrotoxicity in porcine proximal tubular cells: mitochondrial dysfunction by inhibition of complexes I to IV of the respiratory chain. J Pharmacol Exp Ther. 1997;280:638–49.

30. Fard AA, Ahangarpour A, Gharibnaseri MK, Jalali T, Rashidi I, Ahmadzadeh M. Effects of hydrogen sulfide on oxidative stress, tnf-α level and kidney histological changes in cisplatin nephrotoxicity in rat. J Physiol Pharmacol Adv. 2013;3(3):57–65.

31. Ahangarpour A, Fard AA, Gharibnaseri MK, Jalali T, Rashidi I. Hydrogen sulfide ameliorates the kidney dysfunction and damage in cisplatin-induced nephrotoxicity in rat. Vet Res Forum. 2014;5(2):121–7.

32. Fard AA, Ahangarpour A, Gharibnaseri KM, Ahmadizadeh M, Rashidi I, Jalali T. Effects of exogenous and endogenous hydrogen sulfide on plasma renin and erythropoietin in cisplatin-induced nephrotoxicity in rats. URMIAMJ. 2015;26(6):459–66.

33. Le Trionnaire S, Perry A, Szczesny B, et al. The synthesis and functional evaluation of a mitochondrially-targeted hydrogen sulfide donor, (10-oxo-10-(4-(3-thioxo-3H-1,2-dithiol-5yl) phenoxy)decyl)triphenylphosphonium bromide (AP39). MedChemComm. 2014;5:728–36.

34. Ahmad A, Olah G, Szczesny B, Wood ME, Whiteman M, Szabo C. AP39, a mitochondrially-targeted hydrogen sulfide donor, exerts protective effects in renal epithelial cells subjected to oxidative stress *in vitro* and in acute renal injury *in vivo*. Shock. 2016;45:88–97.

35. Dhillon AS, Hagan S, Rath O, et al. MAP kinase signaling pathways in cancer. Oncogene. 2007;26:3279–90.

36. Ramesh G, Reeves WB. TNF-α mediates chemokine and cytokine expression and renal injury in cisplatin nephrotoxicity. J Clin Invest. 2002;110:835–42.

37. Ramesh G, Kimball SR, Jefferson LS, Reeves WB. Endotoxin and cisplatin synergistically stimulate TNF-α production by renal epithelial cells. Am J Physiol. 2007;292:812–9.

38. Faubel S, Lewis EC, Reznikov L, et al. Cisplatin-induced acute renal failure is associated with an increase in the cytokines interleukin (IL)-1beta, IL-18, IL-6, and neutrophil infiltration in the kidney. J Pharmacol Exp Ther. 2007;322:8–15.

39. Faubel S, Lewis EC, Reznikov L, et al. Cisplatin-induced acute renal failure is associate with an increase in the cytokines interleukin (IL)-1beta, IL-18, IL-6, and neutrophil infiltration in the kidney. J Pharmacol Exp Ther. 2007;322:8–15.

40. Lu LH, Oh DJ, Dursun B, He Z, Hoke TS, Faubel S, Edelstein CL. Increased macrophage infiltration and fractalkine expression in cisplatin-induced acute renal failure in mice. J Pharmacol Exp Ther. 2008;324:111–7.

41. Kalayarasan S, Prabhu PN, Sriram N, Manikandan R, Arumugam M, Sudhandiran G. Diallyl sulfide enhances antioxidants and inhibits inflammation through the activation of Nrf2 against gentamicin-induced nephrotoxicity in Wister rats. Eur J Pharmacol. 2009;606(1–3):162–71.

42. Li L, Salto-Tellez M, Tan CH, Whiteman M, Moore PK. GYY4137, a novel hydrogen sulfide-releasing molecule, protects against endotoxic shock in the rat. Free Radic Biol Med. 2009;47:103–13.

43. Meng G, Wang J, Xiao Y, Bai W, Xie L, Shan L, Moore PK, Ji Y. GYY4137 protects against myocardial ischemia and reperfusion injury by attenuating oxidative stress and apoptosis in rats. J Biomed Res. 2015;29:203–13.

44. Lee RH, Song JM, Park MY, et al. Cisplatin-induced apoptosis by translocation of endogenous Bax in mouse collecting duct cells. Biochem Pharmacol. 2001;62:1013–23.

45. Jiang M, Wei Q, Wang J, Du Q, Yu J, Zhang L, Dong Z. Regulation of PUMA- alpha by p53 in cisplatin-induced renal cell apoptosis. Oncogene. 2006;25:4056–66.

46. Yin X, Apostolov EO, Shah SV, et al. Induction of renal endonuclease G by cisplatin is reduced in DNase I-deficient mice. J Am Soc Nephrol. 2007;18:2544–53.

47. Wei Q, Dong G, Franklin J, Dong Z. The pathological role of Bax in cisplatin nephrotoxicity. Kidney Int. 2007;72:53–62.

48. Jiang M, Wang CY, Huang S, Yang T, Dong Z. Cisplatin-induced apoptosis in p53-deficient renal cells via the intrinsic mitochondrial pathway. Am J Physiol Renal Physiol. 2009;296:F983–93.

49. Strutynska NA, Dorofeieva NO, Vavilova HL, Sahach VF. Hydrogen sulfide inhibits Ca(2+)-induced mitochondrial permeability transition pore opening in spontaneously hypertensive rats. Fiziol Zh. 2013;59(1):3–10.

50. Goubern M, Andriamihaja M, Nubel T, Blachier F, Bouillaud F. Sulfide, the first inorganic substrate for human cells. JASEB J. 2007;21:1699–706.

51. Modis K, Coletta C, Erdelyi K, Papapetropoulos A, Szabo C. Intramitochondrial hydrogen sulfide production by 3-mercaptopyruvate sulfurtransferase maintains mitochondrial electron transport flow and supports cellular biogenesis. FASEB J. 2013;27:601–11.

52. Kamat PK, Kalani A, Tyagi SC, Tyagi N. Hydrogen sulfide epigenetically attenuates homocysteine-induced mitochondrial toxicity mediated through NMDA receptor in mouse brain endothelial (bEnd3) cells. J Cell Physiol. 2015;230:378–94.

53. Cheng Y, Ndisang JF, Tang G, Cao K, Wang R. Hydrogen sulfide-induced relaxation of resistance mesenteric artery beds of rats. Am J Physiol Heart Circ Physiol. 2004;287:H2316–23.

54. Yan H, Du J, Tang C. The possible role of hydrogen sulfide on the pathogenesis of spontaneous hypertension in rats. Biochem Biophys Res Commun. 2004;313:22–7.

55. Webb GD, Lim LH, Oh VM, et al. Contractile and vasorelaxant effects of hydrogen sulfide and its biosynthesis in the human internal mammary artery. J Pharmacol Exp Ther. 2008;324:876–82.

56. Miglioli PA, Silini R, Carzeri O, Grabocka E, Allerberger F. Antibacterial activity of gentamicin and ciprofloxacin against Gram-negative bacteria: interactions with pig and calf sera. Pharmacol Res. 1999;39(4):321–3.

57. Schentag JJ, Plaut ME, Cerra FB. Comparative nephrotoxicity of gentamicin and tobramycin: pharmacokinetic and clinical studies in 201 patients. Antimicrob Agents Chemother. 1981;19(5):859–66.

58. Raveh D, Kopyt M, Hite Y, Rudensky B, Sonnenblick M, Yinnon AM. Risk factors for nephrotoxicity in elderly patients receiving once-daily aminoglycosides. QJM. 2002;95(5):291–7.

59. Oliveira JF, Silva CA, Barbieri CD, Oliveira GM, Zanetta DM, Burdmann EA. Prevalence and risk factors for aminoglycoside nephrotoxicity in intensive care units. Antimicrob Agents Chemother. 2009;53(7):2887–91.

60. Weir BA, Mazumdar DC. Aminoglycoside nephrotoxicity following single-dose cystoscopy prophylaxis. Ann Pharmacother. 1994;28(2):199–201.

61. Pedraza-Chaverrí J, Maldonado PD, Barrera D, Cerón A, Medina-Campos ON, Hernández-Pando R. Protective effect of diallyl sulfide on oxidative stress and nephrotoxicity induced by gentamicin in rats. Mol Cell Biochem. 2003;254(1–2):125–30.

62. Silan C, Uzun O, Comunoğlu NU, Gokçen S, Bedirhan S, Cengiz M. Gentamicin-induced nephrotoxicity in rats ameliorated and healing effects of resveratrol. Biol Pharm Bull. 2007;30(1):79–83.

63. Soliman KM, Abdul-Hamid M, Othman AI. Effect of carnosine on gentamicin-induced nephrotoxicity. Med Sci Monit. 2007;13(3):BR73–83.
64. Romero F, Pérez M, Chávez M, Parra G, Durante P. Effect of uric acid on gentamicin- induced nephrotoxicity in rats—role of matrix metalloproteinases 2 and 9. Basic Clin Pharmacol Toxicol. 2009;105(6):416–24.
65. Al-Shabanah OA, Aleisa AM, Al-Yahya AA, Al-Rejaie SS, Bakheet SA, Fatani AG, Sayed-Ahmed MM. Increased urinary losses of carnitine and decreased intramitochondrial coenzyme A in gentamicin-induced acute renal failure in rats. Nephrol Dial Transplant. 2010;25(1):69–76.
66. Ateşşahin A, Karahan I, Yilmaz S, Ceribaşi AO, Princci I. The effect of manganese chloride on gentamicin-induced nephrotoxicity in rats. Pharmacol Res. 2003;48(6):637–42.
67. Bledsoe G, Crickman S, Mao J, Xia CF, Murakami H, Chao L, Chao J. Kallikrein/kinin protects against gentamicin-induced nephrotoxicity by inhibition of inflammation and apoptosis. Nephrol Dial Transplant. 2006;21(3):624–33.
68. Polat A, Parlakpinar H, Tasdemir S, Colak C, Vardi N, Ucar M, Emre MH, Acet A. Protective role of aminoguanidine on gentamicin-induced acute renal failure in rats. Acta Histochem. 2006;108(5):365–71.
69. Ozbek E, Cekmen M, Ilbey YO, Simsek A, Polat EC, Somay A. Atorvastatin prevents gentamicin-induced renal damage in rats through the inhibition of p38-MAPK and NF-kappaB pathways. Ren Fail. 2009;31(5):382–92.
70. Lakshmi BVS, Sudhakar M. Protective effect of zingiber officinale on gentamicin-induced nephrotoxicity in rats. Int J Pharmacol. 2010;6:58–62.
71. Laurent G, Carlier MB, Rollman B, Van Hoof F, Tulkens P. Mechanism of aminoglycoside-induced lysosomal phospholipidosis: in vitro and in vivo studies with gentamicin and amikacin. Biochem Pharmacol. 1982;31(23):3861–70.
72. Sandhu JS, Sehgal A, Gupta O, Singh A. Aminoglycoside nephrotoxicity revisited. J Indian Acad Clin Med. 2007;8:331–3.
73. Wahl SM, Hunt DA, Wakefield LM, McCartney-Francis N, Wahl LM, Roberts AB, Sporn MB. Transforming growth factor type beta induces monocyte chemotaxis and growth factor production. Proc Natl Acad Sci U S A. 1987;84(16):5788–92.
74. Tang WW, Feng L, Mathison JC, Wilson CB. Cytokine expression, upregulation of intercellular adhesion molecule-1, and leukocyte infiltration in experimental tubulointerstitial nephritis. Lab Invest. 1994;70(5):631–8.
75. Ali BH. Gentamicin nephrotoxicity in humans and animals: some recent research. Gen Pharmacol. 1995;26(7):1477–87.
76. El Mouedden M, Laurent G, Mingeot-Leclercq MP, Taper HS, Cumps J, Tulkens PM. Apoptosis in renal proximal tubules of rats treated with low doses of aminoglycosides. Antimicrob Agents Chemother. 2000;44(3):665–75.
77. Geleilete TJ, Melo GC, Costa RS, Volpini RA, Soares TJ, Coimbra TM. Role of myofibroblasts, macrophages, transforming growth factor-beta endothelin, angiotensin-II, and fibronectin in the progression of tubulointerstitial nephritis induced by gentamicin. J Nephrol. 2002;15(6):633–42.
78. Walker PD, Barri Y, Shah SV. Oxidant mechanisms in gentamicin nephrotoxicity. Ren Fail. 1999;21(3–4):433–42.
79. Maldonado PD, Barrera D, Rivero I, Mata R, Medina-Campos ON, Hernández-Pando R, Pedraza-Chaverrí J. Antioxidant S-allylcysteine prevents gentamicin-induced oxidative stress and renal damage. Free Radic Biol Med. 2003;35(3):317–24.
80. Wang Z, Liu L, Mei Q, Liu L, Ran Y, Zhang R. Increased expression of heat shock protein 72 protects renal proximal tubular cells from gentamicin-induced injury. J Korean Med Sci. 2006;21(5):904–10.
81. Balakumar P, Chakkarwar VA, Kumar V, Jain A, Reddy J, Singh M. Experimental models for nephropathy. J Renin Angiotensin Aldosterone Syst. 2008;9(4):189–95.

82. Pedraza-Chaverrí J, González-Orozco AE, Maldonado PD, Barrera D, Medina-Campos ON, Hernández-Pando R. Diallyl disulfide ameliorates gentamicin-induced oxidative stress and nephropathy in rats. Eur J Pharmacol. 2003;473(1):71–8.
83. Kalayarasan S, Prabhu PN, Sriram N, Manikandan R, Arumugam M, Sudhandiran G. Diallyl sulfide enhances antioxidants and inhibits inflammation through the activation of Nrf2 against gentamicin-induced nephrotoxicity in Wistar rats. Eur J Pharmacol. 2009;606(1–3):162–71.
84. Otunctemur A, Ozbek E, Dursun M, Sahin S, Besiroglu H, Ozsoy OD, Cekmen M, Somay A, Ozbay N. Protective effect of hydrogen sulfide on gentamicin-induced renal injury. Ren Fail. 2014;36(6):925–31.
85. Maldonado PD, Chánez-Cárdenas ME, Pedraza-Chaverrí J. Aged garlic extract, garlic powder extract, S-allylcysteine, diallyl sulfide and diallyl disulfide do not interfere with the antibiotic activity of gentamicin. Phytother Res. 2005;19(3):252–4.
86. Laplace N, Kepenekian V, Friggeri A, Vassal O, Ranchon F, Rioufol C, Gertych W, Villeneuve L, Glehen O, Bakrin N. Sodium thiosulfate protects from renal impairment following hyperthermic intraperitoneal chemotherapy (HIPEC) with cisplatin. Int J Hyperth. 2020;37(1):897–902.
87. Della Colleta Francescato H, Cunha FQ, Costa RS, et al. Inhibition of hydrogen sulfide formation reduces cisplatin-induced renal damage. Nephrol Dial Transplant. 2011;26:479–88.
88. Dam VP, Scott JL, Ross A, Kinobe RT. Inhibition of cystathionine gamma-lyase and the biosynthesis of endogenous hydrogen sulphide ameliorates gentamicin-induced nephrotoxicity. Eur J Pharmacol. 2012;685(1–3):165–73.
89. Francescato HD, Chierice JR, Marin EC, Cunha FQ, Costa RS, Silva CG, Coimbra TM. Effect of endogenous hydrogen sulfide inhibition on structural and functional renal disturbances induced by gentamicin. Braz J Med Biol Res. 2012;45(3):244–9.

Chapter 3
Hydrogen Sulfide as a Potential Future Therapy for Chronic Kidney Disease, Hyperhomocysteinemia, and Management of Polycystic Kidney Disease

George J. Dugbartey

Chronic Kidney Disease

Chronic kidney disease (CKD) is a growing and serious public health burden throughout the world and poses a major threat to the twenty-first-century global health policy. It is associated with increased morbidity, prolonged hospitalization, and higher mortality in addition to increased caregiver burden and higher financial cost. In 1990, CKD was ranked 27th in the global causes of death but rose to 18th in 2012 [1] with a mortality rate of 82% [1]. There is compelling evidence that CKD is most prevalent among ethnic minorities and disadvantaged populations in developed countries [2], and in many developing countries [3]. CKD ultimately

---

This chapter is an expanded version by the same author in the publication titled The smell of renal protection against chronic kidney disease: hydrogen sulfide offers a potential stinky remedy. Pharmacol Rep. 2018;70(2):196–205.

G. J. Dugbartey (✉)
Department of Pharmacology and Toxicology, School of Pharmacy, College of Health Sciences, University of Ghana, Accra, Ghana

Department of Physiology and Pharmacology, Accra College of Medicine, Accra, Ghana

Division of Urology, Department of Surgery, London Health Sciences Center, Western University, London, ON, Canada

Multi-Organ Transplant Program, London Health Sciences Center, Western University, London, ON, Canada

Matthew Mailing Center for Translational Transplant Studies, London Health Sciences Center, Western University, London, ON, Canada
e-mail: gdugbart@uwo.ca

G. J. Dugbartey, A. Sener, *Hydrogen Sulfide in Kidney Diseases*,
https://doi.org/10.1007/978-3-031-44041-0_3

progresses to end-stage renal disease (ESRD, the terminal stage of CKD), the rate of which is dependent on coexisting pathologies and other risk factors. Although the definition and classification of CKD have evolved over time, recent international guidelines consider CKD as a progressive loss of renal function (decreased glomerular filtration rate) for 3-month duration or more, regardless of the underlying cause [4]. Kidney function declines in the initial stages of the disease with no symptoms, and adaptive mechanisms attempt to compensate for the reduced nephron number. However, complications such as uremia, vascular calcification and mineral bone disease, reduced red blood cell survival, iron deficiency, and anemia due to reduced production of erythropoietin arise as CKD progresses to ESRD for which renal replacement therapy is required [5–7].

Pathophysiology of CKD

The kidney, particularly the renal medulla, is physiologically considered a hypoxic environment due to an arteriovenous oxygen shunt and the complex transport function, which requires oxygen usage [8, 9]. Hence, the renal medulla forms an important pathophysiological basis of CKD and other causes of renal dysfunction in patients with preexisting pathologies. Imaging studies with needle electrodes and visualization of hypoxia-inducible factor activity using luciferase in mice have demonstrated this innately low oxygen tension in the kidney [10]. In addition, blood oxygen level-dependent magnetic resonance imaging showed some correlation between renal hypoxia and severity of CKD in several clinical studies [11]. In line with this, renal hypoxia, especially tubulointerstitial hypoxia, has emerged as a central pathophysiological player in the progression of renal damage in CKD, serving as the "final common pathway" towards ESRD development [12]. As illustrated in Fig. 3.1, tubulointerstitial hypoxia activates signaling cascades that drive several molecular processes such as induction of oxidative and endoplasmic reticulum (ER) stress, inflammation, and tubulointerstitial fibrosis [13–15]. These events in turn further aggravate hypoxia in the tubulointerstitium, forming a pathological vicious cycle of chronic hypoxia and tubulointerstitial injury that results in ESRD, as first proposed in the "chronic hypoxia hypothesis" [16]. Although the importance of CKD is widely appreciated, including improvements in the quality of existing therapies, new therapeutic options are limited, thereby causing increased morbidity, mortality, and poor quality of life among CKD patients. Therefore, instead of preserving glomerular filtration rate in CKD and other renal diseases as a conventional therapy, new treatment regimens should aim at preserving oxygenation in the renal tissue, particularly the renal medulla.

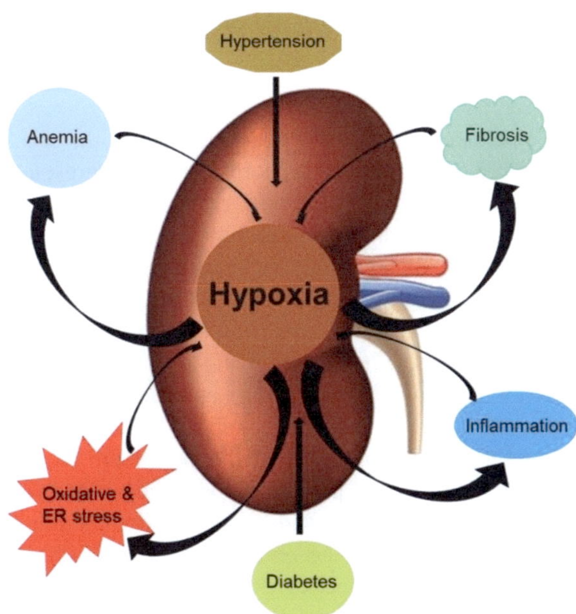

Fig. 3.1 Renal hypoxia as a central pathophysiological player in chronic kidney disease (CKD). Renal hypoxia, particularly tubulointerstitial hypoxia, stimulates induction of tubulointerstitial fibrosis, inflammation, and oxidative and endoplasmic reticulum stress, which in turn promote cellular susceptibility and further aggravate hypoxia, thus forming a pathological vicious cycle in CKD progression to end-stage renal disease. Comorbidities such as hypertension and diabetes also accelerate CKD progression

Hydrogen Sulfide Against CKD

It is now widely accepted among researchers that hydrogen sulfide (H_2S), a gas with malodorous smell and the most recently recognized member of a family of gaseous signaling molecules secondary to nitric oxide (NO) and carbon monoxide (CO), exhibits remarkable therapeutic characteristics. Alteration of its level contributes to various renal pathologies including diabetic and hypertensive nephropathies [17, 18], drug-induced AKI [19, 20], hypothermia-induced acute kidney injury [21–23], as well as ischemia/reperfusion injury in experimental models of renal transplantation [24, 25]. H_2S has also been recently implicated in CKD [26], and several experimental studies regarding its protective mechanisms against CKD are currently underway, with some promising findings reported so far.

H_2S is produced endogenously in the cytoplasm and mitochondria of mammalian cells using L-cysteine and D-cysteine as substrates and catalyzed by the enzymes cystathionine β-synthase (CBS), cystathionine γ-lyase (CSE), 3-mercaptopyruvate sulfurtransferase (3-MST), and D-amino acid oxidase (DAO) [27–29]. Although these H_2S-producing enzymes are expressed in a tissue-specific manner, all four of them are abundantly expressed in various cell types in the kidney [27, 30], thus making the kidney a rich source of endogenous H_2S production. In addition to its endogenous production, H_2S is also applied exogenously via sources such as sodium hydrosulfide (NaHS), sodium sulfide (Na_2S), GYY4137, AP39 and AP123, SG1002, S-propargyl cysteine, sodium thiosulfate, sulfurous mineral water, garlic-derived polysulfide, diallyl disulfide, and diallyl sulfide [31–40]. List of H_2S donors currently under investigation and the results of clinical trials.

H_2S Preserves Medullary Oxygenation and May Prevent Hypoxia in CKD

As mentioned above, oxygen availability in the renal medulla is greatly reduced compared to that in the renal cortex. It is of interest to note that although the kidney receives about 25% of the total cardiac output, the medulla receives only about 10% of the total renal perfusion in functionally normal kidney [9], thus making this region of the kidney highly vulnerable to pathological conditions such as CKD in which hypoxic injury is inevitable. Growing evidence indicates that H_2S is an oxygen sensor and mediates tubulovascular cross talk in the renal medulla [27, 41]. H_2S accumulates in the renal medulla under hypoxic condition and restores oxygen balance by increasing medullary flow and decreasing tubular sodium (Na^+) transport in the medullary thick ascending limb [27]. Also, H_2S induces vasodilation by stimulating the opening of ATP-sensitive potassium (K_{ATP}) channels, the main vascular target of H_2S [42, 43], thereby increasing blood flow in various blood vessels. Although H_2S-induced vasodilation is yet to be studied in the vasa recta, the straight arterioles that supply the renal medulla, K_{ATP} channels have been found in the descending vasa recta pericytes [44]—vascular smooth muscle cells that respond to vasoactive agents and regulate medullary perfusion. This finding suggests that endogenous H_2S may regulate pericyte tone. In addition to increasing medullary blood flow and decreasing tubular Na^+ transport, H_2S (at high concentrations) inhibits mitochondrial respiration, an oxygen-consuming process, via reversible antagonism at complex IV of the mitochondrial respiratory chain [45], thus reducing the energy required for tubular transport function. This mechanism may help preserve medullary oxygenation. Moreover, it has been shown that under hypoxic conditions, the cytosolic H_2S-producing enzymes, CBS and CSE, translocate to the mitochondria and, together with 3-MST, stimulate mitochondrial H_2S production [46, 47]. Furthermore, H_2S at low concentrations (i.e., low micromolar concentrations) stimulates cellular respiration and hence ATP production, by donating electron at the level of coenzyme Q in the mitochondrial electron transport chain between complexes I and III [46, 48], which may provide some energy for tubular Na^+ transport, thereby preventing ATP-depleted tubular injury. In conclusion, although the effect of H_2S in the renal medulla is understudied in CKD models, available data indicate that H_2S is an oxygen sensor and its stimulation improves medullary blood flow and oxygenation during hypoxia (Fig. 3.2), and hence may protect against CKD and its associated complications.

H_2S Stabilizes HIF Pathway and May Prevent CKD Progression

Hypoxia-inducible factor (HIF) is a well-known transcription factor whose activation induces the expression of many protective genes in hypoxia-adaptive response in various pathophysiological processes in renal diseases [49]. It comprises α and β

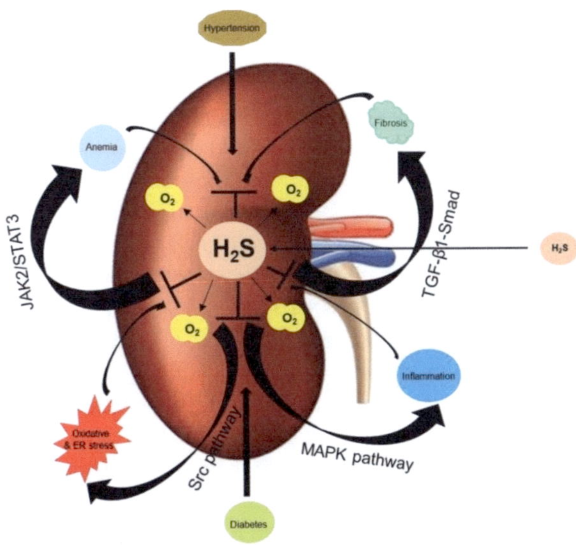

Fig. 3.2 Protective mechanisms of hydrogen sulfide (H₂S) against chronic kidney disease (CKD). Endogenous H₂S accumulates in the renal medulla under hypoxic conditions and functions as an oxygen sensor that restores oxygen balance and increases blood flow in the renal medulla, thereby reducing hypoxia. This effect is boosted by exogenous H₂S supplementation. H₂S also exhibits antioxidant, anti-inflammatory, anti-fibrotic, and anemia-relieving characteristics via various cellular and molecular mechanisms, all of which inhibit the pathological vicious cycle induced by hypoxia and protect the kidney against the pathogenesis and progression of CKD

subunits of which HIF-1α and HIF-2α are isoforms of the α subunit. In response to renal hypoxia, HIF-1α is primarily expressed in the tubular epithelial cells, where it mediates hypoxia adjustment while HIF-2α is limited to the endothelial and interstitial cells [50, 51]. There is currently an ongoing debate regarding the effect of HIF on CKD pathophysiology. Pharmacological activation of the HIF pathway has been shown to be protective against hypoxic injury in the tubulointerstitium of rats with nephritis [52] as well as in obese, hypertensive diabetic type 2 rat model [53] and in rat remnant kidney model of CKD [54–56]. Moreover, it has been well established that HIF accumulates at certain stages of CKD, which protects against hypoxic injury [57, 58]. Arguing against these encouraging findings, renal hypoxia is rather aggravated in many CKD patients, with declining renal function, which progresses to ESRD. This suggests impairment of the HIF system in CKD. Indeed, activation of renal HIF was found to be suboptimal in CKD even in the face of profound renal hypoxia in rats and in immortalized rat proximal tubular cells exposed to hypoxic conditions [59, 60]. In addition, impairment in cellular adaptation to hypoxia has been reported in chronic diabetic condition in which HIF-1α was deregulated [61, 62]. Moreover, an inappropriate and prolonged activation of HIF was found to initiate and promote renal fibrosis in CKD [63, 64] and contributed to angiotensin II-induced glomerular injury and hypertensive CKD via induction of vasoactive factors [65]. These divergent results suggest that the effect of HIF on the pathophysiology of CKD may depend on the pathological context.

Considering the experimental evidence that the HIF system is activated to suboptimal levels in CKD, its stabilization holds a promising novel therapeutic target in CKD and its associated complications. H_2S has been reported to stabilize the HIF system in pathologies and under hypoxic conditions, although its effect in CKD has not been described extensively. In experimental ulcerative colitis, for example, garlic-derived diallyl disulfide, a natural source of H_2S, was found to stabilize the expression of colonic HIF-1α, upregulate hypoxia-responsive genes, and reduce the extent and severity of colitis, as loss of CSE (H_2S-producing enzyme) reduced HIF-1α stabilization and aggravated the disease [66]. The authors further observed that compared to control mice and rats, diallyl disulfide maintained HIF-1α level even at a later stage of the disease when HIF-1α level was expected to decline, and thus improved recovery from the disease. Since the HIF system is impaired in CKD, this finding suggests that addition of garlic to diets of CKD patients could help stabilize the HIF system and may contribute to renal protection and prevent CKD progression. Besides, garlic has been reported to improve diabetic and hypertensive conditions (two leading causes of CKD and its progression to ESRD) in preclinical and clinical studies [67, 68]. The finding also supports that of a previous study in which low H_2S concentrations (via NaHS at 300 µM) upregulated and stabilized HIF-1α mRNA and proteins and also increased transcriptional activity of HIF-1α in vascular smooth muscle cells under hypoxic condition [69], suggesting that H_2S may have an important protective role via the HIF pathway against hypoxia in the vascular system. It is, however, important to point out that the HIF pathway is regulated primarily at the posttranslational level. Therefore, the finding that H_2S influences HIF mRNA suggests its interaction with an HIF transcriptional regulator upstream, and therefore, further investigation is needed in order to provide greater insights into this mechanism. In addition to the findings of Flannigan et al. [66], the slow-releasing H_2S donor, GYY4137, was reported to prevent degradation (and induce accumulation) of HIF-1α under normoxic and hypoxic conditions in THP-1 macrophages, human monocytic *cell* line derived from an acute monocytic leukemia patient [70]. Notwithstanding these effects of H_2S, Kai et al. [71] reported that high H_2S concentrations (via NaHS at 1 mM) downregulated and destabilized HIF-1α protein accumulation and its target gene expression in cultured cells and in mice exposed to hypoxic conditions. Since NaHS at 10–100 µM is widely used to reflect physiologically relevant concentration of H_2S in various studies [72, 73], one could argue that such a high concentration (1 mM) of H_2S is clearly outside the physiological range of endogenous H_2S and therefore may be cytotoxic in the long term. However, one study claims that NaHS at 10–100 µM downregulates HIF-1α protein levels in established human cell lines under both hypoxic and hypoxia-mimetic conditions [74]. This contradictory finding warrants further investigations since it is likely that the effects of H_2S on the HIF pathway are dose dependent. Overall, H_2S upregulates and stabilizes the HIF pathway under hypoxic condition and therefore should be considered in CKD prevention and/or retardation of its progression to ESRD.

H₂S Stimulates EPO Production and May Prevent Anemia of CKD and ESRD

Anemia is a common clinical problem among CKD patients. It decreases oxygen delivery to the kidney and further aggravates tubulointerstitial hypoxia, thereby accelerating decline in renal function [75, 76]. A number of factors are attributed to the development of anemia. However, since the 1950s, reduced production of erythropoietin (EPO, a hormone of renal origin that promotes erythrogenesis in response to tissue hypoxia) has been the most notable factor in CKD patients [77, 78]. Hence, EPO-stimulating agents (and adjuvant iron therapy) are often prescribed to ESRD patients with anemia [7]. However, a major concern in the prescription of EPO-stimulating agents is the development of drug resistance and other side effects such as increased systemic inflammation at later stages of treatment [79, 80]. Therefore, novel and alternative modes of intervention have become imperative in the treatment of anemia of CKD and ESRD.

Recent reports indicate that H_2S can induce EPO synthesis, and thus prevent the development of anemia of CKD and ESRD. In an experiment to investigate the effect of H_2S on EPO production during hypoxia, CSE knockout mice showed markedly reduced levels of EPO, hemoglobin, and HIF-responsive genes following 72 h of exposure to hypoxia compared to wild-type mice [81]. In the same study, exogenous H_2S supplementation reversed and restored the levels of EPO, hemoglobin, and HIF-regulated genes. In addition, pharmacological inhibition of H_2S resulted in significantly lower levels of EPO, HIF-1α, HIF-2α, as well as CBS protein levels in renal and haptic cell lines exposed to hypoxia, all of which were increased above hypoxic and normoxic levels following H_2S treatment [81]. These findings suggest that blocking endogenous H_2S production inhibits the HIF pathway during hypoxia as well as its target genes including EPO. These findings also suggest that endogenous H_2S and its exogenous donors should be further explored as an alternative to the conventional therapies for anemia of CKD.

The anemia-relieving effect of H_2S has also been implicated in inflammation-anemia relationship following the discovery of hepcidin, the master regulator of iron homeostasis. In a mouse model of anemia of inflammation (AI), formerly known as "anemia of chronic diseases," common in patients with chronic inflammation, Wang et al. [82] recently reported high levels of serum hepcidin and compromised erythrocyte membrane integrity. This finding supports clinical evidence that disturbance in iron homeostasis occurs in CKD and ESRD patients under hemodialysis, as high serum hepcidin levels as well as increased markers of inflammation and reduced iron absorption and mobilization were observed in these patients, thus presenting lower levels of iron and transferrin (carrier for iron in the bloodstream) [83, 84]. The study by Wang et al. [82] also found that the novel water-soluble H_2S donor, S-propargyl cysteine, suppressed production of hepatic hepcidin and corrected lipopolysaccharide-driven hypoferremia (iron deficiency in blood). They further observed that S-propargyl cysteine administration reduced serum hepcidin level, improved transferrin saturation, and maintained erythrocyte membrane integrity via inhibition of JAK2/STAT3 activation, leading to improvement in chronic AI. Interestingly, pharmacological inhibition of H_2S reversed all these effects. This result was consistent with another AI model in which CSE knockout mice were used [85], thus further elucidating the anemia-relieving effect of H_2S. On the whole, H_2S has the potential to maintain acceptable EPO and iron levels, and therefore could serve as a remedy for anemia of CKD and other anemia-related diseases (Fig. 3.2).

H_2S Inhibits Fibrosis and Inflammatory Response in CKD and Prevents Its Progression

Renal fibrosis, including glomerulosclerosis and tubulointerstitial fibrosis, is a common pathological hallmark of progressive renal diseases with diverse etiologies. It is characterized by injury and death of renal parenchymal cells and influx and maturation of inflammatory cells in the interstitium, which accounts for the general inflammatory response commonly associated with CKD progression [14, 15, 86]. There is also fibroblast proliferation and myofibroblast transdifferentiation, excessive accumulation and deposition of extracellular matrix (ECM), and fibrogenesis [15]. The development of tubulointerstitial fibrosis in CKD is driven by chronic hypoxia, leading to excessive scarring, which in turn aggravates hypoxia and further contributes to CKD progression [12, 87]. In fact, studies have shown that tubulointerstitial fibrosis is the most reliable predictor of CKD progression to ESRD [87, 88]. Due to their high metabolic activity and oxygen demand, renal tubular epithelial cells become vulnerable and suffer hypoxic injury in CKD, and in response secrete pro-fibrotic and pro-inflammatory agents such as fibroblast growth factor-2, transforming growth factor-β (TGF-β), and tumor necrosis factor-alpha (TNF-α). These factors in turn activate the tubular epithelial cells and renal fibroblasts into myofibroblasts, which produce excess ECM proteins such as collagen and matrix metalloproteinases (MMPs) in the injured interstitium [87, 88]. Additionally, the activated epithelial cells undergo a phenotypic change referred to as epithelial-to-mesenchymal transition (EMT), which further contributes to ECM accumulation and tubular atrophy, thereby extending the distance between the capillaries and nearby tubular cells, leading to endothelial dysfunction and capillary rarefaction. This, in turn, impairs oxygen delivery and further aggravates tubulointerstitial hypoxia, thus forming a pathological vicious cycle [88, 89].

Against this background, suppressing renal fibroblast activation and EMT inhibition are of utmost interest to reverse renal fibrosis and inflammation in CKD and other renal pathologies. Growing evidence indicates that H_2S exhibits anti-fibrotic characteristics that inhibit fibrosis in CKD. Evidence from clinical studies shows that plasma H_2S and H_2S-producing enzymes in circulating leukocytes are significantly reduced in chronic hemodialysis and uremic patients due to transcriptional deregulation of genes encoding for H_2S-producing enzymes [90, 91]. This suggests that uremic toxin of CKD impairs endogenous H_2S system. Interestingly, the reduction in H_2S and H_2S-producing enzymes is associated with increased cardiovascular risk factors and mortality, mediated by activation of the pro-inflammatory molecules, vascular cell adhesion molecule-1, and intercellular adhesion molecule-1 [91]. These reports were in agreement with experimental findings in which Aminzadeh and Vaziri [26] observed significantly reduced plasma H_2S concentration as well as reduced renal H_2S-producing capacity and H_2S-producing enzymes in rats with CKD caused by 5/6 nephrectomy, the mainstay of studies of progressive renal disease. In a mouse model of CKD characterized by hyperhomocysteinemia (a human recessive genetic disorder due to CBS deficiency and a known risk factor for cardiovascular diseases), proteinuria, and reduced plasma H_2S, heterozygous $CBS^{+/-}$ mice showed markedly increased activities of MMP-2 and MMP-9, which form one of the early events of ECM remodeling in renal fibrosis [92]. In the same study, the authors further observed that H_2S supplementation increased plasma H_2S level, normalized urinary protein secretion and MMP activities, and prevented apoptotic cell death. Along the same train of thought, exogenous H_2S administration also attenuated increased production of collagen, ECM, and expression of α-smooth muscle actin (a fibrotic marker) and also decreased macrophage infiltration in the interstitium and expression of TNF-α and other pro-inflammatory cytokines, thereby inhibiting renal fibrosis and inflammation in a rat model of unilateral urethral obstruction (UUO) [15, 86], an experimental model commonly used for progressive renal interstitial fibrosis without confounding causative factors (Fig. 3.2). In another model of UUO-induced renal fibrosis, Jung et al. [93] observed decreased renal CBS, CSE, and H_2S concentration in a time-dependent manner, which negatively correlated with tubulointerstitial fibrosis after UUO in mice. Interestingly, all these effects were reversed following H_2S treatment. This result was consistent with another rat model of UUO in which H_2S supplementation upregulated CBS and CSE mRNA and protein expressions in the kidney and plasma H_2S level and significantly reduced the degree of tubulointerstitial fibrosis [94].

Several *in vitro* studies have demonstrated the mechanisms underlying the anti-fibrotic effect of H_2S in various tissues. In the kidney, for example, H_2S treatment suppressed cultured renal fibroblast proliferation by reducing DNA synthesis and expression of proliferation-related proteins such as proliferating cell nuclear antigen and c-Myc within the cells [15]. In addition, H_2S inhibited quiescent renal fibroblast and renal tubular epithelial cell transdifferentiation into myofibroblast by blocking TGF-β1-Smad and mitogen-activated protein kinase signaling pathways [15, 93], two major signaling pathways implicated in renal fibrosis. Moreover, Jung et al. [93] also reported inhibition of UUO-induced activation of nuclear factor-kappa B (a transcriptional regulator of inflammatory genes) following H_2S administration, suggesting that the anti-fibrotic effect of H_2S is associated with a decline in renal inflammation in CKD. H_2S also inhibited TGF-β1-induced renal EMT in HK-2 cells (renal tubular epithelial cells) via ERK-dependent and β-catenin-dependent pathways [95]. Similar anti-fibrotic mechanisms of H_2S were observed in lung and cardiac fibroblasts, and hepatic and pancreatic stellate cells in humans and animals, in which H_2S suppressed the activation of proliferation-related genes, protein kinases, signaling pathways, and ion channels [96–100]. Furthermore, as with HK-2 cells, H_2S also attenuated TGF-β1-induced EMT of A549 cells (human alveolar epithelial cells) by decreasing the expression of vimentin (a mesenchymal marker) and TGF-β1-induced Smad2/3 phosphorylation and increasing the levels of E-cadherin (an epithelial marker) [101]. Interestingly, pharmacological inhibition of H_2S in the A549 cells resulted in induction of EMT, characterized by decreased E-cadherin level, increased vimentin expression, and appearance of fibroblast-like morphology. Several studies have also reported inhibition of the TGF-β1-Smad pathway by H_2S, leading to decreased TGF-β1 and collagen synthesis and accumulation, suppression of proliferation and hypertrophy of mesangial cells, and ultimately mitigation of renal ECM remodeling in diabetic and hypertensive rat models [40].

It is also of interest to note that the effect of H_2S on renal fibrosis extends to intrarenal renin-angiotensin-aldosterone system (RAAS), a system of hormones involved in the regulation of plasma sodium concentration and arterial blood pressure and abnormally activated in diabetic and nondiabetic patients with CKD. Angiotensin II (Ang II), a component of the RAAS and a well-known activator of fibrotic and inflammatory pathways, induces stimulation of collagen synthesis in cultured murine renal proximal tubular cells and collecting duct cells via TGF-β1-Smad-dependent and -independent signaling pathways [102, 103]. Also, renin has been implicated in the progression of renal fibrosis in a mouse model of UUO, as renin inhibition with aliskiren (an antihypertensive agent) attenuated UUO-induced renal fibrosis and inflammation [104]. Recent reports indicate that H_2S suppresses the levels and activities of renin and Ang II. In a rat model of renovascular hypertension, H_2S administration reduced levels of serum Ang II via downregulation of intracellular cyclic adenosine monophosphate (cAMP, a second messenger that regulates renin release) and reversed Ang II-induced hypertension, proteinuria, and renal injury [105]. In a subsequent *in vitro* study, the authors further observed that H_2S treatment of renin-containing As4.1 cells (renal tumor cell line) and renin-rich juxtaglomerular cells strongly reduced synthesis, release, and activity of renin by suppressing cAMP production [106], thus inhibiting the initial and rate-limiting step in the RAAS cascade. Laggner et al. [107] also found that H_2S directly inhibits the activity of angiotensin-converting enzyme (ACE, a zinc-containing vasoconstrictor) in human endothelial cells by interfering with zinc in the active center of the enzyme, leading to attenuation of hypertension. Clinical studies have shown that RAAS inhibition with ACE inhibitors (ACEis) and Ang II receptor blockers (ARBs), the primary medications for renal fibrosis and cardiovascular conditions, does not sufficiently achieve the expected renal protection in CKD patients, thereby causing many patients to still progress to ESRD or die from cardiovascular causes [108, 109]. Therefore, administration of H_2S donors or in combination with ACEi and ARB could exert a complementary action to ACEi and ARB and may increase the efficacy of RAAS inhibition and improve renal protection. Taken together, these pieces of experimental evidence indicate that H_2S is a very potent anti-fibrotic agent that may represent a novel approach in drug development for the treatment of renal fibrosis in CKD and its associated complications.

H₂S Suppresses Oxidative and Endoplasmic Reticulum Stress Associated with CKD

Tubulointerstitial hypoxia in CKD induces increased production of reactive oxygen species (ROS) from mitochondria and ER, which react with various biomolecules, causing increased renal oxygen consumption and decreased oxygen levels. This leads to oxidative and ER stress, which in turn further aggravates renal hypoxia [13]. Oxidative stress has been found to impair renal oxygen sensing due to the lack of increased EPO production as well as heme oxygenase-1 (HO-1, CO-producing enzyme) and vascular endothelial growth factor (VEGF, a protein that promotes angiogenesis and restores blood supply to ischemic tissue) in the kidneys of diabetic rats [110]. Interestingly, impaired mitochondrial respiratory machinery has been reported in CKD patients and has been suggested as both the cause and consequence of overproduction of ROS and enhanced oxidative stress [111]. This might explain the subnormal energy metabolism among CKD population since the mitochondria is the powerhouse of cell. Oxidative and ER stress induces apoptosis of renal tubular epithelial cells and leads to CKD progression [112, 113]. Oxidative stress has been reported in the early stages in CKD patients as renal function declines, as well as in those with ESRD [114]. Ceballos-Picot et al. [115] observed reduced serum levels of glutathione (GSH, the most abundant naturally occurring antioxidant in cells) and activity of glutathione peroxidase (GPx, an antioxidant and component of the glutathione cycle) in the plasma of ESRD patients. Also, lower concentration of serum selenium (another natural antioxidant) and platelet GPx activity were reported in CKD patients as well as increased serum levels of ROS in hemodialysis patients compared to healthy control subjects [116]. Furthermore, CKD is associated with impaired nitric oxide (NO) system (another natural antioxidant system), in which decreased NO and increased concentration of endogenous NO synthase inhibitors were reported [115]. High levels of serum malondialdehyde (MDA, a product of lipid peroxidation in the cell and a marker of oxidative stress) in erythrocytes and severe vitamin deficiency were also found in hemodialysis patients, suggesting shortening of the life span of erythrocytes in CKD patients, which may lead to anemia of ESRD [117]. In addition to this latter clinical observation, some preclinical studies reported that ER stress also suppresses EPO production and induces hepcidin expression, thereby causing hypoferremia in mice under hypoxic condition [118, 119]. This implies that ER stress is related to erythropoiesis, iron metabolism, and anemic conditions.

Despite prophylactic use of antioxidant therapies in the treatment and amelioration of CKD, the outcome has been disappointing so far. Hence, the search for novel antioxidant therapies still continues. H₂S has been established in several experimental disease models as a potent antioxidant, directly scavenging ROS and activating several endogenous antioxidant enzymes, thereby bolstering endogenous antioxidant defense system and preventing oxidative and ER stress (Fig. 3.2). In a rat model of CKD induced by 5/6 nephrectomy, Aminzadeh and Vaziri [26] observed downregulation of glutathione synthase and upregulation of nicotinamide adenine dinucleotide phosphate oxidase (NADPH oxidase, a major source of ROS in the kidney) in the remnant kidney and markedly increased plasma MDA at 6 weeks after renal ablation. Interestingly, this was associated with markedly reduced renal H_2S-producing capacity and renal CBS in the CKD rats compared to control group, while renal CSE and 3-MST expressions were reduced at 12 weeks post-renal ablation in the CKD group. Although the authors did not consider the effect of H_2S treatment in their study, other studies reported significantly reduced levels of MDA and ROS and increased activities of endogenous antioxidants such as GPx and superoxide dismutase (SOD), as well as downregulation of pro-apoptotic proteins and upregulation of anti-apoptotic proteins following H_2S administration, thus contributing to renal protection in a rat model of chronic renal failure [120]. This report supports that of another chronic renal failure model, in which exogenous H_2S supplementation normalized hyperhomocysteinemia-induced increased renal ROS production, reduced glutathione-to-oxidized glutathione ratio, and partly prevented renal damage in heterozygous $CBS^{+/-}$ mice [92]. In addition, mice subjected to UUO and treated with H_2S during surgery reversed the decreases in renal CBS and CSE expressions and renal H_2S concentrations and also markedly reduced UUO-induced oxidative stress, with preservation of endogenous antioxidant enzymes including catalase and SOD expressions as well as GSH level compared to sham group, leading to renal protection against UUO-induced oxidative damage [93]. This observation was confirmed by recent studies of other UUO models in rats in which the levels and activities of renal GSH, NO, and SOD were markedly increased while renal MDA levels significantly decreased following 10–14 days of UUO induction and H_2S administration in comparison with sham-operated group [86, 121]. Studies have shown that H_2S inhibits ROS-induced oxidative stress by enhancing homocysteine transport for GSH synthesis in cells using cysteine as a substrate and suppressing the activity of NADPH oxidase [122]. In addition, H_2S regulates the activity of nuclear factor erythroid 2-related factor 2 (Nrf2, a transcriptional regulator of oxidative stress) signaling, thereby inducing antioxidant enzyme expression [123]. Moreover, the mitochondrially targeted H_2S donor, AP39, stimulates mitochondrial respiration and generates mitochondrial sulfide and persulfide [124], which act to maintain mitochondrial function during periods of hypoxia and, therefore, could protect against mitochondrial impairment in CKD patients.

Apart from combating oxidative stress, H_2S has also been reported to inhibit ER stress. In rat model of vascular calcification, a common complication in CKD, Yang et al. [125] reported that H_2S treatment inhibited ER stress in calcified aortic tissues via activation of Akt signaling pathway (a pathway that promotes survival and growth in response to extracellular signals), leading to alleviation of vascular calcification and phenotype transformation of vascular smooth muscle cells. This supports results from previous clinical studies in which sodium thiosulfate, a major oxidation product of H_2S, improved calciphylaxis (a syndrome of vascular calcification) in patients with ESRD [126, 127]. Other studies have also shown that H_2S suppresses ER stress-induced endothelial-to-mesenchymal transition via suppression of Src pathway and ameliorated cardiac fibrosis [128]. In summary, H_2S

protects against the damaging effects of oxidative and ER stress associated with CKD (Fig. 3.2) and should be further explored, as it may constitute a unique target for antioxidant therapy in CKD and other renal diseases.

H$_2$S Interaction with Other Gasotransmitters in CKD

Studies about interactions among members of the gasotransmitter family (NO, CO, and H$_2$S) in CKD have not been described extensively. However, some data describe this subject in experimental models of hypertensive nephropathy (one of the leading causes of CKD) and renal transplantation (a replacement therapy for CKD and ESRD). In line with previous studies [129–131], the gasotransmitters interact with one another and exhibit a mutual adaptation between them, compensating for one another when the level of one of these gases is altered. In a rat model of Ang II-induced hypertension, for example, pharmacological inhibition of H$_2$S increased blood pressure but upregulated renal expression of HO-1 (CO-producing enzyme), leading to increased CO production and renal protection [132]. Also, Wesseling et al. [133] observed enhanced H$_2$S production and NO metabolites in renal tissue following inhibition of HO-1. In the same study, the authors also observed that depletion of NO increased blood pressure, causing renal injury and loss of renal function in rats after 4 weeks of NO depletion but without any effect on other gasotransmitters [133]. In contrast to this latter observation, Wesseling et al. [134] reported that chronic (21 days) inhibition of NO did not only cause hypertension and renal injury but also downregulated CSE and upregulated HO-1 levels. Interaction between H$_2$S and NO also protected the kidney against ischemia-reperfusion injury in experimental renal transplantation [135, 136]. In conclusion, the three gasotransmitters interact with and compensate for one another under pathological conditions when the level of the other is depleted.

Hyperhomocysteinemia in CKD

Homocysteine (Hcy) is a nonessential non-proteinogenic sulfur-containing amino acid and a homologue of cysteine. It is synthesized from the essential diet-derived amino acid, methionine, through transmethylation, a biological reaction that requires the transfer of methyl group from one compound to another. The metabolism of Hcy is regulated by two important pathways: remethylation back to methionine, a process which requires vitamins B6, B9 (folate), and B12, and CBS-mediated transsulfuration to cystathionine, which occurs primarily in the kidney [137–139]. The involvement of CBS in the metabolism of Hcy implies simultaneous H$_2$S production and further suggests that impairment in renal transsulfuration pathway could lead to increased plasma Hcy levels. Factors such as diet, lifestyle, medications, and genetic factors can increase Hcy levels, while vitamin B6, B9, and B12 supplementation can reduce its level [140, 141]. Normal plasma Hcy level is <10 μmol/L. However, elevated levels, called hyperhomocysteinemia (HHcy, >15 μmol/L), have attracted significant clinical attention in CKD and ESRD patients due to impaired intrarenal metabolism and renal clearance [142–147]. Thus, HHcy is caused by deficiencies in vitamins B6, B9, and B12 as well as decreased CBS activity or expression [148, 149]. HHcy impairs GFR and is considered a causative factor in arterial and glomerular sclerosis due to its associated ROS generation and inflammation [138].

Hydrogen Sulfide Against Hyperhomocysteinemia in CKD

Recent data from *in vitro* and *in vivo* studies indicate that HHcy impairs endogenous H_2S system by inhibiting the expressions and activities of H_2S-producing enzymes (CBS, CSE, and 3-MST) and contributing to endothelial dysfunction in the vasculature by enhancing inflammation, free radical production, and autophagy in the endothelial cells [150–152]. In the kidney, HHcy was associated with glomerular damage in uninephrectomized $CBS^{+/-}$ mice, which was characterized by increased MMP-2 and -9 activities, collagen deposition, glomerular infiltration with macrophages, increased ICAM-1 and VCAM-1 expression, apoptotic cells, increased proteinuria, upregulation of NADPH oxidase expression, and ROS production in the renal cortex. These pathological changes corresponded with decreased plasma H_2S level [153, 154]. Interestingly, $CBS^{+/-}$ mice which received 30 μmol/L of NaHS in drinking water for 8 weeks showed reversal of the HHcy-associated renal damage along with increased plasma H_2S level [153, 154]. These findings suggest that H_2S administration attenuates HHcy-associated renal damage through its antioxidant, anti-inflammatory, anti-apoptotic, and anti-fibrotic properties. Considering that HHcy induces chronic inflammation in glomeruli and causes glomerulosclerosis in CKD patients, extracellular signal-regulated kinase 1/2 (ERK1/2) and c-Jun NH_2-terminal kinase (JNK1/2) were identified as two major inflammatory pathways that contribute to inflammation in an in vitro model of HHcy-induced glomerular inflammation using mouse glomerular mesangial cells [155]. However, treatment with H_2S as well as CBS/CSE double-gene transfer to mouse glomerular mesangial cells inhibited ERK1/2 and JNK1/2 signaling pathways and attenuated Hcy-induced mesangial inflammation [155]. In an *ex vivo* model to investigate the effect of elevated Hcy level on renovascular function, the same salutary effects were obtained by the same authors following H_2S triple-gene therapy (CBS/CSE/3-MST), which inhibited high Hcy level-induced renal microvascular impairment and vasoconstriction in renal arteries *ex vivo* and induced vasodilation by upregulating the expressions of CD31 (a marker for vascular differentiation) and vascular endothelial growth factor (VEGF, activator of vasodilation) while downregulating the expression of endostatin (antiangiogenic factor) via Akt/$FoxO_3$ signaling pathways [150].

This suggests that H_2S preserves renovascular function and plays a key role in preventing renovasculopathy induced by HHcy.

In addition, a previous study also showed significant downregulation of renal CBS mRNA and protein, which resulted in HHcy and subsequent development of arterial and glomerular sclerosis in a rat model of salt-sensitive hypertension [149]. A subsequent study by the same group using HHcy-treated mouse mesangial cells showed that treatment with 250 μM GYY4137 downregulated mRNA and protein expressions of pro-apoptotic caspases, MMP-2, -9, and -14, collagen I and IV, and fibronectin; inhibited ROS production; prevented loss of mitochondrial membrane potential; and increased mitochondrial ATP production, leading to attenuation of HHcy-induced mesangial cell damage and ECM remodeling [156]. In the same study, the authors found that the mechanism underlying the protection of mesangial cells by GYY4137 involves regulation of Akt/FOXO1 pathway [156], a pathway that participates in oxidative stress, inflammation, and apoptosis. The GYY4137-induced renal protection also involves modulation of caveolin-1, endothelial nitric oxide synthase (eNOS), tissue inhibitors of metalloproteinase, and connexins in HHcy mice [157]. Similar to the effects by GYY4137 and the triple-gene therapy [150], Pushpakumar et al. [158] also reported that NaHS administration along with transfection of triple genes (CBS, CSE, and 3-MST) attenuated homocysteinylation of eNOS, downregulated caveolin-1 protein expression, and reduced ECM remodeling in a genetic model of HHcy-induced hypertensive nephropathy in mice, thereby restoring systolic blood pressure and GFR. Collectively, HHcy is associated with CKD and ESRD, and H_2S supplementation could be considered a potential future therapy for HHcy-associated CKD and ESRD and other HHcy-related diseases.

Autosomal Dominant Polycystic Kidney Disease

Autosomal dominant polycystic kidney disease (ADPKD) is an inherited life-threatening multisystemic disorder of the renal tubules due to mutations in polycystin 1 (PKD1) or polycystin 2 (PKD2) genes [159]. It presents with the development and continued growth of multiple kidney cysts that results in loss of renal function, in addition to several extrarenal manifestations. Its prevalence increases with increasing human population. Chronic pain in the flank or loin usually occurs due to large cysts that compress surrounding structures, and rapture of the cysts into the renal collecting system results in hematuria [160, 161]. ADPKD is a serious form of CKD and the most common genetic cause of ESRD and cardiovascular diseases, contributing significantly to premature mortality of ADPKD patients globally [162, 163]. Unfortunately, ADPKD is incurable, and treatment is limited to pharmacological (e.g., antihypertensive agents and vasopressin receptor antagonists) and non-pharmacological (e.g., lifestyle and nutritional therapy) management of complications to retard disease progression [164–166], while patients who progress to ESRD require renal replacement therapy (dialysis or transplantation) [167, 168].

Inflammation Contributes to Vascular Endothelial Dysfunction in ADPKD and Its Progression to ESRD

It is well established that vascular endothelial dysfunction precedes renal and cardiovascular pathology in ADPKD and correlates with disease severity [169–172]. Systemic inflammation is a major pathological process that has been implicated in vascular dysfunction and renal injury in clinical and preclinical models of ADPKD [171–173]. In a rat model of ADPKD, Cowley et al. [174] observed significant upregulation in mRNA and protein expressions of monocyte chemoattractant protein-1 (MCP-1) and osteopontin (mediator of inflammation) in the kidneys of homozygous and heterozygous cystic rats compared to wild-type rats, which correlated positively with progression to ESRD. In addition, immunohistochemical examination with ED-1 antibody revealed accumulation of macrophages in the interstitium of cystic kidneys. This report aligns with a recent study in a clinically relevant mouse model of ADPKD in which marked expression of pro-inflammatory genes such as TNF-α and IL-6 was observed in the kidneys of mice with PKD1 gene mutation and corresponded with reduced GFR and increased blood urea nitrogen levels and blood pressure as well as increased gene and protein expression of markers of kidney injury (KIM-1 and NGAL) relative to control wild-type mice [175]. Consistent with the results of these experimental studies, several clinical studies also reported inflammation in ADPKD patients as observed in significantly increased endothelial cell protein expression of NF-κB and higher plasma levels of IL-6, IL-8, adhesion molecules (ICAM-1 and VCAM-1), serum C-reactive protein (a systemic marker of inflammation and mediator of vascular endothelial injury), and urinary MCP-1, which preceded increased serum creatinine and proteinuria at different stages of ADPKD in comparison with healthy control subjects [171, 176–179]. These clinical observations suggest that inflammation contributes to ADPKD pathogenesis and progression in these patients.

Oxidative Stress Contributes to Vascular Endothelial Dysfunction in ADPKD and Accelerates ESRD Development

In addition to inflammation, oxidative damage is also evident in ADPKD and contributes to vascular dysfunction, which accelerates progression to ESRD. Animal models of ADPKD showed upregulation of renal mRNA of heme oxygenase-1 (HO-1, an inducible marker of oxidative stress) as well as renal and plasma levels of malondialdehyde (MDA, a by-product of lipid peroxidation and indicator of ROS production) and 4-hydroxy-2(E)-nonenal along with downregulation of mRNA and protein expressions of antioxidant enzymes such as glutathione peroxidase, superoxide dismutase (SOD), catalase, and glutathione S-transferase during ADPKD progression, and reduced plasma levels of these antioxidant enzymes in ADPKD mice and rats [180]. As with inflammation, ADPKD patients also showed oxidative damage characterized by markedly elevated levels of plasma and urinary oxidative stress markers such as 13-hydroxyoctadecadienoic acid, prostaglandins (8-epi-$PGF_{2\alpha}$, PGD_2, PGE_2, and 8-isoprostane), and nicotinamide adenine dinucleotide phosphate oxidase 2 (NOX2) and significantly reduced levels of antioxidant enzymes, with increased serum creatinine level and reduced GFR compared to healthy control subjects [171, 172, 176, 179, 181]. Considering that NOX enzymes are abundantly expressed in the vascular wall and produce ROS at physiologically low levels in vascular cells [182], the upregulation of NOX2 observed in ADPKD patients strongly explains the oxidative stress and vascular endothelial dysfunction in these patients [171, 179], as NOX2 is the NOX isoform that has the highest involvement in vascular diseases and its deletion resulted in significantly reduced ROS production while its overexpression markedly increased ROS levels in mice [183]. In summary, vascular oxidative stress is a major player in the development of vascular endothelial dysfunction in ADPKD and partly contributes to progression towards ESRD.

H_2S as an Additional Pharmacological Agent in ADPKD Management

There is a dearth of studies in the literature on the effect of H_2S on ADPKD. The only available study is the one by Lai et al. [179], who recently reported a controlled longitudinal, prospective interventional study involving 33 ADPKD patients who received daily administration of 1.6 g of alpha-lipoic acid (ALA, an endogenous source of H_2S) for 6 months and 26 ADPKD patients with no ALA administration as control group. They observed significant reduction in serum levels of C-reactive protein and pro-inflammatory cytokines (IL-1β, IL-6, and TNF-α), uric acid, as well as plasma NOX2 and renal resistive index (a renal and systemic vascular damage marker), which partly contributed to improvement in vascular endothelial dysfunction, renal function, and cardiovascular risk factors in ALA-treated ADPKD patients compared to ADPKD control subjects [179]. ALA is an organosulfur antioxidant and anti-inflammatory compound that is synthesized from cysteine (an endogenous source of H_2S) by lipoic acid synthase in the mitochondria of kidney and other tissues [184, 185], with beneficial effects in diabetic nephropathy and ESRD patients [186, 187]. Besides its endogenous production, ALA can also be obtained from dietary sources or given as dietary supplement. It is also a licensed drug for the treatment of diabetic neuropathy. Recent preclinical evidence including that from our research group demonstrates that administration of ALA results in H_2S release from sulfane sulfur (precursor of H_2S) in the homogenates of rat kidneys and other tissues and increases expression of H_2S-producing enzymes (CBS, CSE, and 3-MST), leading to increased renal and plasma H_2S levels under pathological conditions [186, 188–191]. This suggests that ALA can be considered an H_2S-storage compound that releases H_2S in response to biological signals. Although endogenous

H_2S level was not measured following administration of ALA in ADPKD patients in the above clinical study, it is possible that the beneficial effect of ALA in this group of patients could be due to increased expression of H_2S-producing enzymes and endogenous H_2S production by ALA along with the potent antioxidant, anti-inflammatory, and other therapeutic properties of H_2S.

Burgeoning evidence also suggests that metabolic dysregulations in ADPKD involve abnormal mitochondrial morphology and function and facilitate cyst formation, as seen in increased vacuolated and fragmented mitochondria in $PKD1^{-/-}$ mutant renal epithclial cell lines, mouse and human kidneys, and decreased viability and exercise endurance along with increased carbon dioxide production [192, 193]. Against this background, the mitochondrial synthesis of ALA and improvement in renal function following its administration in ADPKD patients suggest that ALA may have attenuated pathological events that lead to abnormal renal mitochondrial morphology and function and inhibited cyst formation. Besides, ALA has been reported to increase mitochondrial membrane potential (an indication of improved mitochondrial bioenergetics) and inhibit ROS generation in the mitochondria under pathological conditions [194]. Furthermore, the H_2S-producing enzyme, 3-MST, is a mitochondrial enzyme, which accounts principally for renal mitochondrial H_2S production, while CBS and CSE (cytosolic H_2S-producing enzymes) translocate to the mitochondria to increase endogenous H_2S production in response to specific stressful stimuli. Therefore, the observed improvement in renal function in ALA-treated ADPKD patients may imply that ALA may have facilitated CBS and CSE translocation to the mitochondria to increase renal mitochondrial H_2S production via mechanisms that are activated under stressful conditions such as ADPKD. While this assumption sounds logical and convincing, further studies are needed to validate it.

Conclusion

Renal hypoxia has emerged as a central pathophysiological player, preceding the development of renal dysfunction in experimental models of CKD. Hence, the pathogenesis and progression of CKD can be prevented by preventing renal hypoxia, thus by increasing and preserving medullary oxygenation using hypoxia-oriented therapies. In addition, HHcy has been well established in CKD and ESRD patients. Recent experimental results have established therapeutic characteristics of H_2S including targeting hypoxia and preventing HHcy in the kidney, thus making it a potential alternative treatment strategy against CKD and HHcy and their complications. Also, exogenous H_2S administration in the form of ALA has been shown in one clinical study to be beneficial in ADPKD. Collectively, the fact that H_2S donor drugs such as sodium thiosulfate and ALA are already in clinical use makes H_2S a promising novel therapeutic tool that should be further explored.

References

1. Lozano R, Naghavi M, Foreman K, Lim S, Shibuya K, Aboyans V, et al. Global and regional mortality from 235 causes of death for 20 age groups in 1990 and 2010: a systematic analysis for the Global Burden of Disease Study 2010. Lancet. 2012;380:2095–128.
2. Bruce MA, Beech BM, Crook ED, Sims M, Wyatt SB, Flessner MF, et al. Association of socioeconomic status and CKD among African Americans: the Jackson Heart Study. Am J Kidney Dis. 2010;55(6):1001–8.
3. Obrador GT, Garcia-Garcia G, Villa AR, Rubilar X, Olvera N, Ferreira E, et al. Prevalence of chronic kidney disease in the Kidney Early Evaluation Program (KEEP) Mexico and comparison with KEEP US. Kidney Int Suppl. 2010;116:S2–8.
4. Ognibene A, Grandi G, Lorubbio M, Rapi S, Salvadori B, Terreni A, et al. KDIGO 2012 clinical practice guideline CKD classification rules out creatinine clearance 24 hour urine collection? Clin Biochem. 2016;49(1–2):85–9.
5. Nasrallah MM, El-Shehaby AR, Salem MM, Osman NA, El Sheikh E, Sharaf El Din UA. Fibroblast growth factor-23 (FGF-23) is independently correlated to aortic calcification in haemodialysis patients. Nephrol Dial Transplant. 2010;25(8):2679–85.
6. Houston J, Smith K, Isakova T, Sowden N, Wolf M, Gutiérrez OM. Associations of dietary phosphorus intake, urinary phosphate excretion, and fibroblast growth factor 23 with vascular stiffness in chronic kidney disease. J Ren Nutr. 2013;23(1):12–20.
7. Hung SC, Lin YP, Tarng DC. Erythropoiesis-stimulating agents in chronic kidney disease: what have we learned in 25 years? J Formos Med Assoc. 2014;113(1):3–10.
8. Welch WJ, Baumgärtl H, Lübbers D, Wilcox CS. Nephron pO2 and renal oxygen usage in the hypertensive rat kidney. Kidney Int. 2001;59(1):230–7.
9. Maruno M, Kiyosue H, Tanoue S, Hongo N, Matsumoto S, Mori H, et al. Renal arteriovenous shunts: clinical features, imaging appearance, and transcatheter embolization based on angio-architecture. Radiographics. 2016;36(2):580–95.
10. Safran M, Kim WY, O'Connell F, Flippin L, Günzler V, Horner JW, et al. Mouse model for noninvasive imaging of HIF prolyl hydroxylase activity: assessment of an oral agent that stimulates erythropoietin production. Proc Natl Acad Sci U S A. 2006;103(1):105–10.
11. Inoue T, Kozawa E, Okada H, Inukai K, Watanabe S, Kikuta T, et al. Noninvasive evaluation of kidney hypoxia and fibrosis using magnetic resonance imaging. J Am Soc Nephrol. 2011;22(8):1429–34.
12. Manotham K, Tanaka T, Matsumoto M, Ohse T, Miyata T, Inagi R, et al. Evidence of tubular hypoxia in the early phase in the remnant kidney model. J Am Soc Nephrol. 2004;15:1277–88.
13. Welch WJ, Blau J, Xie H, Chabrashvili T, Wilcox CS. Angiotensin-induced defects in renal oxygenation: role of oxidative stress. Am J Physiol Heart Circ Physiol. 2005;288(1):H22–8.
14. Peyster E, Chen J, Feldman H, Go AS, Gupta J, Mitra N, et al. Inflammation and arterial stiffness in chronic kidney disease: findings from the CRIC study. Am J Hypertens. 2017;30(4):400–8.
15. Song K, Wang F, Li Q, Shi YB, Zheng HF, Peng H, et al. Hydrogen sulfide inhibits the renal fibrosis of obstructive nephropathy. Kidney Int. 2014;85(6):1318–29.
16. Fine LG, Orphanides C, Norman JT. Progressive renal disease: the chronic hypoxia hypothesis. Kidney Int Suppl. 1998;65:S74–8.
17. Dugbartey GJ. Diabetic nephropathy: a potential savior with 'rotten-egg' smell. Pharmacol Rep. 2017;69(2):331–9.
18. Dugbartey GJ. H2S as a possible therapeutic alternative for the treatment of hypertensive kidney injury. Nitric Oxide. 2017;64:52–60.
19. Dugbartey GJ, Bouma HR, Lobb I, Sener A. Hydrogen sulfide: a novel nephroprotectant against cisplatin-induced renal toxicity. Nitric Oxide. 2016;57:15–20.
20. Dugbartey GJ, Peppone LJ, de Graaf IA. An integrative view of cisplatin-induced renal and cardiac toxicities: molecular mechanisms, current treatment challenges and potential protective measures. Toxicology. 2016;371:58–66.

21. Dugbartey GJ, Bouma HR, Strijkstra AM, Boerema AS, Henning RH. Induction of a torpor-like state by 5′-AMP does not depend on H2S production. PLoS One. 2015;10(8):e0136113.
22. Dugbartey GJ, Talaei F, Houwertjes MC, Goris M, Epema AH, Bouma HR, et al. Dopamine treatment attenuates acute kidney injury in a rat model of deep hypothermia and rewarming—the role of renal H2S-producing enzymes. Eur J Pharmacol. 2015;769:225–33.
23. Dugbartey GJ, Hardenberg MC, Kok WF, Boerema A, Carey HV, Staples J, et al. Renal mitochondrial response to low temperature in non-hibernating and hibernating species. Antioxid Redox Signal. 2017;27(9):599–617.
24. Lobb I, Davidson M, Carter D, Liu W, Haig A, Gunaratnam L, et al. Hydrogen sulfide treatment mitigates renal allograft ischemia-reperfusion injury during cold storage and improves early transplant kidney function and survival following allogeneic renal transplantation. J Urol. 2015;194:1806–15.
25. Dugbartey GJ, Bouma HR, Saha MN, Lobb I, Henning RH, Sener A. A hibernation-like state for transplantable organs: is hydrogen sulfide therapy the future of organ preservation? Antioxid Redox Signal. 2018;28(16):1503–15. https://doi.org/10.1089/ars.2017.7127.
26. Aminzadeh MA, Vaziri ND. Downregulation of the renal and hepatic hydrogen sulfide (H2S)-producing enzymes and capacity in chronic kidney disease. Nephrol Dial Transplant. 2012;27:498–504.
27. Xia M, Chen L, Muh RW, Li PL, Li N. Production and actions of hydrogen sulfide, a novel gaseous bioactive substance, in the kidneys. J Pharmacol Exp Ther. 2009;329(3):1056–62.
28. Mikami Y, Shinuya N, Kimura Y, Nagahara N, Ogasawara Y, Kimura H. Thioredoxin and dihydrolipoic acid are required for 3-mercaptopyruvate sulfurtransferase to produce hydrogen sulfide. Biochem J. 2011;439:479–85.
29. Shibuya N, Koike S, Tanaka M, Ishigami-Yuasa M, Kimura Y, Ogasawara Y, et al. A novel pathway for the production of hydrogen sulfide from D-cysteine in mammalian cells. Nat Commun. 2013;4:1366.
30. Yamamoto J, Sato W, Kosugi T, Yamamoto T, Kimura T, Taniguchi S, et al. Distribution of hydrogen sulfide (H2S)-producing enzymes and the roles of the H2S donor sodium hydrosulfide in diabetic nephropathy. Clin Exp Nephrol. 2013;17(1):32–40.
31. Kashfi K, Olso KR. Biology and therapeutic potential of hydrogen sulfide and hydrogen sulfide-releasing chimeras. Biochem Pharmacol. 2013;85:689–703.
32. Caliendo G, Cirino G, Santagada V, Wallace JL. Synthesis and biological effects of hydrogen sulfide (H2S): development of H2S-releasing drugs as pharmaceuticals. J Med Chem. 2010;53:6275–86.
33. Li L, Whiteman M, Guan YY, Neo KL, Cheng Y, Lee SW, et al. Characterization of a novel, water-soluble hydrogen sulfide-releasing molecule (GYY4137): new insights into the biology of hydrogen sulfide. Circulation. 2008;117:2351–60.
34. Gerő D, Torregrossa R, Perry A, Waters A, Le-Trionnaire S, Whatmore JL, et al. The novel mitochondria-targeted hydrogen sulfide (H2S) donors AP123 and AP39 protect against hyperglycemic injury in microvascular endothelial cells in vitro. Pharmacol Res. 2016;113(Pt A):186–98.
35. Benavides GA, Squadrito GL, Mills RW, Patel HD, Isbell TS, Patel RB, et al. Hydrogen sulfide mediates the vasoactivity of garlic. Proc Natl Acad Sci U S A. 2007;104:17977–82.
36. Ginter E, Simko V. Garlic (Allium sativum L.) and cardiovascular diseases. Bratisl Lek Listy. 2010;111:452–6.
37. Snijder PM, Frenay AR, Koning AM, Bachtler M, Pasch A, Kwakernaak AJ, et al. Sodium thiosulfate attenuates angiotensin II-induced hypertension, proteinuria and renal damage. Nitric Oxide. 2014;42:87–98.
38. Polhemus DJ, Li Z, Pattillo CB, Gojon G Sr, Gojon G Jr, Giordano T, et al. A novel hydrogen sulfide prodrug, SG1002, promotes hydrogen sulfide and nitric oxide bioavailability in heart failure patients. Cardiovasc Ther. 2015;33(4):216–26.
39. Safar MM, Abdelsalam RM. H2S donors attenuate diabetic nephropathy in rats: modulation of oxidant status and polyol pathway. Pharmacol Rep. 2015;67(1):17–23.

40. Qian X, Li X, Ma F, Luo S, Ge R, Zhu Y. Novel hydrogen sulfide-releasing compound, S-propargyl-cysteine, prevents STZ-induced diabetic nephropathy. Biochem Biophys Res Commun. 2016;473(4):931–8.
41. Olson KR, Dombkowski RA, Russell MJ, Doellman MM, Head SK, Whitfield NL, et al. Hydrogen sulfide as an oxygen sensor/transducer in vertebrate hypoxic vasoconstriction and hypoxic vasodilation. J Exp Biol. 2006;209(Pt 20):4011–23.
42. Zhao W, Zhang J, Lu Y, Wang R. The vasorelaxant effect of H2S as a novel endogenous gaseous KATP channel opener. EMBO J. 2001;20:6008–16.
43. Sun Y, Huang Y, Zhang R, Chen Q, Chen J, Zong Y, et al. Hydrogen sulfide upregulates KATP channel expression in vascular smooth muscle cells of spontaneously hypertensive rats. J Mol Med. 2015;93:439–55.
44. Cao C, Lee-Kwon W, Silldorff EP, Pallone TL. KATP channel conductance of descending vasa recta pericytes. Am J Physiol Renal Physiol. 2005;289(6):F1235–45.
45. Blackstone E, Morrison M, Roth MB. H2S induces a suspended animation-like state in mice. Science. 2005;308(5721):518.
46. Fu M, Zhang W, Wu L, Yang G, Li H, Wang R. Hydrogen sulfide (H2S) metabolism in mitochondria and its regulatory role in energy production. Proc Natl Acad Sci U S A. 2012;109:2943–8.
47. Teng H, Wu B, Zhao K, Yang G, Wu L, Wang R. Oxygen-sensitive mitochondrial accumulation of cystathionine β-synthase mediated by Lon protease. Proc Natl Acad Sci U S A. 2013;110(31):12679–84.
48. Modis K, Coletta C, Erdelyi K, Papapetropoulos A, Szabo C. Intramitochondrial hydrogen sulfide production by 3-mercaptopyruvate sulfurtransferase maintains mitochondrial electron flow and supports cellular bioenergetics. FASEB J. 2013;27:601–11.
49. Nordquist L, Friederich-Persson M, Fasching A, Liss P, Shoji K, Nangaku M, et al. Activation of hypoxia-inducible factors prevents diabetic nephropathy. J Am Soc Nephrol. 2015;26(2):328–38.
50. Rosenberger C, Mandriota S, Jürgensen JS, Wiesener MS, Hörstrup JH, Frei U, et al. Expression of hypoxia-inducible factor-1alpha and -2alpha in hypoxic and ischemic rat kidneys. J Am Soc Nephrol. 2002;13(7):1721–32.
51. Wiesener MS, Jürgensen JS, Rosenberger C, Scholze CK, Hörstrup JH, Warnecke C, et al. Widespread hypoxia-inducible expression of HIF-2alpha in distinct cell populations of different organs. FASEB J. 2003;17(2):271–3.
52. Tanaka T, Matsumoto M, Inagi R, Miyata T, Kojima I, Ohse T, et al. Induction of protective genes by cobalt ameliorates tubulointerstitial injury in the progressive Thy1 nephritis. Kidney Int. 2005;68(6):2714–25.
53. Ohtomo S, Nangaku M, Izuhara Y, Takizawa S, Strihou CV, Miyata T. Cobalt ameliorates renal injury in an obese, hypertensive type 2 diabetes rat model. Nephrol Dial Transplant. 2008;23(4):1166–72.
54. Tanaka T, Kojima I, Ohse T, Ingelfinger JR, Adler S, Fujita T, et al. Cobalt promotes angiogenesis via hypoxia-inducible factor and protects tubulointerstitium in the remnant kidney model. Lab Invest. 2005;85(10):1292–307.
55. Song YR, You SJ, Lee YM, Chin HJ, Chae DW, Oh YK, et al. Activation of hypoxia-inducible factor attenuates renal injury in rat remnant kidney. Nephrol Dial Transplant. 2010;25(1):77–85.
56. Deng A, Arndt MA, Satriano J, Singh P, Rieg T, Thomson S, et al. Renal protection in chronic kidney disease: hypoxia-inducible factor activation vs. angiotensin II blockade. Am J Physiol Renal Physiol. 2010;299(6):F1365–73.
57. Bernhardt WM, Wiesener MS, Weidemann A, Schmitt R, Weichert W, Lechler P, et al. Involvement of hypoxia-inducible transcription factors in polycystic kidney disease. Am J Pathol. 2007;170(3):830–42.

58. Yu X, Fang Y, Ding X, Liu H, Zhu J, Zou J, et al. Transient hypoxia-inducible factor activation in rat renal ablation and reduced fibrosis with L-mimosine. Nephrology (Carlton). 2012;17(1):58–67.
59. Katavetin P, Miyata T, Inagi R, Tanaka T, Sassa R, Ingelfinger JR, et al. High glucose blunts vascular endothelial growth factor response to hypoxia via the oxidative stress-regulated hypoxia-inducible factor/hypoxia-responsible element pathway. J Am Soc Nephrol. 2006;17(5):1405–13.
60. Rosenberger C, Khamaisi M, Abassi Z, Shilo V, Weksler-Zangen S, Goldfarb M, et al. Adaptation to hypoxia in the diabetic rat kidney. Kidney Int. 2008;73(1):34–42.
61. Liu L, Marti GP, Wei X, Zhang X, Zhang H, Liu YV, et al. Age-dependent impairment of HIF-1alpha expression in diabetic mice: correction with electroporation-facilitated gene therapy increases wound healing, angiogenesis, and circulating angiogenic cells. J Cell Physiol. 2008;217(2):319–27.
62. Catrina SB, Okamoto K, Pereira T, Brismar K, Poellinger L. Hyperglycemia regulates hypoxia-inducible factor-1alpha protein stability and function. Diabetes. 2004;53(12):3226–32.
63. Kimura K, Iwano M, Higgins DF, Yamaguchi Y, Nakatani K, Harada K, et al. Stable expression of HIF-1alpha in tubular epithelial cells promotes interstitial fibrosis. Am J Physiol Renal Physiol. 2008;295(4):F1023–9.
64. Wang Z, Zhu Q, Li PL, Dhaduk R, Zhang F, Gehr TW, et al. Silencing of hypoxia-inducible factor-1α gene attenuates chronic ischemic renal injury in two-kidney, one-clip rats. Am J Physiol Renal Physiol. 2014;306(10):F1236–42.
65. Luo R, Zhang W, Zhao C, Zhang Y, Wu H, Jin J, et al. Elevated endothelial hypoxia-inducible factor-1α contributes to glomerular injury and promotes hypertensive chronic kidney disease. Hypertension. 2015;66(1):75–84.
66. Flannigan KL, Agbor TA, Motta JP, Ferraz JG, Wang R, Buret AG, et al. Proresolution effects of hydrogen sulfide during colitis are mediated through hypoxia-inducible factor-1α. FASEB J. 2015;29(4):1591–602.
67. Padiya R, Khatua TN, Bagul PK, Kuncha M, Banerjee SK. Garlic improves insulin sensitivity and associated metabolic syndromes in fructose fed rats. Nutr Metab (Lond). 2011;8:53.
68. Ried K, Frank OR, Stocks NP. Aged garlic extract reduces blood pressure in hypertensives: a dose-response trial. Eur J Clin Nutr. 2013;67:64–70.
69. Liu X, Pan L, Zhuo Y, Gong Q, Rose P, Zhu Y. Hypoxia-inducible factor-1α is involved in the pro-angiogenic effect of hydrogen sulfide under hypoxic stress. Biol Pharm Bull. 2010;33(9):1550–4.
70. Lohninger L, Tomasova L, Praschberger M, Hintersteininger M, Erker T, Gmeiner BM, et al. Hydrogen sulphide induces HIF-1α and Nrf2 in THP-1 macrophages. Biochimie. 2015;112:187–95.
71. Kai S, Tanaka T, Daijo H, Harada H, Kishimoto S, Suzuki K, et al. Hydrogen sulfide inhibits hypoxia- but not anoxia-induced hypoxia-inducible factor 1 activation in a von Hippel-Lindau- and mitochondria-dependent manner. Antioxid Redox Signal. 2012;16(3):203–16.
72. Yang G, Yang W, Wu L, Wang R. H2S, endoplasmic reticulum stress, and apoptosis of insulin-secreting beta cells. J Biol Chem. 2007;282(22):16567–76.
73. Yang G, Li H, Tang G, Wu L, Zhao K, Cao Q, et al. Increased neointimal formation in cystathionine gamma-lyase deficient mice: role of hydrogen sulfide in α5β1-integrin and matrix metalloproteinase-2 expression in smooth muscle cells. J Mol Cell Cardiol. 2012;52(3):677–88.
74. Wu B, Teng H, Yang G, Wu L, Wang R. Hydrogen sulfide inhibits the translational expression of hypoxia-inducible factor-alpha. Br J Pharmacol. 2012;167(7):1492–505.
75. Astor BC, Muntner P, Levin A, Eustace JA, Coresh J. Association of kidney function with anemia: the Third National Health and Nutrition Examination Survey (1988-1994). Arch Intern Med. 2002;162(12):1401–8.

76. Garrido P, Ribeiro S, Fernandes J, Vala H, Bronze-da-Rocha E, Rocha-Pereira P, et al. Iron-hepcidin dysmetabolism, anemia and renal hypoxia, inflammation and fibrosis in the remnant kidney rat model. PLoS One. 2015;10(4):e0124048.
77. Jacobson LO, Goldwasser E, Fried W, Plzak L. Role of the kidney in erythropoiesis. Nature. 1957;179(4560):633–4.
78. McGonigle RJ, Wallin JD, Shadduck RK, Fisher JW. Erythropoietin deficiency and inhibition of erythropoiesis in renal insufficiency. Kidney Int. 1984;25(2):437–44.
79. Greenwood RN, Ronco C, Gastaldon F, Brendolan A, Homel P, Usvyat L, et al. Erythropoietin dose variation in different facilities in different countries and its relationship to drug resistance. Kidney Int Suppl. 2003;(87):S78-S86.
80. Yilmaz MI, Solak Y, Covic A, Goldsmith D, Kanbay M. Renal anemia of inflammation: the name is self-explanatory. Blood Purif. 2011;32:220–5.
81. Leigh J, Saha MN, Mok A, Champsi O, Wang R, Lobb I, et al. Hydrogen sulfide-induced erythropoietin synthesis is regulated by HIF proteins. J Urol. 2016;196(1):251–60.
82. Wang M, Tang W, Xin H, Zhu YZ. S-propargyl-cysteine, a novel hydrogen sulfide donor, inhibits inflammatory hepcidin and relieves anemia of inflammation by inhibiting IL-6/STAT3 pathway. PLoS One. 2016;11(9):e0163289.
83. Jairam A, Das R, Aggarwal PK, Kohli HS, Gupta KL, Sakhuja V, et al. Iron status, inflammation and hepcidin in ESRD patients: the confounding role of intravenous iron therapy. Indian J Nephrol. 2010;20(3):125–31.
84. Zaritsky J, Young B, Wang HJ, Westerman M, Olbina G, Nemeth E, et al. Hepcidin—a potential novel biomarker for iron status in chronic kidney disease. Clin J Am Soc Nephrol. 2009;4(6):1051–6.
85. Xin H, Wang M, Tang W, Shen Z, Miao L, Wu W, et al. Hydrogen sulfide attenuates inflammatory hepcidin by reducing IL-6 secretion and promoting SIRT1-mediated STAT3 deacetylation. Antioxid Redox Signal. 2016;24(2):70–83.
86. Jiang D, Zhang Y, Yang M, Wang S, Jiang Z, Li Z. Exogenous hydrogen sulfide prevents kidney damage following unilateral ureteral obstruction. Neurourol Urodyn. 2014;33:538–43.
87. Basu RK, Hubchak S, Hayashida T, Runyan CE, Schumacker PT, Schnaper HW. Interdependence of HIF-1α and TGF-β/Smad3 signaling in normoxic and hypoxic renal epithelial cell collagen expression. Am J Physiol Renal Physiol. 2011;300(4):F898–905.
88. Manotham K, Tanaka T, Matsumoto M, Ohse T, Inagi R, Miyata T, et al. Transdifferentiation of cultured tubular cells induced by hypoxia. Kidney Int. 2004;65(3):871–80.
89. Zeisberg EM, Potenta SE, Sugimoto H, Zeisberg M, Kalluri R. Fibroblasts in kidney fibrosis emerge via endothelial-to-mesenchymal transition. J Am Soc Nephrol. 2008;19(12):2282–7.
90. Perna AF, Luciano MG, Ingrosso D, Pulzella P, Sepe I, Lanza D, et al. Hydrogen sulphide-generating pathways in haemodialysis patients: a study on relevant metabolites and transcriptional regulation of genes encoding for key enzymes. Nephrol Dial Transplant. 2009;24(12):3756–63.
91. Feng SJ, Li H, Wang SX. Lower hydrogen sulfide is associated with cardiovascular mortality, which involves cPKCβII/Akt pathway in chronic hemodialysis patients. Blood Purif. 2015;40(3):260–9. Transl Res 2008; 151: 110–117.
92. Sen U, Basu P, Abe OA, Givvimani S, Tyagi N, Metreveli N, et al. Hydrogen sulfide ameliorates hyperhomocysteinemia-associated chronic renal failure. Am J Physiol Renal Physiol. 2009;297(2):F410–9.
93. Jung KJ, Jang HS, Kim JI, Han SJ, Park JW, Park KM. Involvement of hydrogen sulfide and homocysteine transsulfuration pathway in the progression of kidney fibrosis after ureteral obstruction. Biochim Biophys Acta. 2013;1832(12):1989–97.
94. Zhao DA, Liu J, Huang Q, Han ZM. Change in plasma H2S level and therapeutic effect of H2S supplementation in tubulointerstitial fibrosis among rats with unilateral ureteral obstruction. Zhongguo Dang Dai Er Ke Za Zhi. 2013;15(10):903–8.

95. Guo L, Peng W, Tao J, Lan Z, Hei H, Tian L, et al. Hydrogen sulfide inhibits transforming growth factor-β1-induced EMT via Wnt/catenin pathway. PLoS One. 2016;11(1):e0147018.
96. Fang LP, Lin Q, Tang CS, Liu XM. Hydrogen sulfide suppresses migration, proliferation and myofibroblast transdifferentiation of human lung fibroblasts. Pulm Pharmacol Ther. 2009;22(6):554–61.
97. Schwer CI, Stoll P, Goebel U, Buerkle H, Hoetzel A, Schmidt R. Effects of hydrogen sulfide on rat pancreatic stellate cells. Pancreas. 2012;41(1):74–83.
98. Fan HN, Wang HJ, Yang-Dan CR, Ren L, Wang C, Li YF, et al. Protective effects of hydrogen sulfide on oxidative stress and fibrosis in hepatic stellate cells. Mol Med Rep. 2013;7(1):247–53.
99. Pan LL, Liu XH, Shen YQ, Wang NZ, Xu J, Wu D, et al. Inhibition of NADPH oxidase 4-related signaling by sodium hydrosulfide attenuates myocardial fibrotic response. Int J Cardiol. 2013;168(4):3770–8.
100. Sheng J, Shim W, Wei H, Lim SY, Liew R, Lim TS, et al. Hydrogen sulphide suppresses human atrial fibroblast proliferation and transformation to myofibroblasts. J Cell Mol Med. 2013;17(10):1345–54.
101. Fang LP, Lin Q, Tang CS, Liu XM. Hydrogen sulfide attenuates epithelial-mesenchymal transition of human alveolar epithelial cells. Pharmacol Res. 2010;61(4):298–305.
102. Wolf G, Zahner G, Schroeder R, Stahl RA. Transforming growth factor beta mediates the angiotensin-II-induced stimulation of collagen type IV synthesis in cultured murine proximal tubular cells. Nephrol Dial Transplant. 1996;11(2):263–9.
103. Cuevas CA, Gonzalez AA, Inestrosa NC, Vio CP, Prieto MC. Angiotensin II increases fibronectin and collagen I through the β-catenin-dependent signaling in mouse collecting duct cells. Am J Physiol Renal Physiol. 2015;308(4):F358–65.
104. Choi DE, Jeong JY, Lim BJ, Chang YK, Na KR, Shin YT, et al. Aliskiren ameliorates renal inflammation and fibrosis induced by unilateral ureteral obstruction in mice. J Urol. 2011;186(2):694–701.
105. Lu M, Liu YH, Goh HS, Wang JJ, Yong QC, Wang R, et al. Hydrogen sulfide inhibits plasma renin activity. J Am Soc Nephrol. 2010;21(6):993–1002.
106. Lu M, Liu YH, Ho CY, Tiong CX, Bian JS. Hydrogen sulfide regulates cAMP homeostasis and renin degranulation in As4.1 and rat renin-rich kidney cells. Am J Physiol Cell Physiol. 2012;302(1):C59–66.
107. Laggner H, Hermann M, Esterbauer H, Muellner MK, Exner M, Gmeiner BM, et al. The novel gaseous vasorelaxant hydrogen sulfide inhibits angiotensin-converting enzyme activity of endothelial cells. J Hypertens. 2007;25(10):2100–4.
108. Brenner BM, Cooper ME, de Zeeuw D, Keane WF, Mitch WE, Parving HH, et al. Effects of losartan on renal and cardiovascular outcomes in patients with type 2 diabetes and nephropathy. N Engl J Med. 2001;345(12):861–9.
109. Lewis EJ, Hunsicker LG, Clarke WR, Berl T, Pohl MA, Lewis JB, Ritz E, et al. Renoprotective effect of the angiotensin-receptor antagonist irbesartan in patients with nephropathy due to type 2 diabetes. N Engl J Med. 2001;345(12):851–60.
110. Palm F, Cederberg J, Hansell P, Liss P, Carlsson PO. Reactive oxygen species cause diabetes-induced decrease in renal oxygen tension. Diabetologia. 2003;46(8):1153–60.
111. Granata S, Zaza G, Simone S, Villani G, Latorre D, Pontrelli P, et al. Mitochondrial dysregulation and oxidative stress in patients with chronic kidney disease. BMC Genomics. 2009;10:388.
112. Cuttle L, Zhang XJ, Endre ZH, Winterford C, Gobe GC. Bcl-X(L) translocation in renal tubular epithelial cells in vitro protects distal cells from oxidative stress. Kidney Int. 2001;59:1779–88.
113. Kawakami T, Inagi R, Wada T, Tanaka T, Fujita T, Nangaku M. Indoxyl sulfate inhibits proliferation of human proximal tubular cells via endoplasmic reticulum stress. Am J Physiol Renal Physiol. 2010;299(3):F568–76.

114. Locatelli F, Canaud B, Eckardt KU, Stenvinkel P, Wanner C, Zoccali C. Oxidative stress in end-stage renal disease: an emerging threat to patient outcome. Nephrol Dial Transplant. 2003;18(7):1272–80.
115. Ceballos-Picot I, Witko-Sarsat V, Merad-Boudia M, Nguyen AT, Thévenin M, Jaudon MC, et al. Glutathione antioxidant system as a marker of oxidative stress in chronic renal failure. Free Radic Biol Med. 1996;21(6):845–53.
116. Zachara BA, Gromadzinska J, Zbrog Z, Swiech R, Wasowicz W, Twardowska E, et al. Selenium supplementation to chronic kidney disease patients on hemodialysis does not induce the synthesis of plasma glutathione peroxidase. Acta Biochim Pol. 2009;56(1):183–7.
117. Roob JM, Khoschsorur G, Tiran A, Horina JH, Holzer H, Winklhofer-Roob BM. Vitamin E attenuates oxidative stress induced by intravenous iron in patients on hemodialysis. J Am Soc Nephrol. 2000;11(3):539–49.
118. Vecchi C, Montosi G, Zhang K, Lamberti I, Duncan SA, Kaufman RJ, et al. ER stress controls iron metabolism through induction of hepcidin. Science. 2009;325(5942):877–80.
119. Chiang CK, Nangaku M, Tanaka T, Iwawaki T, Inagi R. Endoplasmic reticulum stress signal impairs erythropoietin production: a role for ATF4. Am J Physiol Cell Physiol. 2013;304(4):C342–53.
120. Wu D, Luo N, Wang L, Zhao Z, Bu H, Xu G, et al. Hydrogen sulfide ameliorates chronic renal failure in rats by inhibiting apoptosis and inflammation through ROS/MAPK and NF-κB signaling pathways. Sci Rep. 2017;7(1):455.
121. Dursun M, Otunctemur A, Ozbek E, Sahin S, Besiroglu H, Ozsoy OD, et al. Protective effect of hydrogen sulfide in renal injury in the experimental unilateral ureteral obstruction. IBJU. 2015;41(6):1185–93.
122. Han SJ, Kim JI, Park JW, Park KM. Hydrogen sulfide accelerates the recovery of kidney tubules after renal ischemia/reperfusion injury. Nephrol Dial Transplant. 2015;30:1497–506.
123. Calvert JW, Jha S, Gundewar S, Elrod JW, Ramachandran A, Pattillo CB, et al. Hydrogen sulfide mediates cardioprotection through Nrf2 signaling. Circ Res. 2009;105(4):365–74.
124. Wedmann R, Onderka C, Wei S, Szijártó IA, Miljkovic JL, Mitrovic A, et al. Improved tag-switch method reveals that thioredoxin acts as depersulfidase and controls the intracellular levels of protein persulfidation. Chem Sci. 2016;7(5):3414–26.
125. Yang R, Teng X, Li H, Xue HM, Guo Q, Xiao L, et al. Hydrogen sulfide improves vascular calcification in rats by inhibiting endoplasmic reticulum stress. Oxid Med Cell Longev. 2016;2016:9095242.
126. Burnie R, Smail S, Javaid MM. Calciphylaxis and sodium thiosulphate: a glimmer of hope in desperate situation. J Ren Care. 2013;39(2):71–6.
127. Nigwekar SU, Brunelli SM, Meade D, Wang W, Hymes J, Lacson E Jr. Sodium thiosulfate therapy for calcific uremic arteriolopathy. Clin J Am Soc Nephrol. 2013;8(7):1162–70.
128. Ying R, Wang XQ, Yang Y, Gu ZJ, Mai JT, Qiu Q, et al. Hydrogen sulfide suppresses endoplasmic reticulum stress-induced endothelial-to-mesenchymal transition through Src pathway. Life Sci. 2016;144:208–17.
129. Rodriguez F, Lamon BD, Gong W, Kemp R, Nasjletti A. Nitric oxide synthesis inhibition promotes renal production of carbon monoxide. Hypertension. 2004;43:347–51.
130. Botros FT, Navar LG. Interaction between endogenously produced carbon monoxide and nitric oxide in regulation of renal afferent arterioles. Am J Physiol Heart Circ Physiol. 2006;291:H2772–8.
131. Rong-na L, Xiang-jun Z, Yu-han C, Ling-qiao L, Gang H. Interaction between hydrogen sulfide and nitric oxide on cardiac protection in rats with metabolic syndrome. Zhongguo Yi Xue Ke Xue Yuan Xue Bao. 2011;33:25–32.
132. Oosterhuis NR, Frenay AR, Wesseling S, Snijder PM, Slaats GG, Yazdani S, et al. DL-propargylglycine reduces blood pressure and renal injury but increases kidney weight in angiotensin-II infused rats. Nitric Oxide. 2015;49:56–66.

133. Wesseling S, Fledderus JO, Verhaar MC, Joles JA. Beneficial effects of diminished production of hydrogen sulfide and carbon monoxide on hypertension and renal injury induced by NO withdrawal. Br J Pharmacol. 2015;172(6):1607–19.

134. Wesseling S, Joles JA, van Goor H, Bluyssen HA, Kemmeren P, Holstege FC, et al. Transcriptome-based identification of pro- and antioxidative gene expression in kidney cortex of nitric oxide-dependent rats. Physiol Genomics. 2007;28:158–67.

135. Xu Z, Prathapasinghe G, Wu N, Hwang SY, Siow YL, Karmin O. Ischemia-reperfusion reduces cystathionine-beta-synthase-mediated hydrogen sulfide generation in the kidney. Am J Physiol Renal Physiol. 2009;297:F27–35.

136. Tripatara P, Patel NS, Gallicchio M, Kieswich J, Castiglia S, Benetti E, et al. Generation of endogenous hydrogen sulfide by cystathionine gamma-lyase limits renal ischemia/reperfusion injury and dysfunction. Lab Invest. 2008;88:1038–48.

137. Finkelstein JD. The metabolism of homocysteine: pathways and regulation. Eur J Pediatr. 1998;157(Suppl 2):S40–4.

138. Pin-Lan L, Fan Y, Ningjun L. Hyperhomocysteinemia: association with renal transsulfuration and redox signaling in rats. Clin Chem Lab Med. 2007;45(12):1688–93.

139. Hermann A, Sitdikova G. Homocysteine: biochemistry, molecular biology and role in disease. Biomolecules. 2021;11(5):737.

140. House AA, Eliasziw M, Cattran DC, Churchill DN, Oliver MJ, Fine A, Dresser GK, Spence JD. Effect of B-vitamin therapy on progression of diabetic nephropathy: a randomized controlled trial. JAMA. 2010;303(16):1603–9.

141. Soohoo M, Ahmadi SF, Qader H, Streja E, Obi Y, Moradi H, Rhee CM, Kim TH, Kovesdy CP, Kalantar-Zadeh K. Association of serum vitamin B12 and folate with mortality in incident hemodialysis patients. Nephrol Dial Transplant. 2017;32(6):1024–32.

142. Mizuno T, Hoshino T, Ishizuka K, Toi S, Takahashi S, Wako S, Arai S, Kitagawa K. Hyperhomocysteinemia increases vascular risk in stroke patients with chronic kidney disease. J Atheroscler Thromb. 2023;30(9):1198–209.

143. Shen Z, Zhang Z, Zhao W. Relationship between plasma homocysteine and chronic kidney disease in US patients with type 2 diabetes mellitus: a cross-sectional study. BMC Nephrol. 2022;23(1):419.

144. Shevchuk SV, Postovitenko KP, Iliuk IA, Bezsmertna HV, Bezsmertnyi YO, Kurylenko IV, Biloshytska AV, Baranova IV. The relationship between homocysteine level and vitamins B12, B9 and B6 status in patients with chronic kidney disease. Wiad Lek. 2019;72(4):532–8.

145. van Guldener C, Lambert J, ter Wee PM, Donker AJ, Stehouwer CD. Carotid artery stiffness in patients with end-stage renal disease: no effect of long-term homocysteine-lowering therapy. Clin Nephrol. 2000;53(1):33–41.

146. van Guldener C. Why is homocysteine elevated in renal failure and what can be expected from homocysteine-lowering? Nephrol Dial Transplant. 2006;21(5):1161–6.

147. Nair AP, Nemirovsky D, Kim M, Geer EB, Farkouh ME, Winston J, Halperin JL, Robbins MJ. Elevated homocysteine levels in patients with end-stage renal disease. Mt Sinai J Med. 2005;72(6):365–73.

148. Miller JW, Nadeau MR, Smith D, Selhub J. Vitamin B-6 deficiency vs folate deficiency: comparison of responses to methionine loading in rats. Am J Clin Nutr. 1994;59(5):1033–9.

149. Li N, Chen L, Muh RW, Li PL. Hyperhomocysteinemia associated with decreased renal transsulfuration activity in Dahl S rats. Hypertension. 2006;47(6):1094–100.

150. Sen U, Sathnur PB, Kundu S, Givvimani S, Coley DM, Mishra PK, Qipshidze N, Tyagi N, Metreveli N, Tyagi SC. Increased endogenous H2S generation by CBS, CSE, and 3MST gene therapy improves ex vivo renovascular relaxation in hyperhomocysteinemia. Am J Physiol Cell Physiol. 2012;303:C41–51.

151. Kamat PK, Kalani A, Givvimani S, Sathnur PB, Tyagi SC, Tyagi N. Hydrogen sulfide attenuates neurodegeneration and neurovascular dysfunction induced by intracerebral-administered homocysteine in mice. Neuroscience. 2013;252:302–19.

152. Pushpakumar S, Kundu S, Sen U. Endothelial dysfunction: the link between homocysteine and hydrogen sulfide. Curr Med Chem. 2014;21:3662–72.
153. Sen U, Basu P, Abe OA, Givvimani S, Tyagi N, Metreveli N, Shah KS, Passmore JC, Tyagi SC. Hydrogen sulfide ameliorates hyperhomocysteinemia-associated chronic renal failure. Am J Physiol Renal Physiol. 2009;297(2):F410–9.
154. Sen U, Munjal C, Qipshidze N, Abe O, Gargoum R, Tyagi SC. Hydrogen sulfide regulates homocysteine-mediated glomerulosclerosis. Am J Nephrol. 2010;31(5):442–55.
155. Sen U, Givvimani S, Abe OA, Lederer ED, Tyagi SC. Cystathionine β-synthase and cystathionine γ-lyase double gene transfer ameliorate homocysteine-mediated mesangial inflammation through hydrogen sulfide generation. Am J Physiol Cell Physiol. 2011;300(1):C155–63.
156. Majumder S, Ren L, Pushpakumar S, Sen U. Hydrogen sulphide mitigates homocysteine-induced apoptosis and matrix remodelling in mesangial cells through Akt/FOXO1 signalling cascade. Cell Signal. 2019;61:66–77.
157. John ASP, Sen U. GYY4137 modulates renal remodeling in hyperhomocysteinemia. FASEB J. 2019;33(S1):570–3.
158. Pushpakumar S, Kundu S, Sen U. Hydrogen sulfide protects hyperhomocysteinemia induced renal damage by modulation of caveolin and eNOS interaction. Sci Rep. 2019;9(1):2223.
159. Chapman AB, Devuyst O, Eckardt KU, Gansevoort RT, Harris T, Horie S, Kasiske BL, Odland D, Pei Y, Perrone RD, Pirson Y, Schrier RW, Torra R, Torres VE, Watnick T, Wheeler DC, Conference Participants. Autosomal-dominant polycystic kidney disease (ADPKD): executive summary from a kidney disease: improving global outcomes (KDIGO) controversies conference. Kidney Int. 2015;88(1):17–27.
160. Hajjar K, Bou Chebl R, Kanso M, Abou DG. Autosomal dominant polycystic kidney disease and minimal trauma: medical review and case report. BMC Emerg Med. 2018;18(1):38.
161. Gabow PA, Duley I, Johnson AM. Clinical profiles of gross hematuria in autosomal dominant polycystic kidney disease. Am J Kidney Dis. 1992;20(2):140–3.
162. Cornec-Le Gall E, Alam A, Perrone RD. Autosomal dominant polycystic kidney disease. Lancet. 2019;393(10174):919–35.
163. Lanktree MB, Haghighi A, di Bari I, Song X, Pei Y. Insights into autosomal dominant polycystic kidney disease from genetic studies. Clin J Am Soc Nephrol. 2021;16(5):790–9.
164. Nutahara K, Higashihara E, Horie S, Kamura K, Tsuchiya K, Mochizuki T, Hosoya T, Nakayama T, Yamamoto N, Higaki Y, Shimizu T. Calcium channel blocker versus angiotensin II receptor blocker in autosomal dominant polycystic kidney disease. Nephron Clin Pract. 2005;99(1):c18–23.
165. Meijer E, Gansevoort RT. Vasopressin V2 receptor antagonists in autosomal dominant polycystic kidney disease: efficacy, safety, and tolerability. Kidney Int. 2020;98(2):289–93.
166. Di Iorio BR, Cupisti A, D'Alessandro C, Bellasi A, Barbera V, Di Lullo L. Nutritional therapy in autosomal dominant polycystic kidney disease. J Nephrol. 2018;31(5):635–43.
167. Jacquet A, Pallet N, Kessler M, Hourmant M, Garrigue V, Rostaing L, Kreis H, Legendre C, Mamzer-Bruneel MF. Outcomes of renal transplantation in patients with autosomal dominant polycystic kidney disease: a nationwide longitudinal study. Transpl Int. 2011;24(6):582–7.
168. Yeh SC, Lin YC, Hong YC, Hsu CC, Lin YC, Wu MS. Different effects of iron indices on mortality in patients with autosomal dominant polycystic kidney disease after long-term hemodialysis: a nationwide population-based study. J Ren Nutr. 2019;29(5):444–53.
169. Wang D, Iversen J, Wilcox CS, Strandgaard S. Endothelial dysfunction and reduced nitric oxide in resistance arteries in autosomal-dominant polycystic kidney disease. Kidney Int. 2003;64(4):1381–8.
170. Wang D, Iversen J, Strandgaard S. Endothelium-dependent relaxation of small resistance vessels is impaired in patients with autosomal dominant polycystic kidney disease. J Am Soc Nephrol. 2000;11(8):1371–6.
171. Nowak KL, Wang W, Farmer-Bailey H, Gitomer B, Malaczewski M, Klawitter J, Jovanovich A, Chonchol M. Vascular dysfunction, oxidative stress, and inflammation in autosomal dominant polycystic kidney disease. Clin J Am Soc Nephrol. 2018;13(10):1493–501.

172. Klawitter J, Reed-Gitomer BY, McFann K, Pennington A, Klawitter J, Abebe KZ, Klepacki J, Cadnapaphornchai MA, Brosnahan G, Chonchol M, Christians U, Schrier RW. Endothelial dysfunction and oxidative stress in polycystic kidney disease. Am J Physiol Renal Physiol. 2014;307(11):F1198–206.

173. Andries A, Daenen K, Jouret F, Bammens B, Mekahli D, Van Schepdael A. Oxidative stress in autosomal dominant polycystic kidney disease: player and/or early predictor for disease progression? Pediatr Nephrol. 2019;34(6):993–1008.

174. Cowley BD Jr, Ricardo SD, Nagao S, Diamond JR. Increased renal expression of monocyte chemoattractant protein-1 and osteopontin in ADPKD in rats. Kidney Int. 2001;60(6):2087–96.

175. Pastor-Soler NM, Li H, Pham J, Rivera D, Ho PY, Mancino V, Saitta B, Hallows KR. Metformin improves relevant disease parameters in an autosomal dominant polycystic kidney disease mouse model. Am J Physiol Renal Physiol. 2022;322(1):F27–41.

176. Menon V, Rudym D, Chandra P, Miskulin D, Perrone R, Sarnak M. Inflammation, oxidative stress, and insulin resistance in polycystic kidney disease. Clin J Am Soc Nephrol. 2011;6(1):7–13.

177. Merta M, Tesar V, Zima T, Jirsa M, Rysavá R, Zabka J. Cytokine profile in autosomal dominant polycystic kidney disease. Biochem Mol Biol Int. 1997;41(3):619–24.

178. Zheng D, Wolfe M, Cowley BD Jr, Wallace DP, Yamaguchi T, Grantham JJ. Urinary excretion of monocyte chemoattractant protein-1 in autosomal dominant polycystic kidney disease. J Am Soc Nephrol. 2003;14(10):2588–95.

179. Lai S, Petramala L, Muscaritoli M, Cianci R, Mazzaferro S, Mitterhofer AP, Pasquali M, D'Ambrosio V, Carta M, Ansuini M, Ramaccini C, Galani A, Amabile MI, Molfino A, Letizia C. α-lipoic acid in patients with autosomal dominant polycystic kidney disease. Nutrition. 2020;71:110594.

180. Maser RL, Vassmer D, Magenheimer BS, Calvet JP. Oxidant stress and reduced antioxidant enzyme protection in polycystic kidney disease. J Am Soc Nephrol. 2002;13(4):991–9.

181. Wang D, Strandgaard S, Borresen ML, Luo Z, Connors SG, Yan Q, Wilcox CS. Asymmetric dimethylarginine and lipid peroxidation products in early autosomal dominant polycystic kidney disease. Am J Kidney Dis. 2008;51(2):184–91.

182. Ismaeel A, Brumberg RS, Kirk JS, Papoutsi E, Farmer PJ, Bohannon WT, Smith RS, Eidson JL, Sawicki I, Koutakis P. Oxidative stress and arterial dysfunction in peripheral artery disease. Antioxidants (Basel). 2018;7(10):145.

183. Zhao R, Ma X, Xie X, Shen GX. Involvement of NADPH oxidase in oxidized LDL-induced upregulation of heat shock factor-1 and plasminogen activator inhibitor-1 in vascular endothelial cells. Am J Physiol Endocrinol Metab. 2009;297(1):E104–11.

184. Padmalayam I, Hasham S, Saxena U, Pillarisetti S. Lipoic acid synthase (LASY): a novel role in inflammation, mitochondrial function and insulin resistance. Diabetes. 2000;58:600–8.

185. Szelag M, Mikulski D, Molski M. Quantum-chemical investigation of the structure and the antioxidant properties of α-lipoic acid and its metabolites. J Mol Model. 2012;18:2907–16.

186. Dugbartey GJ, Alornyo KK, Diaba DE, Adams I. Activation of renal CSE/H2S pathway by alpha-lipoic acid protects against histological and functional changes in the diabetic kidney. Biomed Pharmacother. 2022;153:113386.

187. Chang JW, Lee EK, Kim TH, Min WK, Chun S, Lee KU, Kim SB, Park JS. Effects of alpha-lipoic acid on the plasma levels of asymmetric dimethylarginine in diabetic end-stage renal disease patients on hemodialysis: a pilot study. Am J Nephrol. 2007;27:70–4.

188. Dugbartey GJ, Wonje QL, Alornyo KK, Adams I, Diaba DE. Alpha-lipoic acid treatment improves adverse cardiac remodelling in the diabetic heart—the role of cardiac hydrogen sulfide-synthesizing enzymes. Biochem Pharmacol. 2022;203:115179.

189. Dugbartey GJ, Alornyo KK, Adams I, Atule S, Obeng-Kyeremeh R, Amoah D, Adjei S. Targeting hepatic sulfane sulfur/hydrogen sulfide signaling pathway with α-lipoic acid to prevent diabetes-induced liver injury via upregulating hepatic CSE/3-MST expression. Diabetol Metab Syndr. 2022;14(1):148.

190. Bilska A, Dudek M, Iciek M, Kwiecień I, Sokołowska-Jezewicz M, Filipek B, Włodek L. Biological actions of lipoic acid associated with sulfane sulfur metabolism. Pharmacol Rep. 2008;60(2):225–32.
191. Bilska-Wilkosz A, Iciek M, Kowalczyk-Pachel D, Górny M, Sokołowska-Jeżewicz M, Włodek L. Lipoic acid as a possible pharmacological source of hydrogen sulfide/sulfane sulfur. Molecules. 2017;22(3):388.
192. Lin CC, Kurashige M, Liu Y, Terabayashi T, Ishimoto Y, Wang T, Choudhary V, et al. A cleavage product of Polycystin-1 is a mitochondrial matrix protein that affects mitochondria morphology and function when heterologously expressed. Sci Rep. 2018;8(1):2743.
193. Ishimoto Y, Inagi R, Yoshihara D, Kugita M, Nagao S, Shimizu A, Takeda N, Wake M, Honda K, Zhou J, Nangaku M. Mitochondrial abnormality facilitates cyst formation in autosomal dominant polycystic kidney disease. Mol Cell Biol. 2017;37(24):e00337–17.
194. Wang L, Wu CG, Fang CQ, Gao J, Liu YZ, Chen Y, Chen YN, Xu ZG. The protective effect of α-lipoic acid on mitochondria in the kidney of diabetic rats. Int J Clin Exp Med. 2013;6(2):90–7.

Chapter 4
Hydrogen Sulfide for Diabetic Kidney Disease and Focal Segmental Glomerulosclerosis

George J. Dugbartey

Diabetic Kidney Disease

Diabetic kidney disease (DKD) is a major long-term (chronic) microangiopathy that complicates both type 1 and type 2 diabetes mellitus, with a negative impact on the quality of life of diabetic patients [1, 2]. It is defined as a progressive pathological condition of the kidney caused by angiopathy of glomerular capillaries [3]. The angiopathy of these capillaries is characterized by a progressive loss of glomerular filtration surface areas and capillary volume [4, 5]. DKD is currently the leading cause of end-stage renal disease (ESRD) and accounts for 40% of morbidity and mortality among the diabetic population due to its progression to ESRD [1, 2]. According to the US renal data system, DKD is the leading cause of end-stage renal

---

This chapter is an expanded version by the same author in the publication titled Diabetic nephropathy: a potential savior with rotten-egg smell. Pharmacol Rep. 2017;69(2):331–339.

G. J. Dugbartey (✉)
Department of Pharmacology and Toxicology, School of Pharmacy, College of Health Sciences, University of Ghana, Accra, Ghana

Department of Physiology and Pharmacology, Accra College of Medicine, Accra, Ghana

Division of Urology, Department of Surgery, London Health Sciences Center, Western University, London, ON, Canada

Multi-Organ Transplant Program, London Health Sciences Center, Western University, London, ON, Canada

Matthew Mailing Center for Translational Transplant Studies, London Health Sciences Center, Western University, London, ON, Canada
e-mail: gdugbart@uwo.ca

G. J. Dugbartey, A. Sener, *Hydrogen Sulfide in Kidney Diseases*,
https://doi.org/10.1007/978-3-031-44041-0_4

disease and a major contributing factor to morbidity and mortality of diabetic patients throughout the world [6]. Hence, the guideline of the American Diabetes Association suggests an annual test to assess biomarkers of DKD in type 1 diabetic patients with diabetic duration of at least 5 years and in all type 2 diabetic patients starting at diagnosis [7]. Histologically, DKD presents as aberrant expansion of the mesangial matrix and thickening of glomerular basement membrane (GBM) due to excessive production, accumulation, and deposition of extracellular matrix (ECM) within the glomerular, tubulointerstitial, and vascular spaces and ultimately progresses into glomerulosclerosis, tubulointerstitial fibrosis, and vascular remodeling [3, 5, 8].

The ECM consists of several proteins including collagen and elastin. Collagen is the most abundant protein in the ECM and provides structural support to the cells, while elastin provides elasticity to tissues [9, 10]. A fine balance exists between collagen and elastin in healthy kidneys, which allows normal renal function. In DKD, however, the balance between these ECM proteins is disrupted, causing ECM remodeling, thereby contributing to renal vascular impairment and failure [11, 12]. Also, increased activity and levels of matrix metalloproteinase (MMP, a family of calcium-dependent zinc-containing endopeptidases that controls ECM synthesis and degradation, including collagen and elastin), particularly MMP-9, are abundantly expressed in the kidney and serum of type 1 diabetic patients [13, 14] and have been reported to contribute to diabetic renal remodeling [15]. In addition, mesangial cell (MC) proliferation and hypertrophy have been reported in the early pathological features of DKD in several in vitro and in vivo studies [16].

Experimental evidence suggests that although advanced glycation end products and dyslipidemia are associated with organ injury in diabetic patients, hyperglycemia (high blood glucose) or high glucose is likely to be the principal pathological contributor to the development and progression of DKD [17]. Hyperglycemia/high glucose contributes to the development and progression of DKD via multiple molecular mechanisms such as induction of oxidative stress and upregulation of renal transforming growth factor beta-1 (TGF-β1) expression, production of pro-inflammatory cytokines, activation of fibroblasts and renin-angiotensin-aldosterone system (RAAS), and depletion of adenosine triphosphate (ATP) [18–20]. Apart from hyperglycemia, research has shown that hypertension is another major clinical determinant of DKD and that coexistence of hypertension and hyperglycemia accelerates the development and progression of DKD [21, 22]. Other metabolic disorders including proteins and gaseous molecules such as hydrogen sulfide and nitric oxide are also associated with diabetes [23–25]. It is important to note that uncontrolled diabetes can result in fluid buildup, hypertension, albuminuria, elevated serum creatinine and blood urea nitrogen, and eventually renal failure [26]. Despite the expanded knowledge and understanding of the pathogenesis of DKD, the precise mechanism of the pathogenesis and progression of DKD is not fully elucidated. Also, effective therapeutic agents are still lacking, as existing ones such as hypoglycemic agents, antihypertensive drugs, and RAAS inhibitors only slow down the progression of nephropathy but do not prevent it, and thus the number of patients with DKD continues to rise. Hence, novel therapeutic interventions are in high demand to target additional disease mechanisms, which could prevent or ameliorate the progression of DKD. This chapter discusses recent preclinical findings on the molecular mechanisms underlying the pharmacotherapeutic effects of H_2S against DKD development and progression, and its translation from bench to bedside, which could lay the foundation for its future clinical use. A section of the chapter also discusses focal segmental glomerulosclerosis as a mediator of DKD progression to ESRD and H_2S as a potential novel therapy.

Hydrogen Sulfide as an Alternative Pharmacological Agent for Diabetic Kidney Disease

Over the past decades, researchers have reported biological usefulness and therapeutic potentials of endogenous gaseous signaling molecules collectively known as "gasotransmitters." Nitric oxide (NO) was the first identified gasotransmitter followed by carbon monoxide (CO) [27, 28]. Hydrogen sulfide (H_2S), a gas with a distinctive smell of rotten eggs, has recently been identified as the third member of the gasotransmitter family [29]. Although there are differences in the mechanisms of action of these gaseous molecules, thereby ensuring specific functions, cross talk exists between them, which can provide synergistic effects and additional regulatory mechanisms and effects [30, 31]. H_2S has gained notoriety for several centuries for its toxicity and death, especially among industrial workers. The clinical manifestations of its toxicity are dose dependent. At 50–100 ppm, H_2S causes mucosal irritation, headache, dizziness, nausea, vomiting, coughing, breathing difficulty, keratoconjunctivitis, and corneal ulceration [32]. Olfactory paralysis occurs at concentrations between 100 and 150 ppm, and bronchitis and pulmonary edema may result at concentrations approaching 300 ppm. Cardiopulmonary arrest usually occurs at levels >700 ppm, and sudden but reversible loss of consciousness and death occur following acute exposure at concentrations >1000 ppm [32]. The mechanism of H_2S toxicity has been attributed to reversible antagonism at complex IV of the mitochondrial respiratory chain [33]. In the last two decades, however, H_2S has risen above its public image of a deadly "gas of rotten eggs" and has gained attention among researchers as a signaling molecule with physiological relevance and therapeutic potential. Several recent in vitro and in vivo studies have demonstrated that at low micromolar concentrations, H_2S exhibits important therapeutic characteristics that target multiple molecular pathways, thereby preventing the development and progression of several pathologies including DKD [24, 34, 35]. This beneficial effect of H_2S suggests that it may meet the demand for alternative and/or additional therapeutic agent against DKD.

As illustrated in Fig. 4.1, H_2S is endogenously produced by two cytosolic enzymes, cystathionine β-synthase (CBS), and cystathionine γ-lyase (CSE) using homocysteine and L-cysteine as substrates [36]. The mitochondrial enzyme, 3-mercaptopyruvate sulfurtransferase (3-MST), also catalyzes the production of H_2S from L-cysteine and, coupled with the peroxisomal enzyme, D-amino acid oxidase (DAO), produces H_2S from exogenously administered D-cysteine [37]. Although the distribution of these H_2S-producing enzymes is tissue specific, they are abundantly expressed in the kidney [38, 39]. Specifically, they are expressed in

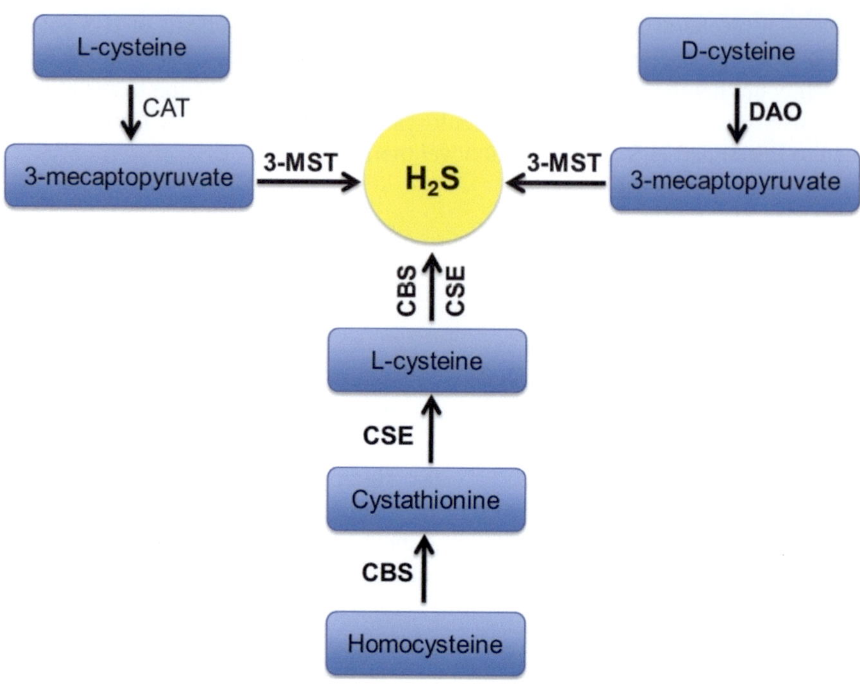

Fig. 4.1 Overview of endogenous hydrogen sulfide (H_2S) production. H_2S is endogenously produced by cystathionine β-synthase (CBS) and cystathionine γ-lyase (CSE) using homocysteine and L-cysteine as substrates. L-cysteine can also be converted to 3-mercaptopyruvate as an intermediate product, a reaction catalyzed by cysteine aminotransferase (CAT). The enzyme 3-mercaptopyruvate sulfurtransferase (3-MST) then produces H_2S from 3-mercaptopyruvate and, coupled with D-amino acid oxidase (DAO), produces H_2S from exogenously administered D-cysteine

the brush border and cytoplasm of epithelial cells of the renal proximal tubules, distal tubules, and peritubular capillaries [24, 36, 37, 40–42]. In the glomeruli, CSE is the main H_2S-producing enzyme expressed by endothelial cells, mesangial cells, and podocytes [40–42]. In fact, about 75% of all renal cells express CSE [40, 42], making the kidney a rich source of endogenous H_2S production. Apart from being generated endogenously, H_2S can also be applied exogenously via H_2S donor compounds such as sodium hydrosulfide (NaHS), sodium sulfide (Na_2S), sodium thiosulfate, GYY4137, AP39, SG1002, S-propargyl cysteine (SPRC, also known as ZYZ-802), sulfurous mineral water, and garlic-derived polysulfide [43–50]. Interestingly, blood H_2S and its H_2S-synthesizing enzymes have recently been reported to be markedly reduced in both diabetic patients and experimental animals compared to nondiabetic control subjects [51–53], suggesting that H_2S may play an important role in diabetic vascular complications, including DKD, and that H_2S restoration could be a target in preventing the progression of DKD. However, the method of plasma H_2S measurement is currently under debate among H_2S researchers.

H₂S Administration Reduces Hyperglycemia-Induced Increase in Renal ROS Production

A growing body of experimental evidence indicates that overproduction of ROS due to hyperglycemia is involved in the pathogenesis of DKD and that oxidative stress is a major denominator in the molecular pathways underlying the development and progression of DKD, as it drives other important pathways in DKD [54–56] (Fig. 4.2). Hyperglycemia and high glucose treatment strongly reduced CSE

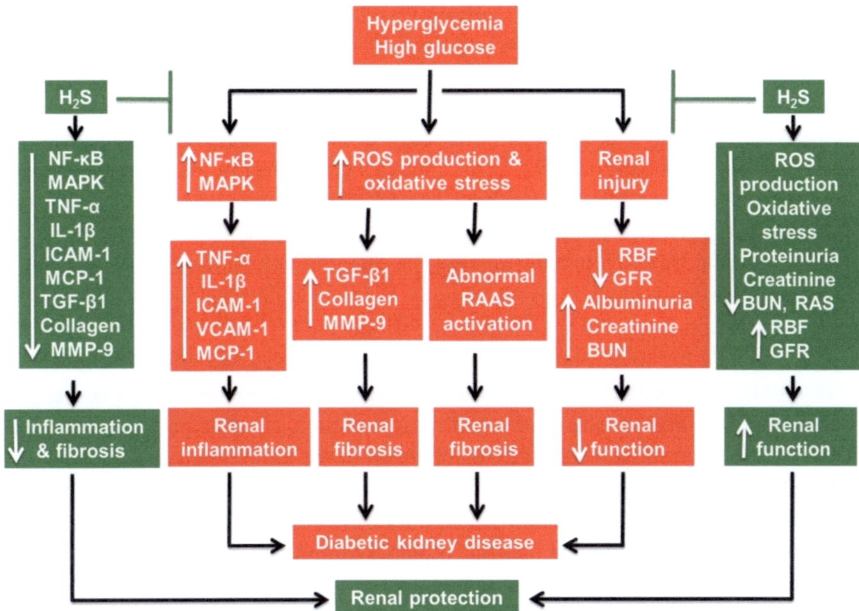

Fig. 4.2 Mechanisms of H₂S protection against diabetic kidney disease. Hyperglycemia or high glucose exposure activates the signaling pathways of nuclear factor kappa-B (NF-κB) and mitogen-activated protein kinase (MAPK), resulting in the production of pro-inflammatory cytokines such as tumor necrosis factor-alpha (TNF-α), interleukin-1β (IL-1β), monocyte chemoattractant protein-1 (MCP-1), intracellular adhesion molecule-1 (ICAM-1), and vascular cell adhesion molecule-1 (VCAM-1) and thus enhances inflammation in diabetic kidneys. Hyperglycemia also induces oxidative stress through increased production of reactive oxygen species (ROS) in mesangial cells and upregulates the expression of transforming growth factor beta-1 (TGF-β1), collagen, and matrix metalloproteinase-9 (MMP-9) in fibrotic kidneys. Excess ROS production also activates components of local renin-angiotensin-aldosterone system (RAAS), leading to mesangial cell proliferation and increased extracellular matrix production and consequently renal fibrosis. Chronic hyperglycemia results in declines in renal blood flow (RBF) and glomerular filtration rate (GFR) as well as elevated albuminuria, serum creatinine, and blood urea nitrogen (BUN). Hydrogen sulfide (H₂S) treatment inhibits all these pathological processes in the diabetic kidney and reverses the hyperglycemic (or high glucose) effects, and thus protects against hyperglycemia-induced diabetic kidney disease

expression in the renal cortex as well as in cultured MCs, leading to reduced endogenous H_2S production, increased ROS generation in MCs, and also decreased activities of naturally occurring antioxidants such as glutathione (GSH) and superoxide dismutase (SOD). This experimental diabetic condition also reduced the transcription factor, nuclear factor erythroid 2-related factor 2 (Nrf-2), which regulates the expression of some antioxidants, and thus increased oxidative stress in diabetic kidneys [45, 48, 57, 58]. Oxidative stress due to excessive ROS production stimulates TGF-β1 in fibrotic kidneys, leading to increase in ECM deposition at the glomerular level [59]. Exogenous H_2S administration in the form of NaHS, SPRC, and sulfurous mineral water lowered blood glucose level, reduced renal ROS production, restored the levels and activities of these endogenous antioxidants as well as the protein levels of their downstream targets in the kidneys of diabetic rats, and prevented the progression of DKD [48, 57, 58]. However, given the low concentrations of H_2S in tissues, its direct interaction with oxidants cannot completely explain its antioxidant effect in DKD [60]. El-Seweidy et al. [61] reported that besides its direct reaction with oxidants, H_2S also enhances GSH level in the heart of diabetic rats, leading to myocardial protection. Several other studies have also shown that H_2S activates SOD, Nrf-2, and catalase in other disease models, thereby enhancing organ protection [62–64]. In addition, H_2S interaction with NO and CO in the mitochondrial respiratory chain might have activated their individual antioxidant activities via activation and opening of adenosine triphosphate (ATP)-sensitive potassium (K_{ATP}) channels [65–67]. Further, H_2S treatment increases NO and GSH levels in heart failure patients [47]. Although the exact mechanism by which H_2S scavenges ROS in DKD is still questionable, as this is common in other pathologies, these pieces of evidence suggest a backup mechanism of the antioxidant activities of H_2S in DKD and in other pathologies.

To further elucidate the antioxidant activity of H_2S under hyperglycemic or high glucose condition, genetic and pharmacological inhibition of endogenous H_2S production by siRNA-induced CSE silencing and PPG elevated ROS generation in high glucose-treated endothelial cells and in experimental diabetic rats [68, 69]. In the same studies, the authors reported that exogenous H_2S supplementation either by pharmacological or by adenoviral overexpression of CSE scavenged ROS and thereby protected against high glucose-induced cell dysfunction and hyperglycemia-induced DKD [68, 69]. Yuan et al. [57] also observed that pharmacological inhibition of H_2S with the CSE inhibitor, DL-propargylglycine (PPG), increased renal ROS production similar to hyperglycemia-induced ROS production. Besides its antioxidant effect, H_2S treatment in the form of sulfurous mineral water may combat the state of hypomagnesemia, which is a modifiable risk factor of DKD, because sulfurous mineral water is rich in magnesium [70]. In summary, administration of H_2S scavenges renal ROS induced by hyperglycemia or high glucose exposure and thus prevents the progression of DKD.

H₂S Supplementation Ameliorates Hyperglycemia-Induced Renal Fibrosis

Hyperglycemia/high glucose is known to upregulate the expression of TGF-β1 in MCs and renal tubular epithelial cells through increased ROS production, leading to MC proliferation and excessive accumulation of ECM and consequently glomerulosclerosis and tubulointerstitial fibrosis [71, 72] (Fig. 4.2). Apart from TGF-β1, hyperglycemia stimulates collagen IV synthesis in the renal cortex, which in turn increases MC proliferation and ECM secretion resulting in glomerular hypertrophy and sclerosis [48, 57]. Such hyperglycemic effect on the kidney also confirms the findings of Ziyadeh et al. [73] and Jiang et al. [74]. It is important to note that the upregulations of TGF-β1 and collagen IV and the consequent glomerulosclerosis and tubulointerstitial fibrosis are in parallel with reduced renal CBS and CSE expression and endogenous H₂S level [40, 48, 57]. Moreover, CSE inhibition with PPG strongly increased renal expressions of the fibrotic proteins TGF-β1 and smooth muscle actin (SMA) [48, 69, 75]. In accord, H₂S treatment restored renal CSE and endogenous H₂S levels; suppressed hyperglycemia-induced cell proliferation; reversed the increases in TGF-β1, collagen synthesis, and accumulation; inhibited renal ECM accumulation, MC proliferation, and hypertrophy; and thus mitigated ECM remodeling in the kidneys of diabetic rats [48, 75]. This remarkable observation is in line with previous studies in which H₂S was reported to reduce hypertrophy of intramyocardial arterioles and cardiac ventricular fibrosis [76]. The mechanism by which H₂S inhibits TGF-β1 synthesis and expression is not completely understood. However, Qian et al. [48] reported that H₂S administration inhibits expression of TGF-β1 and phosphorylation of renal Smad3, a protein involved in the signaling cascade triggered by activation of TGF-β receptor and highly expressed in the kidneys of diabetic patients [77], and thus prevents the progression of renal fibrosis. In addition to TGF-β1 and collagen IV, Zhou et al. [58] also reported that H₂S treatment downregulates the expressions of collagens I and III in renal tissue of diabetic rats and thus prevents the progression of DKD.

At the molecular level, Eid et al. [78] explained that hyperglycemia induces renal hypertrophy in diabetic mice by inhibiting the activity of adenosine monophosphate-activated protein kinase (AMPK), a key enzyme involved in cellular energy homeostasis. Interestingly, it is reported that H₂S inhibited high glucose-induced cellular hypertrophy and cytotoxicity by activating AMPK signaling pathway in renal epithelial cells and in in vitro model of diabetic cardiopathy [40, 79]. As both hypertrophy and renal fibrosis require protein synthesis, which is stimulated by hyperglycemia, H₂S was found to also prevent the development and progression of renal fibrosis and hypertrophy by inhibiting high glucose-induced phosphorylation of proteins such as 4E-BP1 and P70S6 kinase and degradation of PDCD4 [40]. Lee et al. [80] also reported that tadalafil, a phosphodiesterase 5 inhibitor used for the treatment of erectile dysfunction, ameliorated high glucose-induced matrix protein synthesis in mouse podocytes by activating a complex H_2S-NO-AMPK interaction. There are also reports that H_2S attenuates fibrosis by inhibiting the activities of fibroblasts. Although this is yet to be reported in DKD, Sheng et al. [81] observed that H_2S treatment inhibited human atrial fibroblast activities by suppressing potassium channel activity and attenuated cardiac fibrosis.

Hyperglycemia does not only upregulate TGF-β1 and collagen but also induces MMP-9 expression with a decrease in renal CBS and CSE expression, leading to reduced tissue and plasma H_2S levels [15, 75]. As abundance of MMP-9 is associated with ECM deposition and endothelial and renal dysfunction, hyperglycemia-induced MMP-9 expression resulted in pathological remodeling of kidneys of diabetic rats [15, 75]. Interestingly, administration of H_2S increased renal CBS and CSE levels, restored endogenous H_2S production, decreased glucose level, and greatly mitigated MMP-9-induced pathological renal remodeling [75]. Taken together, the glucose-lowering effect of H_2S prevents the development and progression of renal fibrosis in DKD.

Administration of H_2S Inhibits Hyperglycemia-Induced Renal Inflammation

Hyperglycemia-induced inflammation was first described by Cai et al. [82] in which they reported that hyperglycemia activated the transcription factor, nuclear factor kappa-B (NF-κB) in the liver of type 2 diabetic mice. NF-κB is a key mediator of inflammation whose activation leads to downstream pro-inflammatory cytokine production such as tumor necrosis factor alpha (TNF-α), interleukin-6 (IL-6), and IL-1β, which in turn induces persistent and enhanced inflammation, leading to excessive ECM accumulation [83]. In accord, activation of NF-κB by hyperglycemia resulted in production of these cytokines and the ensuing hepatic inflammation [82]. There are now convincing data that hyperglycemia or high glucose exposure induces inflammation and contributes to the progression of DKD (Fig. 4.2). For example, Huang et al. [84] observed that treatment of rat glomerular MCs with high glucose activates NF-κB inflammatory signaling via IκBα sumoylation and ubiquitination. Also, in a streptozotocin (STZ)-induced diabetic rat model, Zhou et al. [58] reported increase in DNA-binding activity of NF-κB in the kidney, suggesting induction of inflammatory pathway. In the same study, the authors further reported that treatment of rat MCs with high glucose also activated the signaling pathways of mitogen-activated protein kinase (MAPK), another key mediator of inflammation.

Against this background, inhibition of NF-κB and MAPK signaling pathways may be of great interest, as it may prove protective against renal inflammation in DKD and other pathologies. H_2S treatment of STZ-induced diabetic rats and rat glomerular MCs under high glucose condition was found to strongly inhibit NF-κB and MAPK signaling pathways and reduced levels of pro-inflammatory cytokines such as TNF-α, intercellular adhesion molecule-1 (ICAM-1), vascular cell adhesion molecule-1 (VCAM-1), and monocyte chemoattractant protein-1 (MCP-1) [58]. This consequently attenuated inflammation in diabetic kidneys and decreased high glucose-induced MC proliferation [58] (Fig. 4.2). However, it is unknown whether NF-κB inhibition by H_2S is via IκBα sumoylation and ubiquitination or via other potential but undefined signaling pathways leading to the reduced cytokine production in DKD. The anti-inflammatory effect of H_2S was also observed in cardiac cells in which exogenous H_2S administration inhibited activation of NF-κB and MAPK signaling pathways and protected cardiomyoblasts against high glucose-induced injury and inflammation including cytotoxicity and apoptosis [85, 86]. In another rat model of STZ-induced DKD, H_2S exhibited its anti-inflammatory property by mitigating macrophage infiltration in diabetic kidneys and downregulated TNF-α, IL-1β, and MCP-1 [48, 87]. Further, H_2S prevented phosphorylation of Stat3, a protein that plays a key role in the regulation of inflammation and thus contributed partly to kidney protection under diabetic setting [48]. This may be another mechanism by which H_2S exerts its anti-inflammatory effect. Studies have shown that in concert with NO and CO, H_2S inhibits the expression of ICAM-1, VCAM-1, and E-selection and thus enhances endothelial health and integrity in other experimental disease models [88]. Whereas these findings are interesting and promising, there are no studies describing the effect of H_2S on other molecules such as Toll-like receptors, adipokines, and nuclear receptors, which are also related to the inflammatory pathways and considered candidates for new molecular targets for DKD treatment. In conclusion, H_2S attenuates renal inflammation induced in a diabetic setting and protects against diabetic kidney injury.

H_2S Supplementation Inhibits High Glucose-Induced RAAS Activation

Renin-angiotensin-aldosterone system (RAAS) has been identified to be a major pathway involved in the development and progression of DKD [89, 90]. Abnormal activation of intrarenal RAAS under hyperglycemic or high glucose condition is associated with glomerular enlargement and secondary glomerulosclerosis, tubular epithelial to mesenchymal transition, interstitial fibroblast proliferation, increased TGF-β1 expression, and ECM deposition [91–93] (Fig. 4.2). In cultured MCs, for example, Xue et al. [93] showed increased expressions of angiotensinogen (AGT), angiotensin-converting enzyme (ACE), and angiotensin II type 1 (AT1) receptor following high glucose treatment. These observations indicate activation of RAAS, which was reversed upon treatment with AT1 receptor blocker. Their reports support earlier reports in which high glucose activated angiotensin II (Ang II) in MCs and also increased myocardial fibrosis [17, 94, 95]. Ang II, the main peptide of RAAS, functions as a growth factor by activating interstitial fibroblasts, tubular cells, and MCs and also promotes synthesis of ECM proteins, making it a potent pro-fibrotic factor. Durvasula et al. [96] found that high glucose directly stimulates podocytes to increase Ang II production and AT1 receptor levels, which in turn promotes podocyte injury through increased intracellular calcium release and influx from extracellular space [97].

Emerging reports also suggest an interaction between excess ROS production and RAAS activation under high glucose conditions. However, the exact mechanism is not fully elucidated. High glucose has recently been reported to cause a shift in the balance between oxidative and reductive species, leading to excessive ROS generation, which activates local RAAS and increases Ang II level. Activation of Ang II in turn stimulates ROS generation by activating AT1 receptor [93, 98]. This pathological vicious cycle leads to MC proliferation and increased ECM production and accumulation [92]. Garrido et al. [99] also reported that Ang II also promotes podocyte injury through increased ROS production, as it activates systems that use NADPH oxidases as substrates for ROS generation. In addition, there is a marked increase in RAAS-related factors (AGT mRNA, AGT protein, and Ang II) and ROS-related factors (4-hydroxy-2-nonenal and heme oxygenase-1) in the kidneys of type 2 diabetic patients with progression of DKD compared to control subjects [100]. In a mouse model of STZ-induced diabetes, overexpression of catalase, an ROS scavenger, attenuated intrarenal AGT expression as well as interstitial fibrosis and apoptosis of proximal tubular cells [101, 102]. This suggests that the changes of RAAS are downstream of ROS. Moreover, inhibition of ROS decreased high glucose-induced increases in RAAS-related factors as well as MC proliferation and ECM production [93].

Currently, therapeutic RAAS inhibitors such as ACE inhibitors and Ang II receptor blockers are used to reduce proteinuria and retard the progression of DKD but unfortunately do not prevent the disease progression [103–105]. It has recently been reported that H_2S does not only possess antioxidant, anti-fibrotic, and anti-inflammatory properties but also has the ability to inhibit RAAS activation, thereby preventing the development and progression of DKD (Fig. 4.2). ROS production and RAAS activation are associated with reduced expression of H_2S-producing enzymes and endogenous H_2S production. Therefore, H_2S supplementation attenuated high glucose-induced ROS production and RAAS activation and reversed MC proliferation and ECM deposition [93]. In addition, Zhou et al. [58] reported that H_2S treatment strongly inhibited RAAS activation and attenuated the development of DKD in STZ-induced diabetic rats. The ability of H_2S to interfere with components of the RAAS has also been observed in hypertension, another major clinical determinant of DKD. Administration of H_2S is reported to inhibit the expression and activity of renin (the rate-limiting enzyme in the formation of Ang II) from juxtaglomerular cells of the kidney and immortalized renin-containing renal tumor cell line by inhibiting the renin stimulator, intracellular cyclic adenosine monophosphate [106, 107]. In addition to renin inhibition, H_2S also decreased Ang II level and ameliorated renovascular hypertension in rats [107]. Furthermore, H_2S treatment inhibited RAAS activation, lowered blood pressure, and attenuated renal fibrosis and proteinuria in salt-sensitive hypertensive rats [108, 109]. It is noteworthy that H_2S interferes with zinc in the active center of ACE and directly inhibits its activity in human endothelial cells and may therefore act as an ACE inhibitor [110]. These important underlying mechanisms may be applicable to RAAS inhibition in DKD. Thus, H_2S prevents the development and progression of DKD not only by scavenging ROS but also by inhibiting the activation of RAAS under high glucose condition.

H_2S Treatment Reverses Renal Functional Changes in DKD

As illustrated in Fig. 4.2, renal functional characteristics such as elevated serum creatinine (sCr), blood urea nitrogen (BUN), and albuminuria and decline in glomerular filtration rate (GFR) are common in patients with DKD [111, 112]. Similar observations were made in rodent models of STZ-induced diabetes [20, 48, 56, 58, 69, 113]. Interestingly, H_2S treatment of STZ-induced diabetic rats significantly reduced sCr and BUN levels as well as proteinuria compared to the group without H_2S treatment and attenuated the progression of DKD [57, 58, 69]. A combined treatment of H_2S and losartan, Ang II receptor antagonist, produced more significant results with increased GSH levels and improved behavioral abnormalities in STZ-treated rats compared to their individual effects. This suggests synergistic effect of both drugs [113]. Moreover, endogenous H_2S inhibition with PPG produced results similar to STZ treatment [113], suggesting that H_2S is important in reversing the biochemical abnormalities induced by STZ. Qian et al. [48] also observed reduced albuminuria, urine volume, and sCr following H_2S treatment, thereby protecting kidneys of diabetic rats against STZ-induced injury.

Currently, there is no available data on the effect of H_2S on GFR in diabetic settings. However, Yamamoto et al. [24] observed vasoconstriction and reduced renal blood flow (RBF) in peritubular capillaries of diabetic mice. In the same study, the authors reported that H_2S treatment increased peritubular capillary diameter and RBF and improved tubulointerstitial microcirculation, suggesting that H_2S may prevent progression of ischemic injury in DKD. There are also reports that H_2S improves RBF and GFR, reduces intrarenal pressure in pre- and post-glomerular arterioles, and enhances renal excretory function in other disease models including hypertension, thereby leading to renal protection [36, 114, 115] (Fig. 4.2). In view of this vasoactivity of H_2S, it is likely that H_2S is involved in the regulation of microcirculation in diabetic kidneys. It is also important to note that RBF and GFR are increased in the initial stages of DKD [5]. However, it still remains to be investigated whether a transient local increase in H_2S production in the glomerular microvasculature contributes to this phenomenon. In summary, administration of H_2S reverses the biochemical abnormalities in DKD and protects the kidney against injury induced by diabetes.

Limitations in the Protective Action of H₂S in Diabetic Kidney Disease

Contrary to the promising effects of H_2S against DKD, Oosterhuis et al. [116] observed reduced proteinuria, blood pressure, sCr, and Ang II-induced hypertensive renal injury in rats following H_2S inhibition with PPG. Also, CSE knockout mice have been reported to be relatively resistant to STZ-induced diabetes, and with delayed development of diabetic status [117]. Moreover, PPG treatment protected wild-type mice from STZ-induced hyperglycemia and hypoinsulinemia [117]. Furthermore, pancreatic CSE expression and H_2S production were significantly higher in Zucker diabetic fatty (ZDF) rats compared to nondiabetic control rats [118]. Interestingly, PPG treatment increased serum insulin level and reduced hyperglycemia, suggesting that abnormally high production of pancreatic H_2S impairs insulin release and results in hyperglycemia in ZDF rats. These conflicting results with those discussed above may be due to differences in experimental models, dose of PPG administered, as well as concentration of H_2S. Moreover, H_2S measurement in some of these studies may be unreliable and overestimated partly due to lack of sensitive measuring technique and partly due to its volatile nature. In addition, since complex interactions exist between the gasotransmitter system, it is also possible that PPG exerts nonspecific effects independent of CSE inhibition. In line with the latter possibility, PPG treatment upregulated heme oxygenase-1, an isoform of CO-producing enzyme, leading to increased CO levels and renal protection in Ang II-induced hypertensive rats [116].

Focal Segmental Glomerulosclerosis in Diabetic Kidney Disease

Described for the first time in 1957 by Arnold Rich [119], focal segmental glomerulosclerosis (FSGS) has become one of the most common forms of acquired glomerular diseases, with a rising global incidence. It is hallmarked histologically by progressive scarring (sclerosis) to parts (segments) of the glomerular capillaries in a minority (focal) of glomeruli along with progressive podocyte depletion [120, 121]. As a compensatory pathological mechanism to regulate glomerular functional integrity, the remaining podocytes undergo hypertrophy, which leads to FSGS progression due to inability of the surviving podocytes to meet the increasing demand of the glomerular volume [122, 123]. Nephrotic syndrome, characterized by proteinuria, hypoalbuminemia, hypercholesterolemia, and peripheral edema, is a clinical picture of FSGS due to the loss of podocytes and their filtration function [124]. Just like DKD, FSGS is also a chronic disease that leads to ESRD. As a mediator of DKD progression to ESRD, FSGS accounts for 4% of all ESRD cases, as 50% of FSGS cases progress to ESRD within 3–8 years [124]. Unfortunately, while pharmacological agents such as antiproteinuric and immunosuppressive drugs are used to manage the disease along with dietary changes, there are currently no approved effective pharmacological treatments for FSGS, as the scarred glomeruli cannot be repaired. The disease can only be treated with renal replacement therapy (dialysis or kidney transplantation), although it can recur in about 40% of patients following kidney transplantation, with an associated increase in posttransplant complications [125–128].

On the basis of etiology, FSGS is classified as primary (idiopathic) and secondary. Primary FSGS occurs with no demonstrable etiology in 80% of FSGS patients, while secondary FSGS accounts for the remaining 20% and could be drug induced, virus induced, or caused by genetic factors and systemic diseases such as diabetes, hypertension, and obesity [129]. As discussed in section "H_2S Supplementation Ameliorates Hyperglycemia-Induced Renal Fibrosis" above, hyperglycemia/high glucose exposure upregulates TGF-β1 expression, stimulates renal cortical synthesis of collagen IV, increases ECM secretion, and through a subsequent series of pathological processes culminates in FSGS development [48, 57, 71, 72]. In a study using human kidney tissues collected from autopsies to determine the mechanisms underlying glomerular hypertrophy in FSGS and DKD, Puelles et al. [130] reported upregulation of the expressions of mammalian target of rapamycin (mTOR) and parietal epithelial cell (PEC) activation-associated genes, while partial pharmacological inhibition of mTOR pathway restored glomerular integrity in their murine model of FSGS. This result corroborated that of previous murine and in vitro models of FSGS by another research group [131]. Taken together, these observations suggest that activation of mTOR pathway is an adaptive process that mediates glomerular hypertrophy in response to podocyte loss in FSGS and that mTOR pathway represents a potential therapeutic target in the treatment or prevention of FSGS.

H_2S as a Potential Therapy for Focal Segmental Glomerulosclerosis

As the search for pharmacological agents for effective treatment of FSGS continues, H_2S is emerging as a potential candidate. There are studies showing that increased expression of the fibrotic proteins, TGF-β1, collagen, and matrix metalloproteinase (MMP)-9, and the resulting ECM deposition along with pathological remodeling in the renal cortex, is associated with decreased renal CBS and CSE expression, thereby leading to reduced renal and plasma H_2S levels [15, 75]. As such, administration of H_2S in the form of NaHS increased renal expression of CBS and CSE, restored endogenous H_2S production, and mitigated pathological renal remodeling induced by MMP-9 [75]. In a genetic model of hyperhomocysteinemia (an important pathogenic factor for glomerular damage), the kidneys of wild-type and heterozygous CBS mice which received 30 µmol/L of NaHS in drinking water for 8 weeks showed significant downregulation of the expression of MMP-2 and -9 and collagen proteins, as well as decreased glomerular depositions and pro-inflammatory markers, which resulted in improved glomerulosclerosis and GFR compared to control mice without NaHS treatment [132]. This finding supports a previous observation in a similar mouse model by the same authors in which FSGS was associated with reduced plasma H_2S level, increased albuminuria, MMP activity, and apoptosis in the renal cortex while the same concentration and route of NaHS administration reversed these pathological changes, with increased plasma H_2S level [133]. Considering that activation of mTOR pathway has been implicated in FSGS development and progression, Lee et al. [134] recently reported that administration of the same concentration of NaHS via the same route increased plasma H_2S level and inhibited insulin/mTOR signaling pathway and MMP activity in the renal cortex, which positively correlated with reduced albuminuria, serum cystatin C, and inflammation and restored AMPK activity, leading to attenuation of glomerulosclerosis and improvement in renal function in aging mice kidneys. While further studies are needed to confirm the inhibitory effect of H_2S with other H_2S donor compounds on mTOR pathway and further investigate other potential mechanisms involved in ameliorating FSGS, results from experimental studies so far show that H_2S supplementation through NaHS administration ameliorates FSGS and improves renal function via mechanisms that include regulation of AMPK/mTOR signaling pathway.

Clinical Application and Future Perspectives

The reduced bioavailability of H_2S and H_2S-producing enzymes as recently observed in both diabetic patients and experimental models of diabetes suggests that H_2S may serve a diagnostic purpose for diabetic patients in the future. At the moment, H_2S itself is not directly used in the clinic since its toxic effects on bystanders seriously hamper the classic form of inhalation. However, its oxidation metabolite, thiosulfate (in the form of sodium thiosulfate), is already being used in the clinic to treat acute cyanide poisoning [135] and calciphylaxis in patients with end-stage renal disease [136, 137]. However, a major concern in the clinical use of thiosulfate is the fact that it is rapidly degraded in the stomach and therefore must be administered intravenously. Given this disadvantage, thiosulfate could be incorporated into gastric acid-resistant capsules and released after leaving the stomach. In agreement with this future direction, hybrids of H_2S donors are currently being designed and synthesized in which sulfide molecules are incorporated into an already existing drug as seen in sulfide-releasing aspirin and S-diclofenac [87, 138, 139] or incorporated into a newly synthesized drug. Although the effects of H_2S donors in human patients have not been described extensively, emerging reports indicate that garlic, a source of natural H_2S donors, improves insulin sensitivity in fructose-induced diabetic rats [140] and reduces blood pressure in patients with uncontrolled arterial hypertension [141], making H_2S a promising antidiabetic and antihypertensive agent for clinical use in the future. This also suggests dietary inclusion of garlic for H_2S treatment in diabetic and FSGS patients. However, the amount of garlic needed to constitute sulfide treatment sufficient to contribute to renal protection in diabetic and FSGS patients is yet to be established. In addition, garlic extract has been reported to antagonize liver X receptor alpha (LXRα), an important protein that regulates cholesterol, triglycerides, and glucose homeostasis [142]. These effects may play a key role in reducing the lipid profile by garlic, which may also account for its potential for the treatment of diabetes and FSGS.

Apart from preclinical studies, recent clinical observations also support the evidence that H_2S contributes to protection against DKD. Excretion of urinary sulfate (partly from cysteine oxidation by cysteine oxidase-dependent pathway and partly from H_2S metabolism) has been associated with a slower decline in GFR and reduced renal failure in type 1 diabetic patients [143]. More recently, van den Born et al. [144] also reported that increased urinary sulfate concentration correlates with reduced risk for renal events in type 2 diabetic patients with nephropathy. However, as human data are scarce in the field of H_2S-related diabetic research, further studies on urinary sulfate excretion in type 2 diabetes are warranted since DKD is more common in type 2 diabetic patients than in their type 1 counterparts. It is important to note that sulfate or sulfur-containing amino acids can also be obtained from diet and, together with thiosulfate, have shown promising predictive values in other disease conditions [145]. Hence, they should be considered in large-scale diabetic and FSGS cohort studies in both urine and plasma samples. In addition, healthy lifestyle habits together with regular physical activity (weight control) and consumption of good-quality diet might enhance vascular function and thereby improve H_2S production. Further, a recent phase I clinical trial of SG1002 (H_2S donor) was safe and well tolerated at all doses administered, increased plasma H_2S and NO bioavailability in both healthy and heart failure subjects, and attenuated increases in cardiac damage markers in the heart failure group [47]. There is currently one clinical trial on clinicaltrials.gov on the effect of N-acetylcysteine on H_2S in chronic kidney disease, chronic kidney failure, and end-stage renal disease. Such trials should be extended to DKD and FSGS as well as other pathologies in order to gain further insight and fully exploit the therapeutic potential of H_2S.

Conclusion

Both DKD and FSGS are chronic renal pathologies that lead to end-stage renal disease and represent major causes of morbidity and mortality of kidney disease patients worldwide. Unfortunately, nephrologists still face the challenge of providing these groups of patients with effective protection against the development and progression of DKD and FSGS since current therapies only retard the progression of both diseases but do not prevent or reverse them. H_2S has overcome its bad reputation and has recently been demonstrated in several in vivo and in vitro studies to possess important therapeutic properties that can prevent the development and progression of DKD and FSGS. Therefore, H_2S may represent an alternative or additional pharmacological approach for DKD and FSGS treatment in the future.

Conflict of Interest None.

References

1. Ritz E, Orth SR. Nephropathy in patients with type 2 diabetes mellitus. N Engl J Med. 1999;341(15):1127–33.
2. Gunzler D, Bleyer AJ, Thomas RL, O'Brien A, Russell GB, Sattar A, et al. Diabetic nephropathy in a sibling and albuminuria predict early GFR decline: a prospective cohort study. BMC Nephrol. 2013;14:124.
3. Kanwar YS, Wada J, Sun L, Xie P, Wallner EI, Chen S, Chugh S, Danesh FR. Diabetic nephropathy: mechanisms of renal disease progression. Exp Biol Med. 2008;233(1):4–11.
4. Steffes MW, Osterby R, Chavers B, Mauer SM. Mesangial expansion as a central mechanism for loss of kidney function in diabetic patients. Diabetes. 1989;38(9):1077–81.
5. Osterby R. Structural changes in the diabetic kidney. Clin Endocrinol Metab. 1986;15(4):733–51.
6. U.S. Renal Data System. USRD 2009 annual data report: atlas of chronic kidney disease and end-stage renal disease in the United States. Bethesda: National Institutes of Health, National Institute of Diabetes and Digestive and Kidney Diseases; 2009.
7. American Diabetes Association. Standards of medical care in diabetes. Diabetes Care. 2013;36(1):S11–66.
8. Hua H, Goldberg HJ, Fantus IG, Whiteside CI. High glucose-enhanced mesangial cell extracellular signal-regulated protein kinase activation and alpha1(IV) collagen expression in response to endothelin-1: role of specific protein kinase C isozymes. Diabetes. 2001;50(10):2376–83.
9. Sterzel RB, Hartner A, Schlotzer-Schrehardt U, Voit S, Hausknecht B, Doliana R, et al. Elastic fiber proteins in the glomerular mesangium in vivo and in cell culture. Kidney Int. 2000;58(4):1588–602.
10. Zeisberg M, Bonner G, Maeshima Y, Colorado P, Muller GA, Strutz F, Kalluri R. Renal fibrosis: collagen composition and assembly regulates epithelial-mesenchymal transdifferentiation. Am J Pathol. 2001;159(4):1313–21.
11. Genovese F, Manresa AA, Leeming DJ, Karsdal MA, Boor P. The extracellular matrix in the kidney: a source of novel non-invasive biomarkers of kidney fibrosis? Fibrogenesis Tissue Repair. 2014;7(1):4.
12. Li SY, Huang PH, Yang AH, Tang DC, Yang WC, Lin CC, et al. Matrix metalloproteinase-9 deficiency attenuates diabetic nephropathy by modulation of podocyte functions and dedifferentiation. Kidney Int. 2014;86(2):358–69.
13. Qing-Hua G, Ju-Ming L, Chang-Yu P, Zhao-Hui L, Xiao-Man Z, Yi-Ming M. The kidney expression of matrix metalloproteinase-9 in the diabetic nephropathy of Kkay mice. J Diabetes Complicat. 2008;22(6):408–12.
14. Gharagozlian S, Svennevig K, Bangstad HJ, Winberg JO, Kolset SO. Matrix metalloproteinases in subjects with type 1 diabetes. BMC Clin Pathol. 2009;9:7.
15. Kundu S, Pushpakumar SB, Tyagi A, Coley D, Sen U. Hydrogen sulfide deficiency and diabetic renal remodeling: role of matrix metalloproteinase-9. Am J Physiol Endocrinol Metab. 2013;304(12):E1365–78.
16. Abboud HE. Mesangial cell biology. Exp Cell Res. 2012;18(9):979–85.
17. Vidotti DB, Casarini DE, Cristovam PC, Leite CA, Schor N, Boim MA. High glucose concentration stimulates intracellular renin activity and angiotensin II generation in rat mesangial cells. Am J Physiol Renal Physiol. 2004;286(6):F1039–45.
18. Kanasaki K, Taduri G, Koya D. Diabetic nephropathy: the role of inflammation in fibroblast activation and kidney fibrosis. Front Endocrinol (Lausanne). 2013;4:7.
19. Reidy K, Kang HM, Hostetter T, Susztak K. Molecular mechanisms of diabetic kidney disease. J Clin Invest. 2014;124(6):2333–40.
20. Lanaspa MA, Ishimoto T, Cicerchi C, Tamura Y, Roncal-Jimenez CA, Chen W, et al. Endogenous fructose production and fructokinase activation mediate renal injury in diabetic nephropathy. J Am Soc Nephrol. 2014;25(11):2526–38.

21. Cooper ME. Interaction of metabolic and haemodynamic factors in mediating experimental diabetic nephropathy. Diabetologia. 2001;44(11):1957–72.
22. Ahmad FU, Sattar MA, Rathore HA, Abdullah MH, Tan S, Abdullah NA, Johns EJ. Exogenous hydrogen sulfide (H2S) reduces blood pressure and prevents the progression of diabetic nephropathy in spontaneously hypertensive rats. Ren Fail. 2012;34(2):203–10.
23. Gougeon R. Insulin resistance and protein metabolism in type 2 diabetes and impact on dietary needs. Can J Diabetes. 2013;37(2):115–20.
24. Yamamoto J, Sato W, Kosugi T, Yamamoto T, Kimura T, Taniguchi S, et al. Distribution of hydrogen sulfide (H2S)-producing enzymes and the roles of the H2S donor sodium hydrosulfide in diabetic nephropathy. Clin Exp Nephrol. 2013;17(1):32–40.
25. Tessari P. Nitric oxide in the normal kidney and in patients with diabetic nephropathy. J Nephrol. 2015;28(3):257–68.
26. Liang S, Li Q, Zhu HY, Zhou JH, Ding R, Chen XM, Cai GY. Clinical factors associated with the diagnosis and progression of diabetic nephropathy. Cell Biochem Biophys. 2014;70(1):9–15.
27. Furchgott RF, Zawadzki JV. The obligatory role of endothelial cells in relaxation of arterial smooth muscle by acetylcholine. Nature. 1980;288(5789):373–6.
28. Wang R. Resurgence of carbon monoxide: an endogenous gaseous relaxing factor. Can J Physiol Pharmacol. 1998;76:1–15.
29. Abe K, Kimura H. The possible role of hydrogen sulfide as an endogenous neuromodulator. J Neurosci. 1996;6(3):1066–71.
30. Hosoki R, Matsuki N, Kimura H. The possible role of hydrogen sulfide as an endogenous smooth muscle relaxant in synergy with nitric oxide. Biochem Biophys Res Commun. 1997;237:527–31.
31. Zhang QY, Du JB, Zhang CY, Tang CS. The regulation of carbon monoxide/heme oxygenase system by hydrogen sulfide in rats with hypoxic pulmonary hypertension. Zhonghua Jie He He Hu Xi Za Zhi. 2004;27(10):659–63.
32. Gabbay DS, De Roos F, Perrone J. Twenty-foot fall averts fatality from massive hydrogen sulfide exposure. J Emerg Med. 2001;20(2):141–4.
33. Blackstone E, Morrison M, Roth MB. H2S induces a suspended animation-like state in mice. Science. 2005;308(5721):518.
34. Kimura H. Hydrogen sulfide: its production, release and functions. Amino Acids. 2011;41(1):113–21.
35. Wang R. Two's company, three's a crowd: can H2S be the third endogenous gaseous transmitter? FASEB J. 2002;16(13):1792–8.
36. Xia M, Chen L, Muh RW, Li PL, Li N. Production and actions of hydrogen sulfide, a novel gaseous bioactive substance, in the kidneys. J Pharmacol Exp Ther. 2009;329(3):1056–62.
37. Shibuya N, Koike S, Tanaka M, Ishigami-Yuasa M, Kimura Y, Ogasawara Y, et al. A novel pathway for the production of hydrogen sulfide from D-cysteine in mammalian cells. Nat Commun. 2013;4:1366.
38. Dugbartey GJ, Talaei F, Houwertjes MC, et al. Dopamine treatment attenuates acute kidney injury in a rat model of deep hypothermia and rewarming—the role of renal H_2S-producing enzymes. Eur J Pharmacol. 2015;769:225–33.
39. Dugbartey GJ, Bouma HR, Strijkstra AM, Boerema AS, Henning HR. Induction of a torpor-like state by 5′-AMP does not depend on H_2S production. PLoS One. 2015;10(8):e0136113.
40. Lee HJ, Mariappan MM, Feliers D, Cavaglieri RC, Sataranatarajan K, Abboud HE, et al. Hydrogen sulfide inhibits high glucose-induced matrix protein synthesis by activating AMP-activated protein kinase in renal epithelial cells. J Biol Chem. 2012;387(7):4451–61.
41. Bos EM, Leuvinink HG, Snijder PM, et al. Hydrogen sulfide-induced hypometabolism prevents renal ischemia/reperfusion injury. J Am Soc Nephrol. 2009;20(9):1901–5.
42. Bos EM, Wang R, Snijder PM, et al. Cystathionine γ-lyase protects against renal ischemia/reperfusion by modulating oxidative stress. J Am Soc Nephrol. 2013;24(5):759–70.

43. Ginter E, Simko V. Garlic (Allium sativum L.) and cardiovascular diseases. Bratisl Lek Listy. 2010;111(8):452–6.
44. Kashfi K, Olson KR. Biology and therapeutic potential of hydrogen sulfide and hydrogen sulfide-releasing chimeras. Biochem Pharmacol. 2013;85(5):689–703.
45. Safar MM, Abdelsalam RM. H2S donors attenuate diabetic nephropathy in rats: modulation of oxidant status and polyol pathway. Pharmacol Rep. 2015;67(1):17–23.
46. Szczesny B, Modis K, Yanagi K, et al. AP39, a novel mitochondria-targeted hydrogen sulfide donor, stimulates cellular bioenergetics, exerts cytoprotective effects and protects against the loss of mitochondrial DNA integrity in oxidatively stressed endothelial cells in vitro. Nitric Oxide. 2014;41:120–30.
47. Polhemus DJ, Li Z, Pattillo CB, Gojon G Sr, Gojon G Jr, Giordano T, Krum H. A novel hydrogen sulfide prodrug, SG1002, promotes hydrogen sulfide and nitric oxide bioavailability in heart failure patients. Cardiovasc Ther. 2015;33(4):216–26.
48. Qian X, Li X, Ma F, Luo S, Ge R, Zhu Y. Novel hydrogen sulfide-releasing compound, S-propargyl-cysteine, prevents STZ-induced diabetic nephropathy. Biochem Biophys Res Commun. 2016;473(4):931–8.
49. Snijder PM, Frenay AR, Koning AM, et al. Sodium thiosulfate attenuates angiotensin II-induced hypertension, proteinuria and renal damage. Nitric Oxide. 2014;42:87–98.
50. Cartar RN, Morton NM. Cysteine and hydrogen sulphide in the regulation of metabolism: insights from genetics and pharmacology. J Pathol. 2016;238(2):321–32.
51. Brancaleone V, Roviezzo F, Vellecco V, De Gruttola L, Bucci M, Cirino G. Biosynthesis of H2S is impaired in non-obese diabetic (NOD) mice. Br J Pharmacol. 2008;155(5):673–80.
52. Jain SK, Bull R, Rains JL, Bass PF, Levine SN, Reddy S, McVie R, Bocchini JA. Low levels of hydrogen sulfide in the blood of diabetes patients and streptozotocin-treated rats causes vascular inflammation? Antioxid Redox Signal. 2010;12(11):1333–7.
53. Dutta M, Biswas UK, Chakraborty R, Banerjee P, Raychaudhuri U, Kumar A. Evaluation of plasma H2S levels and H2S synthesis in streptozotocin induced type-2 diabetes-an experimental study based on Swietenia macrophylla seeds. Asian Pac J Trop Biomed. 2014;4(1):S483–7.
54. Ha H, Lee HB. Reactive oxygen species as glucose signaling molecules in mesangial cells cultured under high glucose. Kidney Int Suppl. 2000;77:S19–25.
55. Kashihara N, Haruna Y, Kondeti VK, Kanwar YS. Oxidative stress in diabetic nephropathy. Curr Med Chem. 2010;17(34):4256–69.
56. Dugbartey GJ, Alornyo KK, N'guessan BB, Atule S, Mensah SD, Adjei S. Supplementation of conventional anti-diabetic therapy with alpha-lipoic acid prevents early development and progression of diabetic nephropathy. Biomed Pharmacother. 2022;149:112818.
57. Yuan P, Xue H, Zhou L, Qu L, Li C, Wang Z, et al. Rescue of mesangial cells from high glucose-induced over-proliferation and extracellular matrix secretion by hydrogen sulfide. Nephrol Dial Transplant. 2011;26(7):2119–26.
58. Zhou X, Feng Y, Zhan Z, Chen J. Hydrogen sulfide alleviates diabetic nephropathy in a streptozotocin-induced diabetic rat model. J Biol Chem. 2014;289(42):28827–34.
59. Zidayeh FN. Mediators of diabetic renal disease: the case for tgf-Beta as the major mediator. J Am Soc Nephrol. 2004;15(1):S55–7.
60. Carballal S, Trujillo M, Cuevasanta E, et al. Reactivity of hydrogen sulfide with peroxynitrite and other oxidants of biological interest. Free Radic Biol Med. 2011;50(1):196–205.
61. El-Seweidy MM, Sadik NA, Shaker OG. Role of sulfurous mineral water and sodium hydro-sulfide as potent inhibitors of fibrosis in the heart of diabetic rats. Arch Biochem Biophys. 2011;506(1):48–57.
62. Kimura Y, Kimura H. Hydrogen sulfide protects neurons from oxidative stress. FASEB J. 2004;18(10):1165–7.
63. Szabo C. Hydrogen sulfide and its therapeutic potential. Nat Rev Drug Discov. 2007;6(11):917–35.

64. Calvert JW, Jha S, Gundewar S, et al. Hydrogen sulfide mediates cardioprotection through Nrf2 signaling. Circ Res. 2009;105(4):365–74.
65. Murphy ME, Brayden JE. Nitric oxide hyperpolarizes rabbit mesenteric arteries via ATP-sensitive potassium channels. J Physiol. 1995;486(Pt 1):47–58.
66. Pareira de Avila MA, Giusti-Paiva A, de Oliveira G, Nascimento C. The peripheral antinociceptive effect induced by the heme oxygenase/carbon monoxide pathway is associated with ATP-sensitive K+ channels. Eur J Pharmacol. 2014;726:41–8.
67. Zhao W, Zhang J, Lu Y, Wang R. The vasorelaxant effect of H(2)S as a novel endogenous gaseous K(ATP) channel opener. EMBO J. 2001;20(21):6008–16.
68. Suzuki K, Olah G, Modis K, Coletta C, Kulp G, Gero D, et al. Hydrogen sulfide replacement therapy protects the vascular endothelium in hyperglycemia by preserving mitochondrial function. Proc Natl Acad Sci U S A. 2011;108(33):13829–34.
69. Dugbartey GJ, Alornyo KK, Diaba DE, Adams I. Activation of renal CSE/H$_2$S pathway by alpha-lipoic acid protects against histological and functional changes in the diabetic kidney. Biomed Pharmacother. 2022;153(2):113386.
70. Barbagallo M, Dominguez LJ, Galioto A, Ferlisi A, Malfa L, Busardo A, Paolisso G. Role of magnesium in insulin action, diabetes and cardio-metabolic syndrome X. Mol Asp Med. 2003;24(1–3):39–52.
71. Nakajima T, Hasegawa G, Kamiuchi K, Fukui M, Yamasaki M, Tominaga M, et al. Differential regulation of intracellular redox state by extracellular matrix proteins in glomerular mesangial cells: potential role in diabetic nephropathy. Redox Rep. 2006;11(15):223–30.
72. Hu C, Sun L, Xiao L, Han Y, Fu X, Xiong X, et al. Insights into the mechanisms involved in the expression and regulation of extracellular matrix proteins in diabetic nephropathy. Curr Med Chem. 2015;22(24):2858–70.
73. Zidayeh FN, Hoffman BB, Han DC, Iglesias-De La Cruz MC, Hong SW, Isono M, et al. Long-term prevention of renal insufficiency, excess matrix gene expression, and glomerular mesangial matrix expansion by treatment with monoclonal antitransforming growth factor-beta antibody in db/db diabetic mice. Proc Natl Acad Sci U S A. 2000;97(14):8015–20.
74. Lee EA, Seo JY, Jiang Z, Yu MR, Kwon MK, Ha H, Lee HB. Reactive oxygen species mediate high glucose-induced plasminogen activator inhibitor-1 upregulation in mesangial cells and in diabetic kidney. Kidney Int. 2005;67(5):1762–71.
75. Kundu S, Pushpakumar S, Sen U. MMP-9- and NMDA receptor-mediated mechanism of diabetic renovascular remodeling and kidney dysfunction: hydrogen sulfide is a key modulator. Nitric Oxide. 2015;46:172–85.
76. Shi YX, Chen Y, Zhu YZ, Huang GY, Moore PK, Huang SH, Yao T, Zhu YC. Chronic sodium hydrosulfide treatment decreases medial thickening of intramyocardial coronary arterioles, interstitial fibrosis, and ROS production in spontaneously hypertensive rats. Am J Physiol Heart Circ Physiol. 2007;293(4):H2093–100.
77. Guo K, Lu J, Kou J, Wu M, Zhang L, Yu H, et al. Increased urinary Smad3 is significantly correlated with glomerular hyperfiltration and a reduced glomerular filtration rate and is a new urinary biomarker for diabetic nephropathy. BMC Nephrol. 2015;16:159.
78. Eid AA, Ford BM, Kasinath BS, Gorin Y, Ghosh-Choudhury G, Barnes JL, Abboud HE. AMP-activated protein kinase (AMPK) negatively regulates Nox4-dependent activation of p53 and epithelial cell apoptosis in diabetes. J Biol Chem. 2010;285(48):37503–12.
79. Wei WB, Hu X, Zhuang XD, Liao LZ, Li WD. GYY4137, a novel hydrogen sulfide-releasing molecule, likely protects against high glucose-induced cytotoxicity by activation of the AMPK/mTOR signal pathway in H9c2 cells. Mol Cell Biochem. 2014;389(1–2):249–56.
80. Lee HJ, Feliers D, Mariappan MM, et al. Tadalafil integrates nitric oxide-hydrogen sulfide signaling to inhibit high glucose-induced matrix protein synthesis in podocytes. J Biol Chem. 2015;290(19):12014–26.
81. Sheng J, Shim W, Wei H, Lim SY, Liew R, Lim TS, et al. Hydrogen sulphide suppresses human atrial fibroblast proliferation and transformation to myofibroblasts. J Cell Mol Med. 2013;17(10):1345–54.

82. Cai D, Yuan M, Frantz DF, Melendez PA, Hansen L, Lee J, Shoelson SE. Local and systemic insulin resistance resulting from hepatic activation of IKK-beta and NF-kappaB. Nat Med. 2005;11(2):183–90.

83. Jiang Q, Liu P, Wu X, Liu W, Shen X, Lan T, et al. Berberine attenuates lipopolysaccharide-induced extracellular matrix accumulation and inflammation in rat mesangial cells: involvement of NF-κB signaling pathway. Mol Cell Endocrinol. 2011;331(1):34–40.

84. Huang W, Xu L, Zhou X, Gao C, Yang M, Chen G, et al. High glucose induces activation of NF-κB inflammatory signaling through IκBα sumoylation in rat mesangial cells. Biochem Biophys Res Commun. 2013;438(3):568–74.

85. Xu W, Wu W, Chen J, Guo R, Lin J, Liao X, Feng J. Exogenous hydrogen sulfide protects H9c2 cardiac cells against high glucose-induced injury by inhibiting the activities of the p38 MAPK and ERK1/2 pathways. Int J Mol Med. 2013;32(4):917–25.

86. Xu W, Chen J, Lin J, Liu D, Mo L, Pan W, Feng J, Wu W, Zheng D. Exogenous H2S protects H9c2 cardiac cells against high glucose-induced injury and inflammation by inhibiting the activation of the NF-κB and IL-1β pathways. Int J Mol Med. 2015;35(1):177–86.

87. Baskar R, Sparatore A, Del Soldato P, Moore PK. Effect of S-diclofenac, a novel hydrogen sulfide releasing derivative inhibit rat vascular smooth muscle cell proliferation. Eur J Pharmacol. 2008;594(1–3):1–8.

88. Mustafa AK, Gadalla MM, Snyder SH. Signaling by gasotransmitters. Sci Signal. 2009;2(68):re2.

89. Ruggenenti P, Cravedi P, Remuzzi G. The RAAS in the pathogenesis and treatment of diabetic nephropathy. Nat Rev Nephrol. 2010;6(6):319–30.

90. Park JH, Jang HR, Lee JH, Lee JE, Huh W, Lee KB, et al. Comparison of intrarenal renin-angiotensin system activity in diabetic versus non-diabetic patients with overt proteinuria. Nephrology (Carlton). 2015;20(4):279–85.

91. Brewster UC, Perazella MA. The renin-angiotensin-aldosterone system and the kidney: effects on kidney disease. Am J Med. 2004;116(4):263–72.

92. Kobori H, Nangaku M, Navar LG, Nishiyama A. The intrarenal renin-angiotensin system: from physiology to the pathobiology of hypertension and kidney disease. Pharmacol Rev. 2007;59(3):251–87.

93. Xue H, Yuan P, Ni J, Li C, Shao D, Liu J, et al. H(2)S inhibits hyperglycemia- induced intrarenal renin-angiotensin system activation via attenuation of reactive oxygen species generation. PLoS One. 2013;8(9):e74366.

94. Amiri F, Shaw S, Wang X, Tang J, Waller JL, Eaton DC, Marrero MB. Angiotensin II activation of the JAK/STAT pathway in mesangial cells is altered by high glucose. Kidney Int. 2002;61(5):1605–16.

95. Asbun J, Manso AM, Villareal FJ. Profibrotic influence of high glucose concentration on cardiac fibroblast functions: effects of losartan and vitamin E. Am J Physiol Heart Circ Physiol. 2005;288(1):H227–34.

96. Durvasula RV, Shankland SJ. Activation of a local renin angiotensin system in podocytes by glucose. Am J Physiol Renal Physiol. 2008;294(4):F830–9.

97. Gloy J, Henger A, Fischer KG, Nitschke R, Bleich M, Mundel P, et al. Angiotensin II modulates cellular functions of podocytes. Kidney Int Suppl. 1998;67:S168–70.

98. Chrissobolis S, Banfi B, Sobey CG, Faraci FM. Role of Nox isoforms in angiotensin II-induced oxidative stress and endothelial dysfunction in brain. J Appl Physiol. 1985;113(2):184–91.

99. Garrido AM, Griendling KK. NADPH oxidases and angiotensin II receptor signaling. Mol Cell Endocrinol. 2009;302(2):148–58.

100. Kamiyama M, Urushihara M, Morikawa T, Konishi Y, Imanishi M, Nishiyama A, Kobori H. Oxidative stress/angiotensinogen/renin-angiotensin system axis in patients with diabetic nephropathy. Int J Mol Sci. 2013;14(11):23045–62.

101. Brezniceanu ML, Liu F, Wei CC, Tran S, Sachetelli S, Zhang SL, et al. Catalase overexpression attenuates angiotensinogen expression and apoptosis in diabetic mice. Kidney Int. 2007;71(9):912–23.

102. Brezniceanu ML, Liu F, Wei CC, Chenier I, Godin N, Zhang SL, et al. Attenuation of interstitial fibrosis and tubular apoptosis in db/db transgenic mice overexpressing catalase in renal proximal tubular cells. Diabetes. 2008;57(2):451–9.
103. Stanton RC. Combination use of angiotensin converting enzyme inhibitors and angiotensin receptor blockers in diabetic kidney disease. Curr Diab Rep. 2013;13(4):567–73.
104. Takebayashi K, Matsumoto S, Aso Y, Inukai T. Aldosterone blockade attenuates urinary monocyte chemoattractant protein-1 and oxidative stress in patients with type 2 diabetes complicated by diabetic nephropathy. J Clin Endocrinol Metab. 2006;91(6):2214–7.
105. Dandona P, Dhindsa S, Ghanim H, Chaudhuri A. Angiotensin II and inflammation: the effect of angiotensin-converting enzyme inhibition and angiotensin II receptor blockade. J Hum Hypertens. 2007;21(1):20–7.
106. Lu M, Liu YH, Goh HS, Wang JJ, Yong QC, Wang R, Bian JS. Hydrogen sulfide inhibits plasma renin activity. J Am Soc Nephrol. 2010;21(6):993–1002.
107. Lu M, Ho CY, Liu YH, Tiong CS, Bian JS. Hydrogen sulfide regulates cAMP homeostasis and renin degranulation in As4.1 and primary cultured juxtaglomerular cells. Am J Physiol Cell Physiol. 2012;302(1):C59–66.
108. Huang P, Chen S, Wang Y, et al. Down-regulated CBS/H_2S pathway is involved in high-salt-induced hypertension in Dahl rats. Nitric Oxide. 2015;46:192–203.
109. Huang P, Shen Z, Liu J, et al. Hydrogen sulfide inhibits high-salt diet-induced renal oxidative stress and kidney injury in Dahl rats. Oxid Med Cell Longev. 2016;2016:2807490.
110. Lag Laggner H, Hermann M, Esterbauer H, et al. The novel gaseous vasorelaxant hydrogen sulfide inhibits angiotensin-converting enzyme activity of endothelial cells. J Hypertens. 2007;25(10):2100–4.
111. Bjornstad P, Cherney DZ, Snell-Bergeon JK, Pyle L, Rewers M, Johnson RJ, Maahs DM. Rapid GFR decline is associated with renal hyperfiltration and impaired GFR in adults with type 1 diabetes. Nephrol Dial Transplant. 2015;30(10):1706–11.
112. Karar T, Alniwaider RA, Fattah MA, Al Tamimi W, Alanazi A, Qureshi S. Assessment of microalbuminuria and albumin creatinine ratio in patients with type 2 diabetes mellitus. J Nat Sci Biol Med. 2015;6(1):S89–92.
113. Kaur M, Sachdevas S, Bedi O, Kaur T, Kumar P. Combined effect of hydrogen sulphide donor and losartan in experimental diabetic nephropathy in rats. J Diabetes Metab Disord. 2015;14:63.
114. Ahmad FU, Sattar MA, Rathore HA, Tan YC, Akhtar S, Jin OH, et al. Hydrogen sulfide and tempol treatments improve the blood pressure and renal excretory responses in spontaneously hypertensive rats. Ren Fail. 2014;36(4):598–605.
115. Sneijder PM, Frenay AR, Konning AM, et al. Sodium thiosulfate attenuates angiotensin II-induced hypertension, proteinuria and renal damage. Nitric Oxide. 2014;42:87–98.
116. Oosterhuis NR, Frenay AR, Wesseling S, et al. DL-propargylglycine reduces blood pressure and renal injury but increases kidney weight in angiotensin-II infused rats. Nitric Oxide. 2015;49:56–66.
117. Yang G, Tang G, Zhang L, Wu L, Wang R. The pathogenic role of cystathionine γ- lyase/hydrogen sulfide in streptozotocin-induced diabetes in mice. Am J Pathol. 2011;179(2):869–79.
118. Wu L, Yang W, Jia X, Yang G, Duridanova D, Cao K, Wang R. Pancreatic islet overproduction of H2S and suppressed insulin release in Zucker diabetic rats. Lab Invest. 2009;89(1):59–67.
119. Rich AR. A hitherto undescribed vulnerability of the juxtamedullary glomeruli in lipoid nephrosis. Bull Johns Hopkins Hosp. 1957;100(4):173–86.
120. Wharram BL, Goyal M, Wiggins JE, Sanden SK, Hussain S, Filipiak WE, et al. Podocyte depletion causes glomerulosclerosis: diphtheria toxin-induced podocyte depletion in rats expressing human diphtheria toxin receptor transgene. J Am Soc Nephrol. 2005;16:2941–52.
121. Woroniecki RP, Kopp JB. Genetics of focal segmental glomerulosclerosis. Pediatr Nephrol. 2007;22:638–44.

122. Wiggins JE, Goyal M, Sanden SK, Wharram BL, Shedden KA, Misek DE, et al. Podocyte hypertrophy, "adaptation," and "decompensation" associated with glomerular enlargement and glomerulosclerosis in the aging rat: prevention by calorie restriction. J Am Soc Nephrol. 2005;16:2953–66.

123. Kriz W. Podocyte hypertrophy mismatch and glomerular disease. Nat Rev Nephrol. 2012;8(11):618–9.

124. D'Agati VD, Kaskel FJ, Falk RJ. Focal segmental glomerulosclerosis. N Engl J Med. 2011;365(25):2398–411.

125. Crosson JT. Focal segmental glomerulosclerosis and renal transplantation. Transplant Proc. 2007;39:737–43.

126. Savin VJ, Sharma M. Plasma "factors" in recurrent nephrotic syndrome after kidney transplantation. Am J Kidney Dis. 2009;54:406–9.

127. Hickson LJ, Gera M, Amer H, Iqbal CW, Moore TB, Milliner DS, Cosio FG, Larson TS, Stegall MD, Ishitani MB. Kidney transplantation for primary focal segmental glomerulosclerosis: outcomes and response to therapy for recurrence. Transplantation. 2009;87(8):1232–9.

128. Pardon A, Audard V, Caillard S, Moulin B, Desvaux D, Bentaarit B, Remy P, Sahali D, Roudot-Thoraval F, Lang P. Risk factors and outcome of focal and segmental glomerulosclerosis recurrence in adult renal transplant recipients. Nephrol Dial Transplant. 2006;21(4):1053–9.

129. D'Agati VD, Fogo AB, Bruijn JA, Jennette JC. Pathologic classification of focal segmental glomerulosclerosis: a working proposal. Am J Kidney Dis. 2004;43(2):368–82.

130. Puelles VG, van der Wolde JW, Wanner N, Scheppach MW, Cullen-McEwen LA, Bork T, et al. mTOR-mediated podocyte hypertrophy regulates glomerular integrity in mice and humans. JCI Insight. 2019;4:e99271.

131. Zschiedrich S, Bork T, Liang W, Wanner N, Eulenbruch K, Munder S, et al. Targeting mTOR signaling can prevent the progression of FSGS. J Am Soc Nephrol. 2017;28:2144–57.

132. Sen U, Munjal C, Qipshidze N, Abe O, Gargoum R, Tyagi SC. Hydrogen sulfide regulates homocysteine-mediated glomerulosclerosis. Am J Nephrol. 2010;31(5):442–55.

133. Sen U, Basu P, Abe OA, Givvimani S, Tyagi N, Metreveli N, Shah KS, Passmore JC, Tyagi SC. Hydrogen sulfide ameliorates hyperhomocysteinemia-associated chronic renal failure. Am J Physiol Renal Physiol. 2009;297(2):F410–9.

134. Lee HJ, Feliers D, Barnes JL, Oh S, Choudhury GG, Diaz V, Galvan V, Strong R, Nelson J, Salmon A, Kevil CG, Kasinath BS. Hydrogen sulfide ameliorates aging-associated changes in the kidney. Geroscience. 2021;43(1):457.

135. Zakharov S, Vaneckova M, Seidl Z, et al. Successful use of hydroxocobalamin and sodium thiosulfate in acute cyanide poisoning: a case report with follow-up. Basic Clin Pharmacol Toxicol. 2015;117(3):209–12.

136. Burnie R, Smail S, Javaid MM. Calciphylaxis and sodium thiosulfate: a glimmer of hope in desperate situation. J Ren Care. 2013;39(2):71–6.

137. Nigweker SU, Brunelli SM, Meade D, et al. Sodium thiosulfate therapy for calcific uremic arteriolopathy. Clin J Am Soc Nephrol. 2013;8(7):1162–70.

138. Sparatore A, Perrino E, Tazzari V, et al. Pharmacological profile of a novel H2S-releasing aspirin. Free Radic Biol Med. 2009;46(5):586–92.

139. Frantzias J, Logan JG, Mollat P, Sparatore A, Del Soldato P, Ralston SH, Idris AI. Hydrogen sulphide-releasing diclofenac derivatives inhibit breast cancer-induced osteoclastogenesis in vitro and prevent osteolysis ex vivo. Br J Pharmacol. 2012;165(6):1914–25.

140. Padiya R, Khatua TN, Bagul PK, Kuncha M, Banerjee SK. Garlic improves insulin sensitivity and associated metabolic syndromes in fructose fed rats. Nutr Metab (Lond). 2011;8:53.

141. Ried K, Frank OR, Stocks NP. Aged garlic extract reduces blood pressure in hypertensives: a dose-response trial. Eur J Clin Nutr. 2013;67(1):64–70.

142. Mohammadi A, Oshanghi EA. Effect of garlic on lipid profile and expression of LXR alpha in intestine and liver of hypercholesterolemic mice. J Diabetes Metab Disord. 2014;13(1):20.

143. Andresdottir G, Bakker SJ, Hansen HP, Parving HH, Rossing P. Urinary sulphate excretion and progression of diabetic nephropathy in type 1 diabetes. Diabet Med. 2013;30(5):563–6.
144. van den Born JC, Frenay AR, Bakker SJ, Pasch A, Hillebrands JL, Lambers Heerspink HJ, van Goor H. High urinary sulfate concentration is associated with reduced risk of renal disease progression in type 2 diabetes. Nitric Oxide. 2016;55–56:18–24.
145. Hayden MR, Tyagi SC, Kolb L, Sowers JR, Khanna R. Vascular ossification-calcification in metabolic syndrome, type 2 diabetes mellitus, chronic kidney disease, and calciphylaxis-calcific uremic arteriolopathy: the emerging role of sodium thiosulfate. Cardiovasc Diabetol. 2005;4:4.

Chapter 5
Hydrogen Sulfide for the Treatment of Hypertensive Nephropathy and Calcium-Based Nephrolithiasis

George J. Dugbartey

Hypertensive Nephropathy

Hypertension is a major public health problem worldwide. It represents a problem of special importance in renal function due to the role of the kidney in fluid and electrolyte balance and blood pressure (BP) regulation. Renal dysfunction, characterized by a decline in renal blood flow (RBF) and glomerular filtration rate (GFR), and impaired tubular function are the results of sustained high BP. This disturbs the fluid and electrolyte balance, with increased fluid and sodium (Na^+) retention in the body and causing further elevation of BP [1]. Elevated BP is also associated with abnormal activation of renin-angiotensin-aldosterone system (RAAS) [1, 2]. Sustained hypertension subjects blood vessel walls to strong pressure, causing

---

This chapter is an expanded version by the same author in the publication titled H₂S as a possible therapeutic alternative for the treatment of hypertensive kidney injury. Nitric Oxide. 2017;64:52–60.

G. J. Dugbartey (✉)
Department of Pharmacology and Toxicology, School of Pharmacy, College of Health Sciences, University of Ghana, Accra, Ghana

Department of Physiology and Pharmacology, Accra College of Medicine, Accra, Ghana

Division of Urology, Department of Surgery, London Health Sciences Center, Western University, London, ON, Canada

Multi-Organ Transplant Program, London Health Sciences Center, Western University, London, ON, Canada

Matthew Mailing Center for Translational Transplant Studies, London Health Sciences Center, Western University, London, ON, Canada
e-mail: gdugbart@uwo.ca

G. J. Dugbartey, A. Sener, *Hydrogen Sulfide in Kidney Diseases*,
https://doi.org/10.1007/978-3-031-44041-0_5

damage to the blood vessels and eventually leading to the development of vascular diseases such as atherosclerosis [3]. Atherosclerosis causes renal artery stenosis, leading to renovascular hypertension and culminating in kidney disease or acceleration of existing kidney injury [3, 4]. According to the US renal data system, hypertension is the second leading cause of end-stage renal disease after diabetes, as it enhances susceptibility to accelerated nephropathy in patients with preexisting renal disease [5]. Despite this disturbing problem, the exact mechanism underlying the pathogenesis of hypertension and its associated nephropathy is not fully understood. Also, the achievement of BP control and preservation of renal function continue to be a global public health issue, as BP remains uncontrolled in a relevant percentage of hypertensive patients. This points to progression of cardiovascular and cardiorenal diseases facilitated by inappropriate therapeutic response to existing antihypertensive drugs. Hence, there is the need to explore novel avenues to expand therapeutic options and increase treatment efficacy.

Hydrogen sulfide (H_2S), the third identified member of a family of gaseous signaling molecules after nitric oxide (NO) and carbon monoxide (CO), has been established to exert multiple therapeutic effects in various experimental disease models including hypertensive nephropathy [6–10]. In this regard, H_2S has been reported to cause vascular smooth muscle relaxation, increase RBF and GFR, and decrease BP in spontaneously hypertensive rats (SHRs) [11, 12]. Therefore, H_2S could be considered a novel therapeutic agent for hypertensive patients as well as those with hypertensive-associated nephropathy. This chapter focuses on current preclinical findings on the effects and mechanisms of H_2S in various models of hypertensive nephropathy. First, renal H_2S production and exogenous sources of H_2S are presented, followed by vascular and antihypertensive effects of H_2S. Next, recent findings on the renal effect of H_2S in hypertension are discussed. Finally, the chapter addresses future direction with the use of H_2S for the treatment of hypertensive patients to reduce cardiovascular and cardiorenal mortalities. A section of the chapter also discusses recent developments about clinical and translational research on calcium-based nephrolithiasis as a risk factor for hypertensive nephropathy, with a further discussion on H_2S as an emerging novel therapy to improve clinical outcome.

Endogenous and Exogenous Sources of H_2S

H_2S Is Constitutively Synthesized in the Kidney

H_2S is a colorless, flammable, water-soluble, and membrane-permeable gas with an obnoxious smell [13]. As illustrated in Fig. 5.1, it is enzymatically synthesized in all mammalian cells through four metabolic pathways that use sulfur-containing amino acids as substrates: (1) desulfhydration of L-cysteine by the cytosolic enzyme cystathionine β-synthase (CBS); (2) desulfhydration of L-cysteine or L-homocysteine by another cytosolic enzyme cystathionine γ-lyase (CSE); (3) transamination of

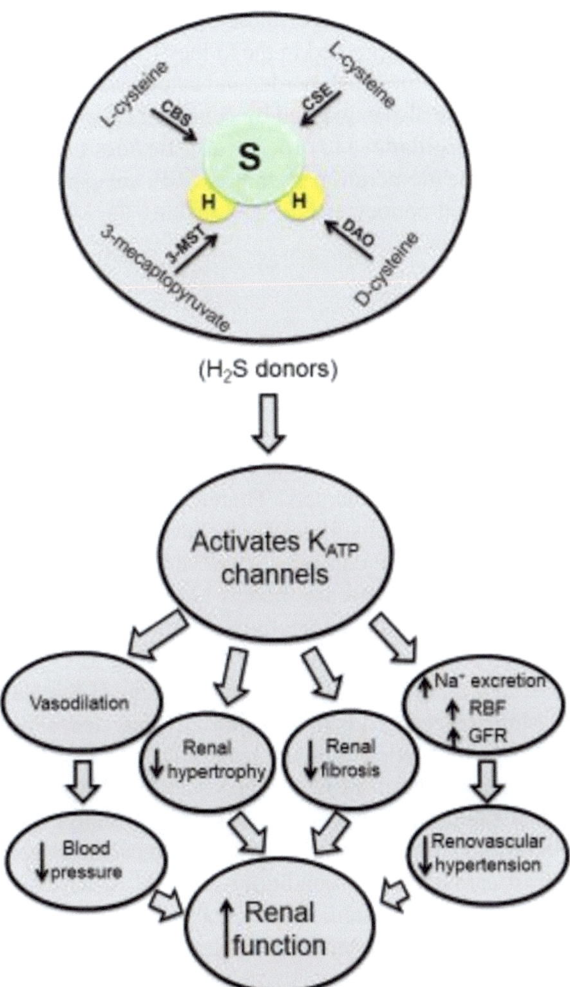

Fig. 5.1 Simplistic view of endogenous H$_2$S production and its effects on hypertension and hypertensive nephropathy. Endogenous H$_2$S is produced enzymatically by cystathionine β-synthase (CBS), cystathionine γ-lyase (CSE), 3-mercaptopyruvate sulfurtransferase (3-MST), and D-amino acid oxidase (DAO). Both endogenous and exogenous H$_2$S stimulate the opening of adenosine triphosphate (ATP)-sensitive potassium (K$_{ATP}$) channels in vascular smooth muscle cells, leading to vasodilation and consequently reduced blood pressure. Activation of K$_{ATP}$ by H$_2$S also attenuates the progression of renal hypertrophy and fibrosis and thus preserves renal function. H$_2$S-induced vasodilation also increases renal sodium (Na$^+$) excretion, renal blood flow (RBF), and glomerular filtration rate (GFR) through K$_{ATP}$ activation and also decreases renin activity, resulting in reduced renovascular hypertension, thereby preserving renal function and integrity

L-cysteine by cysteine aminotransferase to 3-mercaptopyruvate, followed by its desulfhydration to pyruvate catalyzed by the mitochondrial enzyme 3-mercaptopyruvate sulfurtransferase (3-MST); and (4) H$_2$S production from D-cysteine by the peroxisomal enzyme D-amino acid oxidase (DAO) [12, 14–17].

Interestingly, although the expression of these H_2S-synthesizing enzymes is tissue specific, they are abundantly expressed in the kidney [16, 18, 19]. Specifically, they are abundantly expressed in the brush border and cytoplasm of epithelial cells of the proximal tubules. They are also expressed by epithelial cells of the distal tubules as well as the peritubular capillaries [12, 16, 20–23]. Besides the renal tubules, H_2S-producing enzymes in the glomeruli, particularly CSE, are expressed by endothelial cells, mesangial cells, and podocytes [22, 23], making the kidney a rich source of endogenous H_2S production.

H_2S Donor Compounds Augment Endogenous H_2S Level

In addition to its endogenous production, exogenous gaseous H_2S has been used in diverse animal experiments. However, the classic form of inhalation is seriously hampered by toxic effects to bystanders. Therefore, sulfide salts such as sodium hydrosulfide (NaHS) and sodium sulfide (Na_2S) have been developed and function as exogenous H_2S donors. These compounds are widely used as fast-releasing H_2S donors in various experimental disease models [24, 25]. Unfortunately, they offer short-lasting H_2S release and do not sometimes reach their target sites, particularly the mitochondria. Hence, slow-releasing H_2S donors such as GYY4137 have been synthesized and offer a more sustained and longer lasting H_2S release than the sulfide salts [26]. More recently, the mitochondrially targeted slow-releasing H_2S donor, AP39, has been developed and augments mitochondrial H_2S production by 3-MST [27–29]. Further, natural sources of H_2S such as garlic-derived polysulfide, diallyl thiosulfinate (allicin), diallyl trisulfide (DATS), diallyl disulfide (DADS), and diallyl sulfide (DAS) have been suggested and are currently being investigated for the treatment of cardiovascular conditions [30, 31]. Other exogenous sources include SG1002, S-propargyl cysteine (SPRC, also known as ZYZ-802), sodium thiosulfate, and sulfurous mineral water [32–35].

Effect of H_2S on the Cardiovascular System

H_2S Activates K_{ATP} Channels in Vascular Smooth Muscle Cells

Having gained notoriety for several centuries for its toxic effects and high mortality at high concentration, H_2S has overcome its bad reputation and is now recognized among researchers for the past two decades as a gas with important biological benefits and therapeutic potentials, especially in the cardiovascular system and the central nervous system. In the cardiovascular system, it is reported that CSE is the predominant source of H_2S and is expressed in vascular smooth muscle cells (VSMCs) [13, 36]. H_2S has been found to stimulate the opening of adenosine triphosphate (ATP)-sensitive potassium (K_{ATP}) channels by inhibiting phosphorylation of the transcription factors forkhead box O (FOXO1 and FOXO3a) and stimulating their binding activity in VSMCs, resulting in membrane hyperpolarization and reduced voltage-dependent Ca^{2+} influx [30, 37]. This finding was confirmed using a whole-cell and single-channel patch-clamping technique in which the researchers observed activation of K_{ATP} channels and cell membrane hyperpolarization in rat aorta and mesenteric artery smooth muscle cells following exogenous H_2S treatment [38–40]. Also, pharmacological inhibition of endogenous H_2S production with propargylglycine (PAG) decreased whole-cell K_{ATP} currents [36] suggesting that H_2S mediates the activation of K_{ATP} channels. Thus, H_2S stimulates the opening of K_{ATP} channels in VSMCs.

H_2S Induces Vasodilation Following Activation of K_{ATP} Channels

As illustrated in Fig. 5.1, the activation of K_{ATP} channels by H_2S leads to vasodilation [36]. Recently, Chitnis et al. [41] also reported that the treatment of isolated posterior ciliary arteries with GYY4137 induces vasodilation of phenylephrine-induced vasoconstriction. This was supported by the same study showing that administration of the K_{ATP} channel inhibitor, glibenclamide, attenuates the vasodilatory effect of H_2S, suggesting that vasodilation of smooth muscles by H_2S is partly mediated by K_{ATP} channels. This has been suggested to be the primary mechanism by which H_2S reduces hypertension (Fig. 5.1). H_2S is also generated by CSE in perivascular adipose tissues, where it acts as an adipocyte-derived relaxing factor and modulates vascular tone [42]. Apart from CSE, Shibuya et al. [43] recently found that vascular endothelial cells also express 3-MST and produce H_2S, which acts as an endothelium-derived relaxing factor and endothelium-derived hyperpolarizing factor. Intraperitoneal (i.p.) administration of H_2S via the sulfide salt, NaHS, has also been found to upregulate free vascular endothelial growth factor (VEGF) [44]. Further, Zhao et al. [36] demonstrated that endogenous H_2S increases vasodilatory effect of the NO donor, sodium nitroprusside, and enhances NO bioavailability and action in the vasculature, suggesting that enhanced interactions within the gasotransmitter system may reduce BP in hypertensive condition. In summary, activation of K_{ATP} channels by H_2S leads to vasodilation, which implies therapeutic potential in cardiovascular diseases.

Blood Pressure-Lowering Effect of H_2S

Several studies have demonstrated in different hypertensive models that H_2S possesses BP-lowering property. In an SHR model, which mimics essential hypertension in human subjects, i.p. administration of NaHS for 5 weeks in 4-week-old rats ameliorated the increase in BP [45]. NaHS treatment at a lower dose through the same route of administration for 3 consecutive months also reduced systolic and diastolic BP as well as mean arterial pressure in 4-week-old rats [46], suggesting that H_2S at a lower concentration can reduce BP during prolonged treatment. However, it is unknown whether H_2S was reduced prior to the onset of hypertension in this model. Huang et al. [6, 7] also reported BP-lowering effect of H_2S following i.p. injection of NaHS in high-salt-induced hypertensive Dahl rats at 5 weeks old. The same effect was observed in a Dahl rat model of sFlt-induced hypertension [44] and hypertension induced by NO synthase inhibitor [47]. Further, i.p. administration of NaHS and thiosulfate (a major oxidation product of H_2S) in the form of sodium thiosulfate lowered BP and prevented the development of hypertension in a rat model of angiotensin II (Ang II)-induced hypertension [8].

Whereas these findings are exciting and promising, a major drawback in the use of NaHS and other inorganic sulfide salts is their inability to reach stable concentrations in vitro and in vivo, and therefore they could jeopardize safe treatment administration [24, 25, 48]. Therefore, to increase the effectiveness and reliability of H_2S administration in hypertension, Li et al. [26] investigated the effect of the slow-releasing H_2S donor, GYY4137, in an SHR model. In their study, intravenous (i.v.) administration of GYY4137 resulted in a slowly developing fall in BP in both control and SHR groups following 2 days of treatment and persisted after 14 days of treatment. The authors further reported that cessation of GYY4137 treatment caused a slow return of BP to pretreatment values of both groups 14 days after GYY4137 therapy was stopped, with BP of SHR group being well controlled within this time period. In the same study, i.v. administration of NaHS caused immediate and transient and dose-dependent fall in BP. This finding supports the evidence that GYY4137 offers a more sustained H_2S release than the sulfide salt and could therefore be a preferred option in reducing BP in SHR. Other H_2S donors such as organic diallyl polysulfides in garlic have also been reported to exert sustained BP-reducing effect in SHR and 2-kidney, 1-clip (2K1C) models of hypertension [49, 50]. In summary, exogenous H_2S treatment reduces BP increase.

Malfunction of Endogenous H_2S System in Hypertension

Increasing experimental evidence indicates that hypertension is associated with reduced H_2S-producing enzymes as well as endogenous H_2S levels and therefore contributes to the pathogenesis of hypertension. In a high-salt-induced hypertension model in Dahl rats, for example, Huang et al. [7] observed reduced CBS expression and endogenous H_2S content in renal tissue. The authors further reported decreased CSE and 3-MST mRNA expressions [6, 7], suggesting that malfunction of the endogenous H_2S system under high-salt insult contributes to the pathogenesis and development of salt-sensitive hypertension. Weber et al. [51] also reported that low H_2S is associated with CKD-mediated renovascular hypertension and exacerbates hypertension in metabolic and epigenetic hypermethylation diseases. To further elucidate the roles of H_2S in the pathogenesis and development of hypertension, Yang et al. [11] observed endothelial dysfunction and development of hypertension in 10-week-old CSE knockout mice. Additionally, pharmacological inhibition of both CBS and CSE with aminooxyacetic acid (AOAA) and PAG together reduced endogenous H_2S level and increased BP in normotensive rats [45, 52, 53]. Also, plasma and urinary H_2S concentrations as well as vascular CSE expression and activity have been reported to be reduced in SHR model and in hypertension induced by NO synthase inhibitor [9, 54]. Further, d'Emmanuele et al. [55] reported significant reduction in CBS and CSE expressions in mesenteric arterial bed and carotid artery in parallel with reduced plasma H_2S in a rat model of dexamethasone-induced hypertension.

The role of endogenous H_2S in hypertension has also been reported in humans with essential hypertension. Chen et al. [56] observed marked decrease in plasma H_2S in 25 children with essential hypertension in comparison with 66 normotensive control subjects. In addition, plasma H_2S concentration was found to be significantly lower in patients suffering from grade II and grade III hypertension compared to normotensive subjects [57]. Further, plasma levels of H_2S were markedly reduced in women with preeclampsia (a hypertensive syndrome in 4–7% of pregnant women characterized by proteinuria) compared to normal pregnant women [58]. In association with this observation, human placental CSE mRNA expression decreased under preeclamptic condition [58]. Moreover, inhibition of CSE activity (with PAG) ex vivo in human placental explants strongly decreased placental growth factors and blocked the invasion of trophoblasts [58]. In a mouse model of preeclampsia, inhibition of CSE decreased plasma H_2S level, leading to induction of maternal hypertension and placental abnormalities in 10-week-old pregnant mice [58]. Interestingly, these effects were ameliorated following i.p. injection of GYY4137 [58], suggesting that endogenous H_2S could lower BP in preeclamptic women and promote healthy fetal growth and that malfunction of the CSE/H_2S system may contribute to the pathogenesis of preeclampsia and fetal developmental abnormalities. However, it is not known in all these studies whether the reduced expression of H_2S-producing enzymes and endogenous H_2S level occur before or after the rise in BP during the pathogenesis of hypertension. Although this requires further investigation, the findings, so far, imply that reduction in the expression of H_2S-producing enzymes and endogenous H_2S contributes to the development and progression of hypertension.

Contrary to these exciting and encouraging findings, Oosterhuis et al. [59] recently reported that inhibition of CSE with PAG reduced BP in a rat model of Ang II-induced hypertension. Some studies also suggested that H_2S can exert vasoconstriction effect [13, 60]. This discrepancy may be due to the dose of PAG administered as well as concentration of H_2S and its interaction with endothelial NO synthase as posited by Ali et al. [61]. Moreover, H_2S measurement in some of these studies may be questionable partly due to lack of sensitive technique and partly due to its volatile nature. Also, contrary to the observation of Wang et al. [58] and

Holwerda et al. [62] reported that placental CSE mRNA expression did not change in severe preeclampsia although placental CBS mRNA expression decreased significantly. This contradictory finding may be due to differences in the severity of preeclampsia and possibly lack of significant results due to small sample size. Together, these refuting observations warrant rigorous and thorough investigations. In conclusion, H_2S plays important roles in the regulation of BP, and its deficiency contributes to the pathogenesis and development of hypertension.

Effect of H_2S in Hypertensive Nephropathy

H_2S Enhances Renal Tubular Function in Salt-Induced Hypertensive Nephropathy

Hypertension is known to have a direct negative impact on renal Na^+ handling, as the renal tubules play a major role in the long-term regulation of BP [1]. Recent reports indicate that H_2S improves renal Na^+ handling under hypertensive condition (Fig. 5.1). In an in vitro study of salt-sensitive hypertension as a classical model of cardiac remodeling, renal hypertrophy, and injury, for example, treatment with NaHS prevented H_2O_2-induced activation of epithelial sodium channels (ENac) in A6 distal nephron cells and thus prevented Na^+ reabsorption [63]. As the Na^+ pump (Na^+/K^+-ATPase) is the principal driving force for active Na^+ reabsorption along the nephron, H_2S treatment has been found to inhibit Na^+/K^+-ATPase activity in renal tubular epithelial cells, thereby increasing Na^+ excretion and preserving renal tubular function in chronic salt-loaded rats [64]. This finding is consistent with that of Xia et al. [12], who reported that H_2S does not only inhibit Na^+/K^+-ATPase activity but also inhibits the activity of Na^+/K^+-$2Cl^-$ cotransporter, another major renal sodium transporter, and increases urinary sodium excretion. Although these effects of H_2S may suggest reduction in BP, as stimulation of Na^+/K^+-ATPase mediates development and progression of hypertension, it is however not known if these effects were due to vasodilation and increases in GFR by H_2S. In conclusion, H_2S preserves renal tubular function by inhibiting ENac and Na^+/K^+-ATPase activities and increasing Na^+ excretion in salt-induced hypertension.

H_2S Increases RBF and GFR in Hypertensive Nephropathy

The renal effect of H_2S is also observed in other models of hypertension in which H_2S treatment improved RBF. Ahmad et al. [9] recently reported reduced RBF in 4-week-old SHR compared to control rats. In the same study, treatment with NaHS did not only lower BP but also improved RBF and renal excretory function. In addition, combined NaHS and the antioxidant, tempol, caused a larger effect compared to each agent alone. Such BP-lowering effect and improvement of RBF could partially be explained by the ability of H_2S to activate K_{ATP} channels and cause vasodilation (Fig. 5.1), as has been demonstrated in several studies [12, 36]. In a study to investigate renoprotective properties of sulfide-containing compounds, Sneijder et al. [10] showed that i.p. administration of NaHS and thiosulfate restores levels of H_2S-producing enzymes, decreases hypertension and proteinuria, and thus preserves renal function in rats under Ang II-induced hypertension. In a subsequent study, the authors further reported that NaHS treatment reduced intrarenal pressure in an ex vivo-isolated perfused kidney. This latter observation supports previous finding in which intrarenal arterial infusion of NaHS increased RBF and GFR and decreased intrarenal pressure in pre- and post-glomerular arterioles [12]. Although GFR is a better predictor of renal function than RBF in experimental and clinical studies, the finding that H_2S increases GFR in other experimental models is promising and should be investigated under hypertensive condition. It should be noted that since all four endogenous H_2S-producing enzymes are abundantly expressed in the kidney [12, 14–16], exogenous H_2S administration may have activated their respective pathways, leading to the restoration of the levels and activities of these enzymes and the observed protection against hypertensive renal injury. Another interesting hypertensive model is sFlt1-induced hypertension in which i.p. injection of NaHS markedly attenuated sFlt1-induced hypertension, proteinuria, and glomerular endotheliosis in rats by stimulating VEGF synthesis and expression in the kidney podocytes [44]. The mechanism underlying the increased VEGF synthesis and expression by H_2S has not been established. However, matrix metalloproteinases may play a role since they are known to modulate intracellular VEGF release. Taken together, H_2S does not only preserve renal function in salt-induced hypertension but also enhances RBF and preserves renal function in other models of hypertension.

H_2S Disrupts the Rate-Limiting Step in RAAS Activation in Renovascular Hypertension

The kidney contains all the components of RAAS. Abnormal activation of RAAS is commonly associated with the development and progression of hypertension, as it contributes partly to Na^+ retention and vasoconstriction of both afferent and efferent arterioles, resulting in reduced RBF [1, 65, 66]. A recent report indicates that H_2S has the ability to block renin release and thus interfere with the initial steps in the activation of RAAS, leading to BP control [51] (Fig. 5.2). In a Dahl rat model of high-salt-induced hypertension, i.p. administration of NaHS inhibited activation of RAAS in renal tissue and lowered BP [7]. In addition, NaHS treatment inhibited renin expression, activity, and release from juxtaglomerular cells of the kidney and also reduced Ang II level, thereby attenuating renovascular hypertension in rats

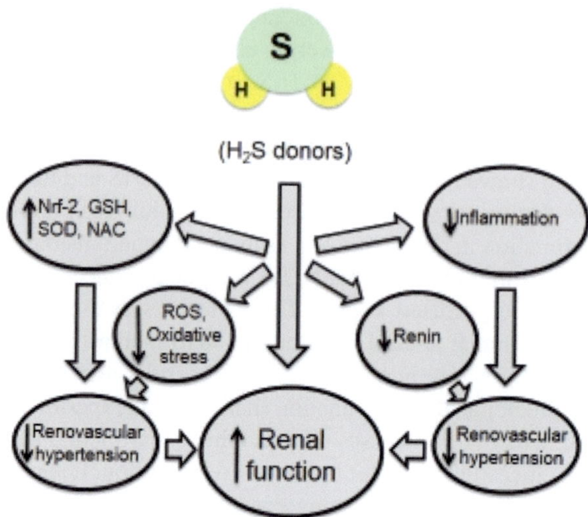

Fig. 5.2 H₂S bolsters endogenous antioxidant defense system and suppresses inflammation and renin activity in hypertensive nephropathy. H₂S acts as a scavenger of reactive oxygen species (ROS) and also activates endogenous antioxidant enzymes including nuclear factor erythroid 2-related factor 2 (Nrf-2), glutathione (GSH), superoxide dismutase (SOD), and N-acetylcysteine (NAC), all of which attenuate oxidative stress-induced renal injury. H₂S also suppresses ROS-induced inflammation in hypertension and renin activity, leading to reduced renovascular hypertension. These effects of H₂S taken together lower blood pressure and hence preserve renal function

[67]. In a follow-up study, the authors confirmed their in vivo observation with an in vitro study in which NaHS treatment of immortalized renin-containing renal tumor cell line (As4.1 cells) and renin-expressing juxtaglomerular cells reduced both synthesis and release of renin via downregulation of intracellular cyclic adenosine monophosphate, a second messenger that regulates renin release [67, 68]. NaHS treatment also reduced plasma Ang II level, strongly downregulated tissue expression of Ang II type 1 receptor in 2K1C rats, and attenuated renovascular hypertension [69]. It is also important to note that H₂S is able to directly inhibit the activity of angiotensin-converting enzyme (ACE, a zinc-containing vasoconstrictor) in human endothelial cells by interfering with zinc in the active center of the enzyme [70], which may also suggest its ability to cause vasodilation apart from K_{ATP} channel activation, and hence attenuates hypertension.

Moreover, as renin and other components of the RAAS are mediators of proteinuria [71], H₂S treatment inhibited RAAS activation in the kidney, and thus ameliorated proteinuria, leading to improvement in renal function and structure in rats under high-salt-induced hypertension [6, 7]. Thus, the specific inhibition of the rate-limiting step in RAAS activation and further inhibition of ACE might prevent the abnormal activation of RAAS and reduce the amount of excreted proteinuria associated with hypertension, thereby attenuating hypertensive renal injury and other complications of hypertension.

H_2S Reduces ROS-Induced Oxidative Stress in Hypertensive Nephropathy

Increased ROS generation causes oxidative stress, and this has been reported to contribute partly to the development and progression of hypertension by increasing renal vasoconstriction, renin release, and Na^+ and volume retention and reducing NO activities [72–75]. Excess production of ROS is associated with increased renal vascular resistance in genetic hypertension in SHR, renovascular hypertension in 2K1C Goldblatt model, and reduced renal mass model of chronic kidney injury as well as rat and mouse models of Ang II-induced hypertension [69, 76–80]. Sakamoto et al. [81] reported that ROS also causes proteinuria, which may partly account for the proteinuria in Ang II-induced hypertensive rats observed by Sneijder et al. [10] and in sFlt1-induced hypertension [44]. Treatment of Ang II-induced hypertensive rats with NaHS and thiosulfate did not only lower BP but also reduced renal ROS production and oxidative stress and attenuated Ang II-induced hypertensive renal injury [8, 10]. In a 2K1C rat model of renovascular hypertension, i.p. administration of NaHS increased tissue level of superoxide dismutase (SOD) and markedly reduced the level of malondialdehyde (MDA, an indicator of ROS production and oxidative stress) by inhibiting the activity of nicotinamide adenine dinucleotide phosphate oxidase (ROS-producing enzyme), thereby contributing to a fall in BP and renal protection [69]. In addition, administration of NaHS (i.p.) to 5-week-old Dahl rats under high-salt-induced hypertension also decreased the activities and contents of ROS indicators and oxidative injury in the kidney, resulting in renal protection [6]. In another study, NaHS and tempol treatments decreased renal ROS production and reduced the damaging effects of oxidative stress, leading to improved BP and renal function [9]. These pieces of evidence suggest H_2S as an ROS scavenger. It is, however, important to point out that in addition to scavenging ROS, H_2S also activates several endogenous antioxidants such as glutathione, catalase, N-acetylcysteine, and nuclear factor erythroid 2-related factor 2 (Nrf-2) [7, 82–87] and thus bolters the endogenous antioxidant defense system against the damaging effects of oxidative stress (Fig. 5.2). To conclude, H_2S has an antioxidant property, which decreases ROS production and ROS-induced renal injury, and reduces the development and progression of hypertension.

H_2S Suppresses Renal Inflammation in Hypertensive Nephropathy

Oxidative stress in the kidney also plays a role in the pathogenesis of renal inflammation in hypertension. Infusion of sodium resulted in increased BP, oxidative stress, and levels of early inflammatory markers such as transcription factor, nuclear factor kappa-B (NF-κB), TGF-β1, chemokine ligand 5 (RANTES), and Ang II in rat proximal tubules [88]. Additionally, increased ROS production caused accumulation of macrophages and other inflammatory cells in the kidney in a rat model of Ang II-induced hypertension [10, 89]. Sen and Packer [90] explained that activation of NF-κB by ROS promotes the expression of genes including those encoding adhesion molecules and thus enhances influx of inflammatory cells in tissues. In keeping with this interaction between ROS and inflammation, attempts to reduce ROS production should also decrease inflammation. In line with this, H_2S significantly decreased ROS production and influx of inflammatory cells in the kidneys of Ang II-induced hypertensive rats [10]. In an SHR model, Zhao et al. [52] reported that H_2S inhibited the activation of mitogen-activated protein kinase signaling pathway (phosphorylated ERK1/2), leading to attenuation of Ang II-induced inflammation in 4-week-old rats. Although the authors did not report on the role of ROS production, it is possible that H_2S attenuated ROS production, thereby leading to reduced inflammation in this model.

The anti-inflammatory effect of H_2S has also been reported in other studies. As NF-κB is a key mediator and early marker of inflammation, H_2S treatment blocked its activation, thereby inhibiting inflammation in a rat model of gentamicin-induced AKI [87]. This implies inhibition of several downstream pro-inflammatory pathways including inhibition of the expression of leukocyte adhesion molecules [90]. In this regard, H_2S does not only block NF-κB activation but also prevents the "rolling" and subsequent adhesion of leukocytes to the endothelium by inhibiting the expression of leukocyte adhesion molecules [91], a property that also prevents the development of atherosclerosis. The authors further observed that the inhibition of leukocyte adhesion molecules was likely through the activation of K_{ATP} channels by H_2S, as K_{ATP} channel inhibitor (glibenclamide) reversed the leukocyte inhibitory effect of H_2S and increased leukocyte adherence [91]. Taken together, besides being an ROS scavenger, H_2S also suppresses the induction of inflammation in hypertension, thereby attenuating hypertensive renal nephropathy.

H_2S Attenuates the Progression of Fibrosis in Hypertensive Nephropathy

The development and progression of hypertension are associated with multiple factors including disequilibrium in the synthesis and degradation of collagen. This results in excessive collagen accumulation within tissues and increase in collagen volume fraction, leading to the development of fibrosis [45, 52, 92, 93] and thereby contributing to complications of hypertension. Reports indicate that renin drives the development of renal fibrosis via stimulation of transforming growth factor beta-1 (TGF-β1) [94, 95].

Recent studies have identified H_2S as an anti-fibrotic agent in hypertension (Fig. 5.1). Guo et al. [96] reported that H_2S inhibits the expression and activity of TGF-β1 and its receptors in the renal tubular epithelial cells via both ERK-dependent and Wnt/catenin-dependent pathways and thus prevents the development of renal fibrosis. In addition, treatment of high-salt-induced hypertensive Dahl rats with NaHS (i.p.) reversed renal collagen remodeling by preventing excessive collagen deposition and accumulation in kidney tissues and decreasing concentration of renal collagen, thereby protecting the kidney from further injury [6, 7]. Matrix metalloproteinase (MMP) and tissue inhibitor of MMP (TIMP) are extracellular matrix (ECM) proteins whose members participate in tissue remodeling and also perform other functions. In a mouse model of Ang II-induced hypertension and renovascular remodeling, Pushpakumar et al. [97] observed increased expression and activity of MMP-9 in TIMP-2 knockout mice compared to wild-type mice. This was associated with marked reduction in RBF, increased peri-glomerular and vascular collagen deposition, and decreased elastin content, suggesting increased wall-to-lumen ratio. The expressions and activities of MMP-9, -2, and -13 were also increased in a model of Dahl salt-sensitive hypertensive nephropathy, while the levels of TIMPs were similar to control rats [98]. This was reversed following administration of the MMP inhibitor, GM6001, leading to reduced collagen deposition and increased elastin in intrarenal vessels, which indicates reduced renal fibrosis. Although the effect of H_2S on MMPs and TIMPs has not been studied extensively in hypertensive kidney injury, there are reports indicating that abundance of MMP-9 is associated with reduced renal CBS and CSE expressions and endogenous H_2S level, ECM deposition, and endothelial dysfunction as well as pathological renal remodeling in a rat model of diabetic nephropathy [99, 100]. In this regard, administration of H_2S restored renal CBS and CSE levels as well as endogenous H_2S production and reversed MMP-9-induced pathological renal remodeling [100]. The anti-fibrotic effect of H_2S is also observed in hypertensive cardiomyopathy, in which NaHS treatment reduced structural remodeling in the aorta and collagen accumulation in the myocardium during the onset and progression of hypertension in an SHR model [45, 52]. Also, NaHS treatment strongly attenuated left ventricular remodeling and cardiac fibrosis in SHR [46]. Further, Huang et al. [7] observed aortic structural remodeling in high-salt-induced hypertension, which was reversed following NaHS administration. As fibrosis is commonly found in association with cardiac hypertrophy and heart failure, Sneijder et al. [8] reported marked reduction in the extent and severity of cardiac fibrosis and cardiac hypertrophy following NaHS and thiosulfate treatments, thus protecting the heart against Ang II-induced hypertension. Interestingly, NaHS administration inhibited myocardial collagen but had no effect on myocardial MMP-13 and TIMP-1 expressions in SHRs [101].

Currently, it is not clear if the anti-fibrotic effect of H_2S is a direct effect or via the reduction of BP. However, there are studies suggesting that the attenuation of fibrosis and hypertrophy by H_2S is partly due to its ability to stimulate the opening of K_{ATP} channels as already discussed [102, 103]. In addition, the anti-fibrotic effect of H_2S in hypertension may be partly due to its ability to inhibit the activities of hypertensive stimuli such as Ang II, which is also a potent pro-fibrotic factor [103], and also the ability of H_2S to interfere with pro-fibrotic pathways as observed in other disease models [96, 104]. Thus, H_2S treatment attenuates the progression of renal fibrosis and other complications of hypertension.

Cross Talk Between H$_2$S and Other Gasotransmitters in Hypertensive Nephropathy

It is an established fact that hypertensive nephropathy is associated with decreased levels of members of the gasotransmitter family such as NO and H$_2$S and their synthesizing enzymes in the kidney [10, 105–109]. Interestingly, whereas mice with deletion of endothelial nitric oxide synthase (eNOS, NO-producing enzyme) and CSE were hypertensive, mice with deletion of heme oxygenase-1 (HO-1, CO-producing enzyme) did not develop hypertension but increased their sensitivity to hypertensive stimuli and to nephrotoxins (e.g., cisplatin) and increased renal injury [110–114]. It is important to note that these gasotransmitters interact with one another and exhibit a mutual adaptation between them when the level of one of these gases is altered [115–117]. In Ang II-induced hypertensive rats, for example, pharmacological inhibition of H$_2$S increased BP but upregulated renal HO-1 expression, leading to increased CO production and renal protection [118]. Also, inhibition of HO-1 enhanced H$_2$S production and NO metabolites in renal tissue. In the same study, the authors further observed that depletion of NO increased BP followed by renal injury and loss of renal function in rats after 4 weeks of NO depletion but had no effect on the other gases [119]. However, Wesseling et al. [120] observed that chronic (21 days) inhibition of NO did not only cause hypertension and renal injury but also resulted in decreased CSE and increased HO-1 levels, suggesting that the effect of NO depletion on the other gases is concentration dependent and that these gases compensate for one another when one or more is depleted. Zhao et al. [36] also showed that increased production of endogenous H$_2$S increases vasodilatory effect of sodium nitroprusside (NO donor) and enhances bioavailability and action of NO in the vasculature, which suggests enhanced interaction within the gasotransmitter family and reduction of BP under hypertensive condition. In conclusion, the three gasotransmitters interact with and compensate for one another, and depletion of one or more leads to development of hypertension and nephropathy.

Calcium-Based Nephrolithiasis

Nephrolithiasis, also known as renal calculi or kidney stones, is characterized by accumulation of freely mobile insoluble mass of tiny mineral crystals or salts in the renal collecting system, which are usually made up of calcium salts, uric acid, and cysteine [121]. These insoluble crystals, referred to as stones, obstruct proper flow of urine. Nephrolithiasis is a global issue, ranking third (15%) among urological diseases in terms of prevalence, and places a significant economic burden on the public healthcare system along with increasing morbidity [122–124]. It affects all ages, races, and genders; is associated with systemic diseases including hypertension; and increases the risk of adverse health outcomes such as hypertensive nephropathy. Clinically, nephrolithiasis presents as acute abdominal or flank pain with nausea and emesis. Hematuria is seen in 90% of cases, but its absence does not preclude the occurrence of nephrolithiasis [122–124]. Although the underlying cause of nephrolithiasis determines its rate of recurrence, a recent study reported a 31% average recurrence rate within 10 years after its onset, and it contributes to severe complications [125].

About 85% of cases of nephrolithiasis are composed of calcium, which bind to either oxalate or phosphate to form crystals (stones) [126]. Hypercalciuria is the greatest risk factor for the development of nephrolithiasis of calcium origin, which is idiopathic in most cases [127]. Idiopathic hypercalciuria is commonly defined as urinary excretion of calcium higher than 250 mg/day in women and 300 mg/day in men. It is an important genetic factor in the formation of nephrolithiasis but is strongly influenced by endogenous and environmental factors such as diet, decreased fluid intake, or relative dehydration. Intestinal hyperabsorption of calcium, increased bone resorption, and renal calcium leak contribute significantly to idiopathic hyper-calciuria [128] (Fig. 5.3). Calcium oxalate (CaOx) nephrolithiasis is the most common type of calcium-based nephrolithiasis encountered in clinical practice. Oxalate is derived from dietary sources in addition to its endogenous production from hepatic oxidation of glyoxylic acid (GA) by glycolic acid oxidase (GAO) and

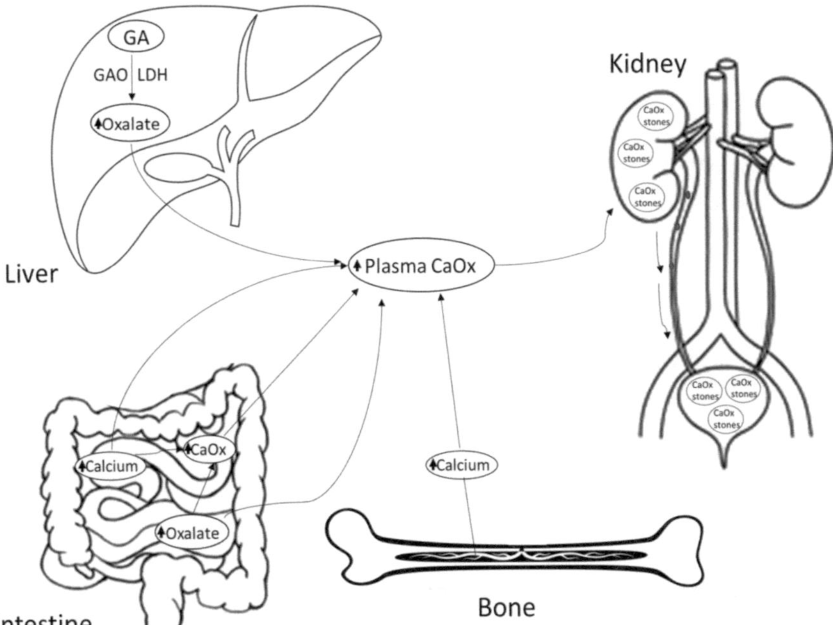

Fig. 5.3 Idiopathic hypercalciuria and hyperoxaluria in calcium oxalate (CaOx) nephrolithiasis. Intestinal hyperabsorption of calcium, increased bone resorption, and renal calcium leak contribute significantly to idiopathic hypercalciuria, while hepatic overproduction of oxalate from glyoxylic acid (GA) by glycolic acid oxidase (GAO) and lactate dehydrogenase (LDH) as well as enteric hyperoxaluria and altered renal tubular transport of oxalate increase plasma and urinary oxalate levels and thus increase the risk of CaOx lithogenesis

lactate dehydrogenase (LDH). Under normal physiological conditions, about 5–10% dietary oxalate is absorbed by the intestine, while majority of urine oxalate has hepatic origin [129, 130]. Like idiopathic hypercalciuria, hyperoxaluria is also a heritable trait, resulting from genetic causes of hepatic overproduction (primary hyperoxaluria), intestinal hyperabsorption of oxalate (enteric hyperoxaluria), and altered renal tubular transport (oxalate leak), all of which increase plasma and urinary oxalate levels, thereby increasing the risk of CaOx nephrolithiasis development and other adverse renal outcomes [129–131] (Fig. 5.3). There are two forms of CaOx, namely CaOx monohydrate (COM) and CaOx dihydrate (COD). While COM is nonpathogenic and associated with low pH, COD is pathogenic under high urinary pH, which together with hypercalciuria is a risk factor for stone growth [132–134].

H₂S Attenuates Calcium-Based Nephrolithiasis

Although most cases of calcium-based nephrolithiasis are managed with hydration therapy along with analgesia, and medications such as potassium citrate to aid stone passage and reduce its formation in the kidney, incidence and recurrence of calcium-based nephrolithiasis have remained high over the past 30 years. This suggests the need to design or identify new pharmacological approaches for an effective treatment. H_2S has recently emerged to possess antilithiatic property, inhibiting calcium-based lithogenesis. In an in vitro study to investigate the antilithiatic property of H_2S in urine obtained from healthy human subjects and recurrent CaOx nephrolithiasis volunteers, treatment with 1.75 mmol/L of NaHS and 3.5 mmol/L of sodium thiosulfate (clinically viable H_2S donor drug) prevented CaOx lithogenesis through pH changes and calcium complex formation [135]. Using a rat model of CaOx nephrolithiasis, Lai et al. [136] observed that administration of diallyl thiosulfinate, diallyl disulfide, and diallyl trisulfide (natural sources of H_2S) increased connexin 43 expression and gap junction function in the kidney, prevented CaOx crystal accumulation and adhesion between CaOx crystals and renal cells, and improved the impairment of proximal tubular cells associated with CaOx nephrolithiasis. These findings indicate that H_2S possesses potent antilithiatic property, with the potential for the treatment of the most common type of nephrolithiasis encountered in clinical practice.

Besides CaOx nephrolithiasis, the antilithiatic property of H_2S has also been reported in nephrocalcinosis, a generalized deposition of calcium in the renal cortex or medulla before the opening into the renal collecting system. In patients with extensive nephrocalcinosis, supplementation of alkalinization therapy with sodium thiosulfate prevented further calcium deposition and preserved renal function with no observable clinical symptoms or adverse effects [137, 138]. In addition, two doses of 5 mM daily administration of sodium thiosulfate prevented recurrent calcium nephrolithiasis in 24 out of 25 patients, while the other patient's result was due to a genetic abnormality [139]. Using genetic hypercalciuric rats to mimic human version of calcium phosphate lithogenesis, eating sodium thiosulfate-supplemented food for 18 weeks significantly lowered urine pH and calcium phosphate supersaturation, leading to reduction in calcium phosphate lithogenesis [140]. Although intracellular levels of H_2S were not measured following administration of the H_2S donors in the above studies, and the molecular mechanisms underlying the antilithiatic effect of H_2S were not studied, it is likely that plasma and renal H_2S levels were reduced in nephrolithiasis and that administration of the H_2S donors increased endogenous H_2S production, suppressed the pathway in the hepatic production of oxalate, and reduced intestinal hyperabsorption of oxalate and calcium and bone resorption, thereby reducing lithogenesis. These hypotheses warrant future investigations. Taken together, the observations from the above experimental and clinical studies show that H_2S exhibits protective effect against calcium-based nephrolithiasis through its antilithiatic property.

Clinical Application and Future Direction in the Use of H_2S Donor Compounds

H_2S has emerged as an important gaseous signaling molecule that diffuses rapidly across cellular membranes, leading to universal biological benefits and therapeutic impression. Currently, H_2S itself is not used in the clinic. However, its major oxidation product, thiosulfate (in the form of sodium thiosulfate), is already being used in the clinic to treat acute cyanide poisoning [141] and calcific uremic arteriolopathy (i.e., calciphylaxis) in patients suffering from end-stage renal disease [142, 143] and has been shown clinically to be effective against calcium-based nephrolithiasis [135, 137–139]. Although the effects of thiosulfate on BP in human subjects have not been studied extensively, the observation that thiosulfate has antihypertensive and renoprotective effects similar to other H_2S-releasing compounds makes it a promising source of H_2S for clinical use. However, one drawback in the therapeutic application of thiosulfate is the fact that it is rapidly degraded in the stomach and, therefore, must be administered intravenously. Considering this challenge, thiosulfate could be incorporated into gastric acid-resistant capsules and released after leaving the stomach. In line with this direction, hybrids of H_2S donors are currently being designed in which sulfide molecules are incorporated into an already existing drug as seen in sulfide-releasing aspirin [144]. Another option is to incorporate these sulfide molecules into a newly synthesized drug. In addition, a recent report indicates that garlic, a natural source of H_2S donors, reduces BP in patients with uncontrolled hypertension [145] and prevents CaOx nephrolithiasis in rats [136]. This makes H_2S a promising antihypertensive and antilithiatic agent for therapeutic use. This also suggests addition of garlic to diets of patients with hypertension and calcium-based nephrolithiasis. However, the amount of garlic needed to constitute sulfide treatment sufficient to reduce BP or hypertensive nephropathy and prevent calcium-based nephrolithiasis is yet to be established.

To facilitate the clinical use of H_2S, a recent human phase I safety and tolerability study revealed increased blood sulfide and thiosulfate concentrations and elevated H_2S concentrations in exhaled breath within the first 5 min of Na_2S intravenous administration [146]. This suggests that measurement of H_2S in exhaled breath offers a great idea on a detectable route of elimination following administration of H_2S donors and may serve a diagnostic purpose together with plasma H_2S in the future. Finally, there are currently two cardiovascular H_2S trials and one renal H_2S trial on clinicaltrials.gov. However, the majority of the cardiovascular and renal studies involving H_2S have been investigated and established in rodent models. Although these rodent models provide a good and strong foundation, their clinical relevance is lacking. Therefore, it will be expedient to move a step further to rigorously confirm the therapeutic effects of H_2S in larger animal models before making a complete transition to the clinic.

Conclusion

Hypertensive nephropathy and calcium-based nephrolithiasis are well-known major global health problems in which the kidney is an important target. Despite their negative impacts on renal function, conventional therapies do not sufficiently achieve the desired therapeutic effects in a significant subset of patients. Although recent studies have reported reduced H_2S level in hypertension, which lowers BP, thereby ensuring renal protection following administration, it is not known whether those patients with resistant hypertension have lower levels of H_2S. Moreover, endogenous H_2S level has not been measured in patients with calcium-based nephrolithiasis. Nevertheless, the therapeutic properties of H_2S make it a possible alternative for the treatment of hypertensive nephropathy and calcium-based nephrolithiasis.

Conflict of Interest None.

References

1. Ramkumar N, Stuart D, Mironova E, Bugay V, Wang S, Abraham N, et al. Renal tubular epithelia cell prorenin receptor regulates blood pressure and sodium transport. Am J Physiol Renal Physiol. 2016;311:F186–94.
2. Gregori M, Tocci G, Giammarioli B, Befani A, Ciavarella GM, Ferrucci A, Paneni F. Abnormal regulation of renin angiotensin aldosterone system is associated with right ventricular dysfunction in hypertension. Can J Cardiol. 2014;30:188–94.
3. Glass CK, Witztum JL. Atherosclerosis: the road ahead. Cell. 2001;104:503–16.
4. Guo H, Kalra PA, Gilbertson DT, Liu J, Chen SC, Collins AJ, Foley RN. Atherosclerotic renovascular disease in older US patients starting dialysis, 1996 to 2001. Circulation. 2007;115:50–8.

5. U.S. Renal Data System. USRD 2009 annual data report: atlas of chronic kidney disease and end-stage renal disease in the United States. Bethesda: National Institutes of Health, National Institute of Diabetes and Digestive and Kidney Diseases; 2009.

6. Huang P, Shen Z, Liu J, Huang Y, Chen S, Yu W, et al. Hydrogen sulfide inhibits high-salt diet-induced renal oxidative stress and kidney injury in Dahl rats. Oxid Med Cell Longev. 2016;2016:2807490.

7. Huang P, Chen S, Wang Y, Liu J, Yao Q, Huang Y, et al. Down-regulated CBS/H_2S pathway is involved in high-salt-induced hypertension in Dahl rats. Nitric Oxide. 2015;46:192–203.

8. Sneijder PM, Frenay AR, de Boer RA, Pasch A, Hillebrands JL, Leuvenink HG, van Goor H. Exogenous administration of thiosulfate, a donor of hydrogen sulfide, attenuates angiotensin II-induced hypertensive heart disease in rats. Br J Pharmacol. 2015;172:1494–504.

9. Ahmad FU, Sattar MA, Rathore HA, Tan YC, Akhtar S, Jin OH, et al. Hydrogen sulfide and tempol treatments improve the blood pressure and renal excretory responses in spontaneously hypertensive rats. Ren Fail. 2014;36:598–605.

10. Sneijder PM, Frenay AR, Konning AM, Bachtler M, Pasch A, Kwakernaak AJ, et al. Sodium thiosulfate attenuates angiotensin II-induced hypertension, proteinuria and renal damage. Nitric Oxide. 2014;42:87–98.

11. Yang G, Wu L, Jiang B, Yang W, Qi J, Cao K, et al. H_2S as a physiological relaxant: hypertension in mice with deletion of cystathionine γ-lyase. Science. 2008;322:587–90.

12. Xia M, Chen L, Muh RW, Li PL, Li N. Production and action of hydrogen sulfide, a novel gaseous bioactive substance in the kidneys. J Pharmacol Exp Ther. 2009;329:1056–62.

13. Polhemus DJ, Lefer DJ. Emergence of hydrogen sulfide as an endogenous gaseous signaling molecule in cardiovascular disease. Circ Res. 2014;114:730–7.

14. Mikami Y, Shinuya N, Kimura Y, Nagahara N, Ogasawara Y, Kimura H. Thioredoxin and dihydrolipoic acid are required for 3-mercaptopyruvate sulfurtransferase to produce hydrogen sulfide. Biochem J. 2011;439:479–85.

15. Modis K, Coletta C, Erdelyi K, Papapetropoulos A, Szabo C. Intramitochondrial hydrogen sulfide production by 3-mercaptopyruvate sulfurtransferase maintains mitochondrial electron transport flow and supports cellular biogenesis. FASEB J. 2013;27:601–11.

16. Shibuya N, Koike S, Tanaka M, Ishigami-Yuasa M, Kimura Y, Ogasawara Y, et al. A novel pathway for the production of hydrogen sulfide from D-cysteine in mammalian cells. Nat Commun. 2013;4:1366.

17. Kimura H. The physiological role of hydrogen sulfide and beyond. Nitric Oxide. 2014;41:4–10.

18. Dugbartey GJ, Talaei F, Houwertjes MC, Goris M, Epema AH, Bouma HR, Henning RH. Dopamine treatment attenuates acute kidney injury in a rat model of deep hypothermia and rewarming—the role of renal H_2S-producing enzymes. Eur J Pharmacol. 2015;769:225–33.

19. Dugbartey GJ, Bouma HR, Strijkstra AM, Boerema AS, Henning HR. Induction of a torpor-like state by 5′-AMP does not depend on H_2S production. PLoS One. 2015;10(8):e0136113.

20. Yamamoto J, Sato W, Kosugi T, Yamamoto T, Kimura T, Taniguchi S, et al. Distribution of hydrogen sulfide (H2S)-producing enzymes and the roles of the H2S donor sodium hydrosulfide in diabetic nephropathy. Clin Exp Nephrol. 2013;17(1):32–40.

21. Bos EM, Leuvinink HG, Snijder PM, et al. Hydrogen sulfide-induced hypometabolism prevents renal ischemia/reperfusion injury. J Am Soc Nephrol. 2009;20(9):1901–5.

22. Lee HJ, Mariappan MM, Feliers D, Cavaglieri RC, Sataranatarajan K, Abboud HE, et al. Hydrogen sulfide inhibits high glucose-induced matrix protein synthesis by activating AMP-activated protein kinase in renal epithelial cells. J Biol Chem. 2012;387(7):4451–61.

23. Bos EM, Wang R, Snijder PM, et al. Cystathionine γ-lyase protects against renal ischemia/reperfusion by modulating oxidative stress. J Am Soc Nephrol. 2013;24(5):759–70.

24. Caliendo G, Cirino G, Santagada V, Wallace JL. Synthesis and biological effects of hydrogen sulfide (H2S): development of H2S-releasing drugs as pharmaceuticals. J Med Chem. 2010;53:6275–86.

25. Kashfi K, Olso KR. Biology and therapeutic potential of hydrogen sulfide and hydrogen sulfide-releasing chimeras. Biochem Pharmacol. 2013;85:689–703.

26. Li L, Whiteman M, Guan YY, Neo KL, Cheng Y, Lee SW, et al. Characterization of a novel, water-soluble hydrogen sulfide-releasing molecule (GYY4137): new insights into the biology of hydrogen sulfide. Circulation. 2008;117:2351–60.

27. Zhao FL, Fang F, Qiao PF, Yan N, Gao D, Yan Y. AP39, a mitochondria-targeted hydrogen sulfide donor, supports cellular bioenergetics and protects against Alzheimer's disease by preserving mitochondrial function in APP/PS1 mice and neurons. Oxid Med Cell Longev. 2016;2016:8360738.

28. Szczesny B, Modis K, Yanagi K, Coletta C, Le Trionnaire S, Perry A, et al. AP39, a novel mitochondria-targeted hydrogen sulfide donor, stimulates cellular bioenergetics, exerts cytoprotective effects and protects against the loss of mitochondrial DNA integrity in oxidatively stressed endothelial cells in vitro. Nitric Oxide. 2014;41:120–30.

29. Ahmad A, Olah G, Szczesny B, Wood ME, Whiteman M, Szabo C. AP39, a mitochondrially-targeted hydrogen sulfide donor, exerts protective effects in renal epithelial cells subjected to oxidative stress in vitro and in acute renal injury in vivo. Shock. 2016;45:88–97.

30. Benavides GA, Squadrito GL, Mills RW, Patel HD, Isbell TS, Patel RB, et al. Hydrogen sulfide mediates the vasoactivity of garlic. Proc Natl Acad Sci U S A. 2007;104:17977–82.

31. Ginter E, Simko V. Garlic (Allium sativum L.) and cardiovascular diseases. Bratisl Lek Listy. 2010;111:452–6.

32. Polhemus DJ, Li Z, Pattillo CB, Gojon G Sr, Gojon G Jr, Giordano T, Krum H. A novel hydrogen sulfide prodrug, SG1002, promotes hydrogen sulfide and nitric oxide bioavailability in heart failure patients. Cardiovasc Ther. 2015;33(4):216–26.

33. Qian X, Li X, Ma F, Luo S, Ge R, Zhu Y. Novel hydrogen sulfide-releasing compound, S-propargyl-cysteine, prevents STZ-induced diabetic nephropathy. Biochem Biophys Res Commun. 2016;473(4):931–8.

34. Snijder PM, Frenay AR, Koning AM, et al. Sodium thiosulfate attenuates angiotensin II-induced hypertension, proteinuria and renal damage. Nitric Oxide. 2014;42:87–98.

35. Safar MM, Abdelsalam RM. H2S donors attenuate diabetic nephropathy in rats: modulation of oxidant status and polyol pathway. Pharmacol Rep. 2015;67(1):17–23.

36. Zhao W, Zhang J, Lu Y, Wang R. The vasorelaxant effect of H_2S as a novel endogenous gaseous K_{ATP} channel opener. EMBO J. 2001;20:6008–16.

37. Sun Y, Huang Y, Zhang R, Chen Q, Chen J, Zong Y, et al. Hydrogen sulfide upregulates KATP channel expression in vascular smooth muscle cells of spontaneously hypertensive rats. J Mol Med. 2015;93:439–55.

38. Tang G, Wu L, Liang W, Wang R. Direct stimulation of K_{ATP} channels by exogenous and endogenous hydrogen sulfide in vascular smooth muscle cells. Mol Pharmacol. 2005;68:1757–64.

39. Liu YH, Yan CD, Bian JS. Hydrogen sulfide: a novel signaling molecule in the vascular system. J Cardiovasc Pharmacol. 2011;58:560–9.

40. Wang R. Signaling pathways for the vascular effects of hydrogen sulfide. Curr Opin Nephrol Hypertens. 2011;20:107–12.

41. Chitnis MK, Njie-Mbye YF, Opare CA, Wood ME, Whiteman M, Ohia SE. Pharmacological actions of the slow release hydrogen sulfide donor GYY4137 on phenylephrine-induced tone in isolated bovine ciliary artery. Exp Eye Res. 2013;116:350–4.

42. Fang L, Zhao J, Chen Y, Ma T, Xu G, Tang C, Liu X, Geng B. Hydrogen sulfide derived from periadventitial adipose tissue is a vasodilator. J Hypertens. 2009;27:2174–85.

43. Shibuya N, Mikami Y, Kimura Y, Nagahara N, Kimura H. Vascular endothelium expresses 3-mercaptopyruvate sulfurtransferase and produces hydrogen sulfide. J Biochem. 2009;146:623–6.

44. Holwerda KM, Burke SD, Faas MM, Zsengeller Z, Stillman IE, Kang PM, et al. Hydrogen sulfide attenuates sFlt1-induced hypertension and renal damage by upregulating vascular endothelial growth factor. J Am Soc Nephrol. 2014;25:717–25.

45. Yan H, Du J, Tang C. The possible role of hydrogen sulfide on the pathogenesis of spontaneous hypertension in rats. Biochem Biophys Res Commun. 2004;313:22–7.

46. Shi YX, Chen Y, Zhu YZ, Huang GY, Moore PK, Huang SH, Yao T, Zhu YC. Chronic sodium hydrosulfide treatment decreases medial thickening of intramyocardial coronary arterioles, interstitial fibrosis, and ROS production in spontaneously hypertensive rats. Am J Physiol Heart Circ Physiol. 2007;293:H2093–100.
47. Zhong G, Chen F, Chen Y, Tang C, Du J. The role of hydrogen sulfide generation in the pathogenesis of hypertension in rats induced by inhibition of nitric oxide synthase. J Hypertens. 2003;21:1879–85.
48. DeLeon ER, Stoy GF, Olson KR. Passive loss of hydrogen sulfide in biological experiments. Anal Biochem. 2011;421:459–88.
49. Elkayam A, Peleg E, Grossman E, Shabtay Z, Sharabi Y. Effects of allicin on cardiovascular risk factors in spontaneously hypertensive rats. Isr Med Assoc J. 2013;15:170–3.
50. Al-Qattan KK, Thomson M, Al-Mutawa'a S, Al-Hajeri D, Drobiova H, Ali M. Nitric oxide mediates the blood pressure-lowering effect of garlic in the two-kidney, one-clip model of hypertension. J Nutr. 2006;136:774S–6S.
51. Weber GJ, Pushpakumar S, Tyagi SC, Sen U. Homocysteine and hydrogen sulfide in epigenetic, metabolic and microbiota related renovascular hypertension. Pharmacol Res. 2016;113(Pt A):300–12.
52. Zhao X, Zhang LK, Zhang CY, Zeng XY, Yan H, Jin HF, Tang CS, Du JB. Regulatory effect of hydrogen sulfide on vascular collagen content in spontaneously hypertensive rats. Hypertens Res. 2008;31:1619–30.
53. Roy A, Khan AH, Islam MT, Prieto MC, Majid DS. Interdependency of cystathionine γ-lyase and cystathionine β-synthase in hydrogen sulfide-induced blood pressure regulation in rats. Am J Hypertens. 2012;25:74–81.
54. Wagner CA. Hydrogen sulfide: a new gaseous signal molecule and blood pressure regulator. J Nephrol. 2009;22:173–6.
55. d'Emmanuele di Villa Bianca R, Mitidieri E, Donnarumma E, Tramontano T, Brancaleone V, Cirino G, Bucci M, Sorrentino R. Hydrogen sulfide is involved in dexamethasone-induced hypertension in rat. Nitric Oxide. 2015;46:80–6.
56. Chen L, Ingrid S, Ding YG, Lui Y, Qi JG, Tang CS, Du JB. Imbalance of endogenous homocysteine and hydrogen sulfide metabolic pathway in essential hypertensive children. Chin Med J. 2007;120:389–93.
57. Sun NL, Xi Y, Yang SN, Ma Z, Tang CS. [Plasma hydrogen sulfide and homocysteine levels in hypertensive patients with different blood pressure levels and complications]. Zhonghua Xin Xue Guan Bing Za Zhi. 2007;35:1145–1148.
58. Wang K, Ahmad S, Cai M, Rennie J, Fujisawa T, Crispi F, et al. Dysregulation of hydrogen sulfide producing enzyme cystathionine γ-lyase contributes to maternal hypertension and placental abnormalities in preeclampsia. Circulation. 2013;127:2514–22.
59. Oosterhuis NR, Frenay AR, Wesseling S, Snijder PM, Slaats GG, Yazdani S, et al. DL-propargylglycine reduces blood pressure and renal injury but increases kidney weight in angiotensin II infused rats. Nitric Oxide. 2015;49:56–66.
60. Koenitzer JR, Isbell TS, Patel HD, Benavides GA, Dickinson DA, Patel RP, et al. Hydrogen sulfide mediates vasoactivity in an O_2-dependent manner. Am J Physiol Heart Circ Physiol. 2007;292:H1953–60.
61. Ali MY, Ping CY, Mok YY, Ling L, Whiteman M, Bhatia M, Moore PK. Regulation of vascular nitric oxide in vitro and in vivo; a new role for endogenous hydrogen sulfide? Br J Pharmacol. 2006;149:625–34.
62. Holwerda KM, Bos EM, Rajakumar A, Ris-Stalpers C, van Pampus MG, Timmer A, et al. Hydrogen sulfide producing enzymes in pregnancy and preeclampsia. Placenta. 2012;33:518–21.
63. Zhang J, Chen S, Liu H, Zhang B, Zhao Y, Ma K, et al. Hydrogen sulfide prevents hydrogen peroxide-induced activation of epithelial sodium channel through a PTEN/PI(3,4,5)P3 dependent pathway. PLoS One. 2013;8:e64304.

64. Ge SN, Zhao MM, Wu DD, Chen Y, Wang Y, Zhu JH, et al. Hydrogen sulfide targets EGFR Cys797/Cys798 residues to induce Na^+/K^+-ATPase endocytosis and inhibition in renal tubular epithelial cells and increase sodium excretion in chronic salt-loaded rats. Antioxid Redox Signal. 2014;21:2061–82.
65. Leong PK, Devillez A, Sandberg MB, et al. Effects of ACE inhibition on proximal tubule sodium transport. Am J Physiol Renal Physiol. 2006;290:F854–63.
66. Welch WJ, Patel K, Modlinger P, Mendonca M, Kawada N, Dennehy K, Aslam S, Wilcox CS. Roles of vasoconstrictor prostaglandins, COX-1 and -2, and AT1, AT2, and TP receptors in a rat model of early 2K,1C hypertension. Am J Physiol Heart Circ Physiol. 2007;293:H2644–9.
67. Lu M, Liu YH, Goh HS, Wang JJ, Yong QC, Wang R, Bian JS. Hydrogen sulfide inhibits plasma renin activity. J Am Soc Nephrol. 2010;21:993–1002.
68. Lu M, Ho CY, Liu YH, Tiong CS, Bian JS. Hydrogen sulfide regulates cAMP homeostasis and renin degranulation in As4.1 and primary cultured juxtaglomerular cells. Am J Physiol. 2012;302:C59–66.
69. Xue H, Zhou S, Xiao L, Guo Q, Liu S, Wu Y. Hydrogen sulfide improves the endothelial dysfunction in renovascular hypertensive rats. Physiol Res. 2015;64(5):663–72.
70. Laggner H, Hermann M, Esterbauer H, Muellner MK, Exner M, Gmeiner BM, Kapiotis S. The novel gaseous vasorelaxant hydrogen sulfide inhibits angiotensin-converting enzyme activity of endothelial cells. J Hypertens. 2007;25:2100–4.
71. Wolf G. Link between angiotensin II and TGF-beta in the kidney. Miner Electrolyte Metab. 1998;24:174–80.
72. Sinha K, Dabla PK. Oxidative stress and antioxidants in hypertension—a current review. Curr Hypertens Rev. 2015;11:132–42.
73. Welch WJ, Ott CE, Guthrie GP Jr, Kotchen TA. Mechanism of increased renin release in the adrenalectomized rat. Adrenal insufficiency and renin. Hypertension. 1983;5:I47–52.
74. Just A, Whitten CL, Arendshorst WJ. Reactive oxygen species participate in acute renal vasoconstrictor responses induced by ETA and ETB receptors. Am J Physiol Renal Physiol. 2008;294:F719–28.
75. Ohsaki Y, O'Connor MT, Ryan RP, Dickinson BC, Chang CJ, et al. Increase of sodium delivery stimulates the mitochondrial respiratory chain H2O2 production in rat medullary thick ascending limb. Am J Physiol Renal Physiol. 2012;302:F95–F102.
76. Kawada N, Imai E, Karber A, Welch WJ, Wilcox CS. A mouse model of angiotensin II slow pressor response: role of oxidative stress. J Am Soc Nephrol. 2002;13:2860–8.
77. Schnackenberg CG, Wilcox CS. Two-week administration of tempol attenuates both hypertension and renal excretion of 8-Iso prostaglandin f2alpha. Hypertension. 1999;33:424–8.
78. Welch WJ, Mendonca M, Aslam S, Wilcox CS. Roles of oxidative stress and ATI receptors in renal hemodynamics and oxygenation in the postclipped 2K,1C kidney. Hypertension. 2003;41:692–6.
79. Welch WJ, Blau J, Xie H, Chabrashvili T, Wilcox CS. Angiotensin II-induced defects in renal oxygenation: role of oxidative stress. Am J Physiol Heart Circ Physiol. 2005;288:H22–8.
80. Wilcox CS. Oxidative stress and nitric oxide deficiency in the kidney: a critical link to hypertension? Am J Physiol Regul Integr Comp Physiol. 2005;289:R913–35.
81. Sakamoto A, Hongo M, Saito K, Nagai R, Ishizaka N. Reduction of renal lipid content and proteinuria by a PPAR-gamma agonist in a rat model of angiotensin II-induced hypertension. Eur J Pharmacol. 2012;682:131–6.
82. Kimura Y, Kimura H. Hydrogen sulfide protects neurons from oxidative stress. FASEB J. 2004;18:1165–77.
83. Szabo C. Hydrogen sulfide and its therapeutic potential. Nat Rev Drug Discov. 2007;6:917–35.
84. Calvert JW, Jha S, Gundewar S, Elrod JW, Ramachandran A, Pattillo CB, Kevil CG, Lefer DJ. Hydrogen sulfide mediates cardioprotection through Nrf2 signaling. Circ Res. 2009;105:365–74.
85. Kimura Y, Goto YI, Kimura H. Hydrogen sulfide increases glutathione production and suppresses oxidative stress in mitochondria. Antioxid Redox Signal. 2010;12:1–13.

86. Shimada S, Fukai M, Wakayama K, Ishikawa T, Kobayahsi N, Kimura T, et al. Hydrogen sulfide augments survival signals in warm ischemia and reperfusion of the mouse liver. Surg Today. 2015;45:892–903.
87. Kalayarasan S, Prabhu PN, Sriram N, Manikandan R, Arumugam M, Sudhandiran G. Diallyl sulfide enhances antioxidants and inhibits inflammation through the activation of Nrf2 against gentamicin-induced nephrotoxicity in Wister rats. Eur J Pharmacol. 2009;606:162–71.
88. Roson MI, Della Penna SL, Cao G, Gorzalczany S, Pandilfo M, Toblli JE, Fernandez BE. Different protective actions of losartan and tempol on the renal inflammatory response to acute sodium overload. J Cell Physiol. 2010;22:41–8.
89. Liu J, Yang F, Yang XP, Jankowski M, Pagano PJ. NAD(P)H oxidase mediates angiotensin II-induced vascular macrophage infiltration and medial hypertrophy. Arterioscler Thromb Vasc Biol. 2003;23:776–82.
90. Sen CK, Packer L. Antioxidant and redox regulation of gene transcription. FASEB J. 1996;10:709–20.
91. Zanardo RC, Brancaleone V, Distrutti E, Fiorucci S, Cirino G, Wallace JL. Hydrogen sulfide is an endogenous modulator of leukocyte-mediated inflammation. FASEB J. 2006;20:2118–20.
92. Varo N, Etayo JC, Zalba G, Beaumont J, Iraburu MJ, Montiel C, et al. Losartan inhibits the post-transcriptional synthesis of collagen type I and reverses left ventricular fibrosis in spontaneously hypertensive rats. J Hypertens. 1999;17:107–14.
93. Berk BC, Fujiwara K, Lehoux S. ECM remodeling in hypertensive heart disease. J Clin Invest. 2007;117:568–75.
94. Huang Y, Wongamorntham S, Kasting J, McQuillan D, Owens RT, Yu L, Noble NA, Border W. Renin increases mesangial cell transforming growth factor-beta1 and matrix proteins through receptor-mediated, angiotensin II-independent mechanisms. Kidney Int. 2006;69:105–13.
95. Rodriguez-Vita J, Sabchez-Lopez E, Esteban V, Ruperez M, Egido J, Ruiz-Ortega M. Angiotensin II activates the smad pathway in vascular smooth muscle cells by a transforming growth factor-beta-independent mechanism. Circulation. 2005;111:2509–17.
96. Guo L, Peng W, Tao J, Lan Z, Hei H, Tian L, Pan W, Wang L, Zhang X. Hydrogen sulfide inhibits transforming growth factor-β1-induced EMT via WNT/catenin pathway. PLoS One. 2016;11:e0147018.
97. Pushpakumar S, Kundu S, Pryor T, et al. Angiotensin-II induced hypertension and renovascular remodeling in TIMP2 knockout mice. J Hypertens. 2013;31(11):2270–81.
98. Pushpakumar S, Kundu S, Metreveli N, Tyagi SC, Sen U. Matrix metalloproteinase inhibition mitigates renovascular remodeling in salt-sensitive hypertension. Physiol Rep. 2013;31(11):2270–81.
99. Kundu S, Pushpakumar SB, Tyagi A, Coley D, Sen U. Hydrogen sulfide deficiency and diabetic renal remodeling: role of matrix metalloproteinase-9. Am J Physiol Endocrinol Metab. 2013;304(12):E1365–78.
100. Kundu S, Pushpakumar S, Sen U. MMP-9- and NMDA receptor-mediated mechanism of diabetic renovascular remodeling and kidney dysfunction: hydrogen sulfide is a key modulator. Nitric Oxide. 2015;46:172–85.
101. Sun L, Jin H, Sun L, et al. Hydrogen sulfide alleviates myocardial collagen remodeling in association with inhibition of TGF-β/Smad signaling pathway in spontaneously hypertensive rats. Mol Med. 2015;20:503–15.
102. Gao S, Long CL, Wang RH, Wang H. K_{ATP} activation prevents progression of cardiac hypertrophy to failure induced by pressure overload via protecting endothelial function. Cardiovasc Res. 2009;83:444–56.
103. Huang J, Wang D, Zheng J, Huang X, Jin H. Hydrogen sulfide attenuates cardiac hypertrophy and fibrosis induced by abdominal aortic coarctation in rats. Mol Med Rep. 2012;5:923–8.
104. Xiao T, Zeng O, Luo J, Wu Z, Li F, Yang J. Effects of hydrogen sulfide on myocardial fibrosis in diabetic rat: changes in matrix metalloproteinases parameters. Biomed Mater Eng. 2015;26 Suppl 1:S2033–9.

105. Baylis C, Vallance P. Nitric oxide and blood pressure: effects of nitric oxide deficiency. Curr Opin Nephrol Hypertens. 1996;5:80–8.
106. Baylis C. Nitric oxide deficiency in chronic kidney disease. Am J Physiol Renal Physiol. 2008;294:F1–9.
107. Zatz R, de Nucci G. Effects of acute nitric oxide inhibition on rat glomerular microcirculation. Am J Physiol. 1991;261(2 Pt 2):F360–3.
108. Baylis C, Mitruka B, Deng A. Chronic blockade of nitric oxide synthesis in the rat produces systemic hypertension and glomerular damage. J Clin Invest. 1992;90:278–81.
109. Verhagen AM, Koomans HA, Joles JA. Predisposition of spontaneously hypertensive rats to develop renal injury during nitric oxide synthase inhibition. Eur J Pharmacol. 2001;411:175–80.
110. Ortiz PA, Garvin JL. Cardiovascular and renal control in NOS-deficient mouse models. Am J Physiol Regul Integr Comp Physiol. 2003;284:R628–38.
111. Yang G, Wu L, Jiang B, et al. H$_2$S as a physiologic vasorelaxant: hypertension in mice with deletion of cystathionine gamma-lyase. Science. 2008;322:587–90.
112. Agarwal A, Nick HS. Renal response to tissue injury: lessons from heme oxygenase-1 gene ablation and expression. J Am Soc Nephrol. 2000;11:965–73.
113. Wiesel P, Patel AP, Carvajal IM, et al. Exacerbation of chronic renovascular hypertension and acute renal failure in heme oxygenase-1-deficient mice. Circ Res. 2001;88:1088–94.
114. Shiraishi F, Curtis LM, Truong L, et al. Heme oxygenase-1 ablation or expression modulates cisplatin-induced renal tubular apoptosis. Am J Physiol Renal Physiol. 2000;278:F726–36.
115. Rodriguez F, Lamon BD, Gong W, Kemp R, Nasjletti A. Nitric oxide synthesis inhibition promotes renal production of carbon monoxide. Hypertension. 2004;43:347–51.
116. Botros FT, Navar LG. Interaction between endogenously produced carbon monoxide and nitric oxide in regulation of renal afferent arterioles. Am J Physiol Heart Circ Physiol. 2006;291:H2772–8.
117. Rong-na L, Xiang-jun Z, Yu-han C, Ling-qiao L, Gang H. Interaction between hydrogen sulfide and nitric oxide on cardiac protection in rats with metabolic syndrome. Zhongguo Yi Xue Ke Xue Yuan Xue Bao. 2011;33:25–32.
118. Oosterhuis NR, Frenay AR, Wesseling S, et al. DL-propargylglycine reduces blood pressure and renal injury but increases kidney weight in angiotensin-II infused rats. Nitric Oxide. 2015;49:56–66.
119. Wesseling S, Fledderus JO, Verhaar MC, Joles JA. Beneficial effects of diminished production of hydrogen sulfide and carbon monoxide on hypertension and renal injury induced by NO withdrawal. Br J Pharmacol. 2015;172(6):1607–19.
120. Wesseling S, Joles JA, van Goor H, et al. Transcriptome-based identification of pro- and anti-oxidative gene expression in kidney cortex of nitric oxide-dependent rats. Physiol Genomics. 2007;28:158–67.
121. Spivacow FR, Del Valle EE, Lores E, Rey PG. Kidney stones: composition, frequency and relation to metabolic diagnosis. Medicina (B Aires). 2016;76(6):343–8.
122. Mugiya S, Ito T, Maruyama S, Hadano S, Nagae H. Endoscopic features of impacted ureteral stones. J Urol. 2004;171(1):89–91.
123. Gottlieb M, Long B, Koyfman A. The evaluation and management of urolithiasis in the ED: a review of the literature. Am J Emerg Med. 2018;36(4):699–706.
124. Pfau A, Knauf F. Update on nephrolithiasis: core curriculum 2016. Am J Kidney Dis. 2016;68(6):973–85.
125. Rule AD, Lieske JC, Li X, Melton LJ 3rd, Krambeck AE, Bergstralh EJ. The ROKS nomogram for predicting a second symptomatic stone episode. J Am Soc Nephrol. 2014;25:2878–86.
126. Knoll T, Schubert AB, Fahlenkamp D, Leusmann DB, Wendt-Nordahl G, Schubert G. Urolithiasis through the ages: data on more than 200,000 urinary stone analyses. J Urol. 2011;185(4):1304–11.
127. Levy FL, Adams-Huet B, Pak CY. Ambulatory evaluation of nephrolithiasis: an update of a 1980 protocol. Am J Med. 1995;98(1):50–9.

128. Pak CY, Kaplan R, Bone H, Townsend J, Waters O. A simple test for the diagnosis of absorptive, resorptive and renal hypercalciurias. N Engl J Med. 1975;292(10):497–500.
129. Holmes RP, Goodman HO, Assimos DG. Contribution of dietary oxalate to urinary oxalate excretion. Kidney Int. 2001;59:270–6.
130. Hesse A, Schneeberger W, Engfeld S, von Unruh GD, Sauerbruch T. Intestinal hyperabsorption of oxalate in calcium oxalate stone formers: application of a new test with [13C2]oxalate. J Am Soc Nephrol. 1999;10:S329–33.
131. Knauf F, Velazquez H, Pfann V, Jiang Z, Aronson PS. Characterization of renal NaCl and oxalate transport in Slc26a6−/− mice. Am J Physiol Renal Physiol. 2019;316:F128–33.
132. Manissorn J, Fong-Ngern K, Peerapen P, Thongboonkerd V. Systematic evaluation for effects of urine pH on calcium oxalate crystallization, crystal-cell adhesion and internalization into renal tubular cells. Sci Rep. 2017;7(1):1798.
133. Maruyama M, Sawada KP, Tanaka Y, Okada A, Momma K, Nakamura M, Mori R, Furukawa Y, Sugiura Y, Tajiri R, Taguchi K, Hamamoto S, Ando R, Tsukamoto K, Takano K, Imanishi M, Yoshimura M, Yasui T, Mori Y. Quantitative analysis of calcium oxalate monohydrate and dihydrate for elucidating the formation mechanism of calcium oxalate kidney stones. PLoS One. 2023;18(3):e0282743.
134. Guerra A, Ticinesi A, Allegri F, Pinelli S, Aloe R, Meschi T. Idiopathic calcium nephrolithiasis with pure calcium oxalate composition: clinical correlates of the calcium oxalate dihydrate/monohydrate (COD/COM) stone ratio. Urolithiasis. 2020;48(3):271–9.
135. Vaitheeswari S, Sriram R, Brindha P, Kurian GA. Studying inhibition of calcium oxalate stone formation: an in vitro approach for screening hydrogen sulfide and its metabolites. Int Braz J Urol. 2015;41(3):503–10.
136. Lai Y, Liang X, Zhong F, Wu W, Zeng T, Huang J, Duan X, Li S, Zeng G, Wu W. Allicin attenuates calcium oxalate crystal deposition in the rat kidney by regulating gap junction function. J Cell Physiol. 2019;234(6):9640–51.
137. Agroyannis B, Tzanatos H, Vlahakos DV, Mallas E. Does long-term administration of sodium thiosulphate inhibit progression to renal failure in nephrocalcinosis? Nephrol Dial Transplant. 2001;16(12):2443–4.
138. Agroyannis BJ, Koutsikos DK, Tzanatos HA, Konstadinidou IK. Sodium thiosulphate in the treatment of renal tubular acidosis I with nephrocalcinosis. Scand J Urol Nephrol. 1994;28(1):107–8.
139. Yatzidis H. Absence or decreased endogenous thiosulfaturia: a cause of recurrent calcium nephrolithiasis. Int Urol Nephrol. 2004;36(4):587–9.
140. Asplin JR, Donahue SE, Lindeman C, Michalenka A, Strutz KL, Bushinsky DA. Thiosulfate reduces calcium phosphate nephrolithiasis. J Am Soc Nephrol. 2009;20(6):1246–53.
141. Zakharov S, Vaneckova M, Seidl Z, Diblik P, Kuthan P, Urban P, Navratil T, Pelclova D. Successful use of hydroxocobalamin and sodium thiosulfate in acute cyanide poisoning: a case report with follow-up. Basic Clin Pharmacol Toxicol. 2015;117:209–12.
142. Burnie R, Smail S, Javaid MM. Calciphylaxis and sodium thiosulfate: a glimmer of hope in desperate situation. J Ren Care. 2013;39:71–6.
143. Nigweker SU, Brunelli SM, Meade D, Wang W, Hymes J, Lacson E Jr. Sodium thiosulfate therapy for calcific uremic arteriolopathy. Clin J Am Soc Nephrol. 2013;8:1162–70.
144. Sparatore A, Perrino E, Tazzari V, Giustarini D, Rossi R, Rossoni G, et al. Pharmacological profile of a novel H$_2$S-releasing aspirin. Free Radic Biol Med. 2009;46:586–92.
145. Ried K, Frank OR, Stocks NP. Aged garlic extract reduces blood pressure in hypertensives: a dose-response trial. Eur J Clin Nutr. 2013;67:64–70.
146. Toombs CF, Insko MA, Wintner EA, Deckwerth TL, Usansky H, Jamil K, et al. Detection of exhaled hydrogen sulphide gas in healthy human volunteers during intravenous administration of sodium sulphide. Br J Clin Pharmacol. 2010;69:626–36.

Chapter 6
Hydrogen Sulfide as a Potential Therapy for COVID-19-Associated Nephropathy

George J. Dugbartey, Karl K. Alornyo, Vincent Boima, Sampson Antwi, and Alp Sener

This chapter is a modified version by the same authors in the publication titled Renal Consequences of the Novel Coronavirus Disease 2019 (COVID-19) and Hydrogen Sulfide as a Potential Therapy. Nitric Oxide. 2022; 120:16–25.

G. J. Dugbartey (✉)
Department of Pharmacology and Toxicology, School of Pharmacy, College of Health Sciences, University of Ghana, Accra, Ghana

Department of Physiology and Pharmacology, Accra College of Medicine, Accra, Ghana

Division of Urology, Department of Surgery, London Health Sciences Center, Western University, London, ON, Canada

Multi-Organ Transplant Program, London Health Sciences Center, Western University, London, ON, Canada

Matthew Mailing Center for Translational Transplant Studies, London Health Sciences Center, Western University, London, ON, Canada
e-mail: gdugbart@uwo.ca

K. K. Alornyo
Department of Pharmacology and Toxicology, School of Pharmacy, College of Health Sciences, University of Ghana, Accra, Ghana

V. Boima
Department of Medicine and Therapeutics, University of Ghana Medical School, College of Health Sciences, University of Ghana, Accra, Ghana

S. Antwi
Department of Child Health, School of Medical Sciences, Kwame Nkrumah University of Science and Technology and Komfo Anokye Teaching Hospital, Kumasi, Ghana

A. Sener
Division of Urology, Department of Surgery, London Health Sciences Center, Western University, London, ON, Canada

Multi-Organ Transplant Program, London Health Sciences Center, Western University, London, ON, Canada

Matthew Mailing Center for Translational Transplant Studies, London Health Sciences Center, Western University, London, ON, Canada

Department of Microbiology and Immunology, London Health Sciences Center, Western University, London, ON, Canada
e-mail: alp.sener@lhsc.on.ca

Coronavirus Disease 2019

The global outbreak of the novel coronavirus disease 2019 (COVID-19) caused by severe acute respiratory syndrome coronavirus-2 (SARS-CoV-2) has rapidly evolved into a global pandemic with enormous consequences. It has caused significant mortality and loss of capital, with a struggling global economy to contain the pandemic [1]. This virus, which is the third zoonotic virus next to SARS-CoV and the Middle East respiratory syndrome (MERS-CoV), was first identified in Wuhan, Hubei Province in China, in December 2019, from where it has spread to all countries and territories of the globe [2]. The initial signs of SARS-CoV-2 infection such as pneumonia, multiple-organ failure, and acute respiratory distress syndrome are elicited through the actions of the immune system [1, 2]. Various immunopathological changes in patients with SARS-CoV-2 infection have been documented in which lymphopenia, abnormalities in granulocytes and monocytes in serum, as well as increase in cytokine production have been reported. These pathological changes seen in the upper respiratory tract are due to uncontrollable viral replication, leading to influx of neutrophils, macrophages, and monocytes and elevated production of pro-inflammatory cytokines, the so-called cytokine storm syndrome [1, 2].

Current studies have shown that the kidneys are badly affected during SARS-CoV-2 infection, leading to kidney injury especially in patients with comorbidities, and worsening kidney conditions with increased mortality of COVID-19 patients with preexisting chronic kidney disease, renal cancer, diabetic nephropathy, and end-stage kidney disease as well as dialysis and kidney transplant patients [3–6]. In the search for antiviral agents for the treatment of COVID-19, hydrogen sulfide (H_2S), a gas known for its distinct "rotten-egg" smell and established as the third member of a family of gaseous signaling molecules, is emerging as a potential candidate. In this chapter, we summarize the global impact of COVID-19 on pathological conditions involving the kidney and discuss the emerging role of H_2S as a potential COVID-19 therapy.

Impact of COVID-19 on Kidney Conditions

The global spread of COVID-19 has left nephrologists and their patients with challenging decisions in the treatment and management of kidney conditions such as acute kidney injury, chronic kidney disease, diabetic nephropathy, renal cancer, kidney infarction, end-stage kidney disease, nephrotic syndrome, dialysis, and kidney transplantation. It has been widely reported that SARS-CoV-2 enters its host cell by binding to angiotensin-converting enzyme 2 (ACE2), a cell-surface protein found in a host of tissues and organs including the kidney [7, 8]. In the kidney, ACE2 is mainly expressed in epithelial cells of proximal tubule and glomerular parietal epithelial cells [9]. In addition to ACE2, transmembrane protease serine 2 (TMPRSS2), which is also expressed in the kidney, facilitates the fusion of the virus and cellular membranes by cleaving the spike (S) protein of the virus [10]. In the kidney, colocalization of ACE2 and TMPRSS was found in the podocytes and the proximal straight tubule cells as the host cells for COVID-19 infection due to their increased expression of these proteins [10, 11]. Interestingly, RNA-sequencing data revealed that ACE2 expression in the kidneys was almost 100-fold greater than in the lungs, suggesting that COVID-19-related kidney injury is significantly through ACE2-dependent pathways [12]. ACE2 is an enzyme of the renin–angiotensin–aldosterone system that converts angiotensin II to angiotensin 1–7 and angiotensin 1–9. The latter binds to Mas receptor and suppresses the action of angiotensin II/AT1R system [13–15]. As illustrated in Fig. 6.1, the attachment and proliferation of the virus in the kidneys lead to an increase in kidney function parameters such as creatinine, along with hematuria, proteinuria, and other urine abnormalities. Furthermore, kidney structures such as the glomeruli are also inflamed and destroyed. These changes in the kidneys progressively may lead to renal failure, needing kidney replacement therapy such as dialysis and transplantation in patients with renal manifestations of COVID-19 infection.

COVID-19 Infection and Acute Kidney Injury

Progressive acute kidney injury (AKI) is common among hospitalized COVID-19 patients and is an independent risk factor for mortality. It has been reported that AKI was one of the complications observed in hospitalized COVID-19 patients with its

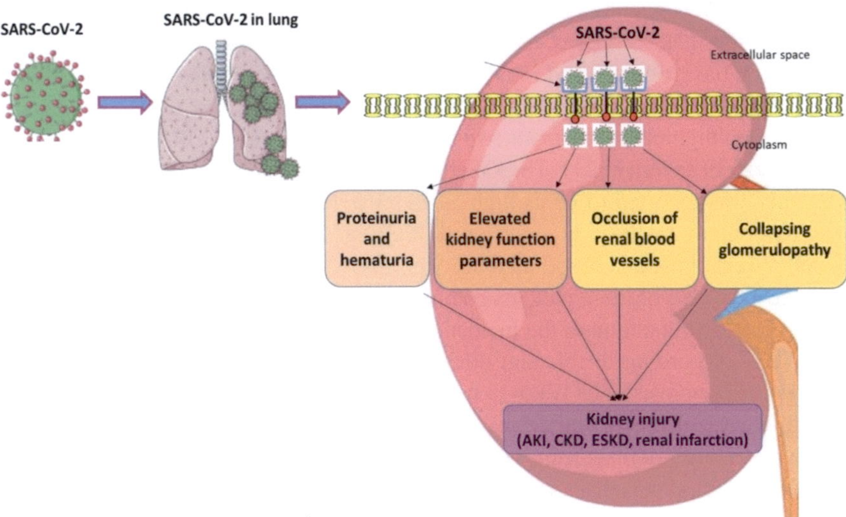

Fig. 6.1 A diagram showing the attachment of SARS-CoV-2 to the ACE2 receptors expressed on the surface of proximal tubule epithelial cells. Invasion of the kidneys by SARS-CoV-2 leads to proteinuria, hematuria, abnormal kidney function parameters (urea, creatinine, uric acid, and albumin), and occlusion of renal arteries and veins as well as collapsing glomerulopathy as a result of local cytokine storm syndrome

occurrence ranging between 0.5 and 80% [16]. The mechanisms underlying COVID-19-associated AKI are unknown. However, proposed mechanisms of kidney injury range from direct viral infection to effects on the renin–angiotensin–aldosterone system, hemodynamic instability, coagulopathy, and cytokine storm. In a systematic review and meta-analysis of outcomes for patients with COVID-19 and AKI among 20 cohorts covering 13,137 hospitalized COVID-19 patients, prevalence of AKI was found to be 17%, out of which 77% experienced severe COVID-19 infection and 52% died [17]. AKI was associated with increased odds of death among COVID-19 patients (pooled odds ratio 15.27, 95% CI 4.82–48.36), although there was considerable heterogeneity across studies and among different regions in the world. About 5% of all patients in the study required the use of kidney replacement therapy. The study concluded that kidney dysfunction was common among patients with COVID-19, and patients who develop AKI have inferior outcomes [17]. A recent multinational observational study of hospitalized COVID-19 patients with AKI also showed significantly high plasma levels of soluble urokinase plasminogen activator receptor (suPAR, an immunological risk factor for AKI and predictive of the need for dialysis) compared to AKI patients without COVID-19 infection [18]. This observation suggests that suPAR may play an important role in the pathophysiology of COVID-19-associated AKI.

Proteinuria and hematuria were common features observed in about 40% of COVID-19 patients on hospital admission [19]. In one observational study of 5449 hospitalized patients, the incidence of AKI was 36.6% with 14.3% of patients requiring dialysis, and this was even higher in patients admitted at the intensive care unit [20]. Autopsy reports from kidneys of COVID-19 deceased patients revealed acute tubular injury and collapsing glomerulopathy as the most prominent damage to the kidneys [21, 22]. Electron microscopy of kidney biopsies revealed viral-like particles in the glomeruli and renal tubules although the particles were not conclusively that of SARS-CoV-2 [19, 22]. The incidence of AKI in COVID-19 patients was also highlighted in 15 separate studies, with an odds ratio (OR) of 18.5% based on COVID-19 severity [21]. The OR for COVID-19 patients with AKI-associated mortality was reported to be as high as 23.95%. In some 710 COVID-19 patients who reported to the hospital, prevalence of elevated markers of renal function such as serum creatinine and blood urea nitrogen (BUN) was 15.5% and 14.1%, respectively, with 26.9% of these patients coming in with microscopic hematuria and 44% having proteinuria although the incidence of AKI in these patients was reported as 3.2% [23]. According to this and other supporting data, AKI is likely associated with worse prognosis in COVID-19 patients and increases their mortality rates [24, 25]. In a related retrospective analysis of medical records from 85 COVID-19-positive patients in Wuhan from January 17 to March 3, 2020, 27.06% of the patients developed AKI especially among the elderly (59–92 years old) [26]. During this study, varying degrees of tubular necrosis, luminal brush border sloughing, and vacuole degeneration were observed in a hematoxylin and eosin staining of 6 kidney samples as well as the presence of CD68$^+$ macrophages, CD8$^+$ T cells, CD4$^+$ T cells, and CD56$^+$ natural killer cells from deceased COVID-19 patients [26]. In conclusion, COVID-19 infection likely accelerates the development of AKI, especially among elderly patients.

COVID-19 Infection and Chronic Kidney Disease

Patients with chronic kidney disease (CKD) are predisposed to COVID-19 [27]. Emerging reports suggest that patients with preexisting kidney injuries got worse after testing positive and being admitted to the hospital for COVID-19. In one study, there was an elevation in markers of renal function, serum D-dimer, and pro-inflammatory cytokines, particularly interleukin-6 as well as neutrophilia [28]. It is currently unclear as to the extent the virus directly damages renal tubular epithelial cells or whether the kidney injury is secondary to the cytokine storm syndrome [12, 29, 30]. In a study involving 1603 patients with COVID-19, 21% presented with increased serum creatinine levels, while 43.5% of them had a previously diagnosed CKD stage 3 or higher and higher mortality rates than those in the non-CKD group [31]. In these CKD patients (n = 146), urea, serum potassium, urinary proteins, D-dimer, procalcitonin, lactate, and troponin levels were elevated, while hemoglobin, platelets, albumin, and estimated glomerular filtration rate were decreased. Mortality was high in COVID-19 patients with elevated serum creatinine (32.4%) and those with previously diagnosed CKD (41.1%) than those with normal serum creatinine levels (5.8%) [31]. In summary, COVID-19 infection appears to damage the kidney and may accelerate the death of patients with CKD.

COVID-19 Infection and Diabetic Nephropathy

COVID-19 patients with comorbidities are more likely to show a more severe clinical picture of the infection with high mortality rate. Most of the available data highlight diabetes mellitus as one exceptional comorbidity associated with more severe COVID-19 and mortality [32]. A survey done in the United Kingdom showed that out of 23,804 patients with COVID-19 dying in hospitals, 1.5% had type 1 diabetes mellitus and 32% had type 2 diabetes mellitus, with 3.5 and 2.03 times the odds of dying compared to patients without diabetes mellitus, respectively [33]. It has been observed that patients with diabetes mellitus have a severe and fatal manifestation of COVID-19 infection with increased ACE2 production in the kidney as an adaptive response to elevated levels of angiotensin I and II, which in effect facilitates the entry of SARS-CoV-2 into host cells [34]. This phenomenon enhances a progressive decline in renal function in diabetic patients characterized by an increase in serum creatinine, uric acid, BUN, and proteinuria and a decrease in estimated glomerular filtration rate [32]. A molecular study revealed that the enhanced progressive decline in renal function in COVID-19 patients with diabetes mellitus could be due to upregulation of genes that influence viral infection pathways in diabetic nephropathy [35]. For example, proximal tubular epithelial cell (PTEC) gene, which is co-expressed with ACE2, may exhibit cellular interplay between mechanisms that enhance viral infection and host immune responses [35]. Thus, COVID-19 increases the severity of the manifestations of diabetes mellitus, which may then contribute to death of the diabetic patient.

COVID-9 Infection and Renal Cancer

Cancer patients undergoing cancer chemotherapy are among those likely to be easily infected with SARS-CoV-2 due to drug-related immunosuppression [36, 37]. Globally, renal cell carcinoma (RCC) represents the sixth and tenth most diagnosed cancer in men and women and accounts for 5% and 3% of all cancers in males and females, respectively [38]. A recent study revealed predominant expression of coronavirus receptors (CoV; DPP4, ANPEP, ENPEP) in clear cell RCC and also in other forms of renal cancers such as papillary and chromophobe subtypes [39]. This finding confirms increased risk of SARS-CoV-2 infection in these groups of patients and has left physicians and other stakeholders to debate whether or not to continue or stop cancer therapy. Considering the risk of cancer progression after stopping or delaying therapy, especially deterioration of metastatic conditions, it is recommended that cancer patients receiving curative treatment should continue their treatment regardless of the potentially high risk of COVID-19 infection during their chemotherapy [40]. However, delaying or minimizing elective surgical procedures in patients with stable cancer as well as in those patients at high risk of ending up in the intensive care units following surgery has been strongly recommended as a strategy to mitigate the COVID-19 crisis [40]. In the light of these strategies, recommendations for the deferment for cytoreductive nephrectomy in patients with RCC in this COVID-19 era and replacement with systemic therapy for patients with intermediate- to poor-risk disease have been made [41]. Current data from a study gives both medical practitioners and patients some hope, as surgery can be safely delayed in a subgroup of patients with RCC to between 3 and 6 months without significant sacrifice in the overall survival [42]. Overall, patients with RCC and other forms of renal cancer, who are undergoing cancer chemotherapy, are at a higher risk of COVID-19 infection, which could further exacerbate their kidney condition.

COVID-19 Infection and Kidney Infarction

An increased risk of the formation of blood clots has previously been noted with SARS and MERS, and this is one proposed cause of prerenal injury in COVID-9 patients [43, 44]. The lodging of thrombi in the renal vessels and kidneys increases the likelihood of kidney damage and possibly kidney death due to kidney infarction. This finding supports the observation that platelet-rich fibrin microthrombi are scattered in peritubular capillaries and tubules in kidneys of deceased COVID-19 patients [45]. In some COVID-19-positive patients, changes in blood coagulation parameters have been observed [46, 47]. Disseminated intravascular coagulopathy (DIC, a condition of overactive clotting factors) is observed in COVID-19 patients, particularly in the critically ill patients. DIC arises from cytokine storm syndrome-induced hemophagocytosis and acute consumptive coagulopathy, which leads to enhanced platelet activation and fibrin and thrombus formation [45]. A cross-sectional study from April 13 to 24 in 2020 revealed elevation of markers of endothelial cells and platelet activation such as von Willebrand factor antigen, coagulation factors, and fibrinolytic enzymes [48]. These coagulation anomalies were reported in a 71-year-old COVID-19-positive patient, who exhibited thromboembolic events such as ascending aortic thrombosis, renal infarction, and a corresponding hypercoagulable state [49]. However, this may seem a little presumptuous given that the coagulation anomalies were reported in only one patient and over a short period (10 days). In a nutshell, COVID-19 infection increases the likelihood of formation of blood clots in the renal vessels and kidney, which may lead to kidney infarction and possibly death of the patient.

COVID-19 Infection and End-Stage Renal Disease

Information on COVID-19 in end-stage renal disease (ESRD) is limited but rapidly evolving. ESRD patients have a higher chance of contracting COVID-19 due to suppression of the immune system, which is associated with ESRD [50, 51]. While there is no evidence-based solution to this concern, patients who are at high risk of progressing to ESRD without immediate treatment are being advised to postpone treatment until their local transmission rates of COVID-19 are low. Further evidence of the impact of COVID-19 on ESRD patients was reported where a higher rate of in-hospital death of COVID-19 patients with ESRD compared to those without ESRD in a retrospective study in the United States [52]. This observation aligned with that of an independent study, where the researchers evaluated clinical characteristics, laboratory measures, and clinical outcomes in 759 hospitalized COVID-19 patients, out of which 45 had ESRD [53]. The authors reported that COVID-19 patients with ESRD had significantly increased leukocyte count, C-reactive protein, lactate dehydrogenase, and ferritin and markedly reduced serum albumin and thrombocytopenia with a higher in-hospital mortality (18%) compared to their counterparts without ESRD (10%) [53]. Another study also reported that COVID-19-positive patients who had ESRD and on dialysis had better outcomes than ESRD patients who were not on dialysis [54]. They attributed their observation to a possible "preconditioning," where underlying chronic inflammation in ESRD patients on dialysis attenuates the inflammatory response from the COVID-19 infection. It is important to note that the spread of COVID-19 in some dialysis centers is on the rise (e.g., Italy), which is partly due to the difficulty in applying social distancing protocols [55], while it is lower in other centers (e.g., Abu Dhabi, United Arab Emirates) due to rapid isolation of COVID-19 patients within their dialysis centers [56]. Taken together, COVID-19 infection worsens kidney condition of ESRD patients and may lead to increased mortality.

COVID-19 Infection and Kidney Transplantation

Kidney transplant patients are currently at a higher risk of COVID-19 infection and its associated mortality, as these patients have a spectrum of kidney diseases and comorbidities such as hypertension, diabetes, and obesity that requires kidney transplantation [57, 58]. Hence, kidney transplant surgeons have been advised to suspend kidney transplantation during this pandemic due to poor outcomes, especially in high-risk older recipients with comorbidities. This unfortunate obstacle to such an important lifesaving procedure is due to possible donor-to-recipient viral transmission or members of the transplant team serving as vectors of the SARS-CoV-2. Suspension of kidney transplantation during the pandemic will have a negative impact on the transplant waiting list, thereby increasing morbidity and mortality [59]. SARS-CoV-2 has a higher tropism for the kidney, where it has been shown to replicate in about 30% of COVID-19 patients [60]. In 12 transplant centers in the United States, Italy, and Spain, Cravedi et al. [61] reported a high COVID-19-related mortality and AKI rate in adult kidney transplant recipients. This observation supports previous findings in which a very high early mortality (28%) was recorded among kidney transplant recipients with COVID-19 in the United States compared to 8–15% of COVID-19 mortality among the general population [62] and dialysis patients on the waiting list for kidney transplantation [63]. The high COVID-19-related mortality in this group of patients is mainly due to advanced age and frailty [63]. In conclusion, patients who have undergone kidney transplantation have a high COVID-19-related mortality risk, which is driven by factors such as immunosuppression therapy, comorbidities, advanced age, and frailty.

A Special Case of COVID-19-Associated Nephropathy in People of African Ancestry

Genetic variants of apolipoprotein L1 (APOL1), which greatly increases the risk of kidney diseases, are found only in people of African descent [64]. The APOL1 alleles became common in sub-Saharan Africa due to protection conferred by these alleles against the pathogen that causes African sleeping sickness (trypanosomiasis). Studies in recent times suggest that black people living in sub-Saharan Africa have high predisposition to kidney disease as do African Americans and that these two groups (African Americans and Black Africans) have common genetic susceptibilities. Two APOL1 susceptibility gene variants (G1 and G2) are linked with hypertension-associated CKD, collapsing focal segmental glomerulosclerosis and HIV-associated nephropathy [65–67]. The APOL1 kidney risk variants encode circulating APOL1, which functions as a trypanolytic factor capable of killing the trypanosome parasites in the human serum [64]. These APOL1 risk variants developed some 10,000 years ago in sub-Saharan Africa where trypanosomiasis was endemic. Thus, APOL1 gene is an innate immunity gene common in people of African ancestry.

Recent studies suggest that people with high/low renal risk alleles for APOL1, who are COVID-19 positive, may have a high risk of developing renal failure, proteinuria, and hematuria. There are six case reports of collapsing glomerulopathy among COVID-19 patients of African ancestry, with severe AKI and nephrotic range proteinuria, two of whom carried APOL1 renal risk genotypes [68–71]. APOL1 coding variants have been associated with collapsing glomerulopathy among individuals with untreated HIV infection or undergoing interferon treatment. There is a high frequency of APOL1 risk genotypes among African Americans (~13%) and West Africans (~25%), with lower frequencies found in East and South Africans [64, 72, 73]. Collapsing glomerulopathy has been described in 24 cases of COVID-19 infection; 23 out of the 24 (95.8%) cases were Africans or African American and 1 was Indian; 18 patients had APOL1 gene variants (12 were G1,G1 and 6 were G1,G2) [16]. This suggests that one of the major risk factors for AKI in patients with COVID-19 infection is black race [74]. Individuals with high renal risk alleles for APOL1 who have COVID-19 infection may be at increased risk of developing AKI, proteinuria, and hematuria and consequent chronic kidney disease. A likely mechanism may be upregulation of APOL1 mediated by cytokines resulting from the SARS-CoV-2 infection. This hypothesis requires investigation. In addition, innate immune response to SARS-CoV-2 infection can drive the APOL1 kidney disease in patients with APOL1 high-risk genotypes. The latter argument is based on a case series of collapsing glomerulopathy linked to interferon therapy [75].

Hydrogen Sulfide as a Potential Therapy Against COVID-19 Infection

A search for antiviral agents is currently underway in the face of the alarming rate of global COVID-19 infections. Just recently, ritonavir-boosted nirmatrelvir was granted emergency use authorization by the US Food and Drug Administration (FDA) for the treatment of mild-to-moderate COVID-19 cases. Prior to this, remdesivir, an orphan antiviral drug originally developed to treat Ebola virus disease and Marburg virus infections (via inhibition of the viral RNA-dependent RNA polymerase), was the only drug approved by the US FDA for the treatment of COVID-19 in symptomatic patients [76]. This antiviral drug was administered along with convalescent plasma. In addition, a host of vaccine candidates have been approved and distributed for global use to curb the spread of SARS-CoV-2.

Endogenous and Exogenous Sources of Hydrogen Sulfide

In the search for antiviral agents for effective treatment of COVID-19, hydrogen sulfide (H_2S), a pungent-smelling gas which gained notoriety for several centuries for its toxicity and death among industrial and agricultural workers, is emerging as a potential candidate drug. Over the last two decades, however, H_2S has moved past its historic notorious label as a gas which was once feared to an intracellular messenger molecule that plays important roles in cellular homeostasis and impacts physiological and pathophysiological conditions, including regulation of the renal system [77]. H_2S possesses important therapeutic properties including antiviral, anti-inflammatory, antithrombotic, and antioxidant properties, which are important for any drug candidate against COVID-19. Endogenous H_2S is produced in mammalian cells by four enzymatic pathways. The first two pathways involve the use of the substrate L-cysteine, a sulfur-containing amino acid, in the presence of two cytosolic enzymes cystathionine β-synthase (CBS) and cystathionine γ-lyase (CSE), while the third pathway uses the mitochondrial enzyme 3-mercaptopyruvate sulfurtransferase (3-MST) and the intermediate product 3-mercaptopyruvate (from L-cysteine). The fourth enzymatic pathway uses D-cysteine, an enantiomer of L-cysteine, and the peroxisomal enzyme D-amino acid oxidase (DAO) [78–81]. Reduced production of endogenous H_2S and expression of these H_2S-producing enzymes have been associated with various pathologies of the organ system including the renal system. Whereas the distribution of these H_2S-producing enzymes is tissue specific, we and others have previously reported that all the four enzymes are abundantly expressed in the glomerular and tubular compartments of the kidney [81–84]. This makes the kidney a richer source of endogenous H_2S production compared to other organs.

In addition to its endogenous production, H_2S is also administered exogenously in its gaseous form (though less ideal) and via H_2S donor compounds. These H_2S donors include water-soluble, fast-releasing but short-lasting H_2S donors such as the inorganic sulfide salts, sodium hydrosulfide (NaHS), and sodium sulfide (Na_2S) [85]. There are also water-soluble, slow- and controlled-releasing, long-lasting H_2S donor GYY4137 [86] and mitochondrially targeted slow-releasing donors AP39 and AP123 [87], which augment mitochondrial H_2S production by 3-MST and provide an effective and longer treatment time in experimental models of kidney diseases including acute kidney injury, chronic kidney disease, diabetic nephropathy, hypertensive kidney injury, renal cancer, drug-induced nephropathy, renal ischemia-reperfusion injury, and kidney transplantation. As already discussed in previous sections, all these renal pathologies are worsened by COVID-19 infection. Also, several organic small-molecule H_2S donors have been developed [88, 89]. While these H_2S donors are limited to only preclinical studies, thiosulfate, a major H_2S oxidation product in the form of sodium thiosulfate (STS), is an FDA-approved drug already in clinical use for the treatment of calciphylaxis in ESRD patients and other clinical situations [90]. Other clinically viable H_2S donor drugs such as ATB-346 (H_2S-generating naproxen molecule) and zofenopril (FDA-approved anti-hypertensive drug that increases H_2S release) are currently in human clinical trials for gastric ulcer, osteoarthritis, chronic pain, cardiovascular diseases, and type 2 diabetes mellitus (www.clinicaltrials.gov).

Antiviral Action of H_2S and Its Underlying Mechanisms in Relation to COVID-19 Infection

Burgeoning evidence shows that H_2S donors such as NaHS and GYY4137 exhibit excellent effects against the family of enveloped RNA viruses of which SARS-CoV-2 is a member [91–94]. Also, natural sources of exogenous H_2S such as diallyl sulfide, diallyl disulfide, and diallyl trisulfide, which are derived from garlic, have been reported to reduce viral load of cytomegalovirus (another enveloped virus) in infected organs of humans and rodents [95]. Furthermore, sinigrin, a precursor of the H_2S donor allyl isothiocyanate, and obtained from the root extract of *Isatis indigotica* plant for Chinese traditional medicine [96], inhibited the function of 3-chymotrypsin-like protease, the main protease of SARS-CoV, which caused the 2002–2004 outbreak of severe acute respiratory syndrome [97].

There are several mechanisms that underlie the antiviral action of H_2S. Firstly, the antiviral activity of H_2S has been suggested to be partly linked to its antioxidant property—activating and increasing the levels of other antioxidants including gluta-thione (GSH), the most abundant naturally occurring antioxidant in the body, which inhibits overproduction of reactive oxygen species (ROS, a destructive mediator in tissue injury) and its consequent oxidative stress [98, 99]. Interestingly, ROS-induced oxidative stress has been associated with viral infection in the kidney [100], impairing the kidney's antioxidant defense system. Moreover, Kim et al. [99] recently predicted in their study involving high-throughput artificial intelligence-based binding affinity that GSH interacts with and possibly inhibits the action of ACE2 and TMPRSS2, the two proteins that facilitate SARS-CoV-2 entry into the kidney. Secondly, findings from a very recent study show that H_2S also exhibits its antiviral activity against SARS-CoV-2 by inhibiting TMPRSS2 in human airway epithelial cells and possibly interfering with ACE2 and potentially blocking the attachment of the virus to these host proteins [101], thereby inhibiting the entry of the virus into the host cell (Fig. 6.2). However, a previous study reported that administration of H_2S via its donor molecule NaHS upregulated carotid ACE2 expression and reduced organ damages in a mouse model of carotid artery ligation [102]. These

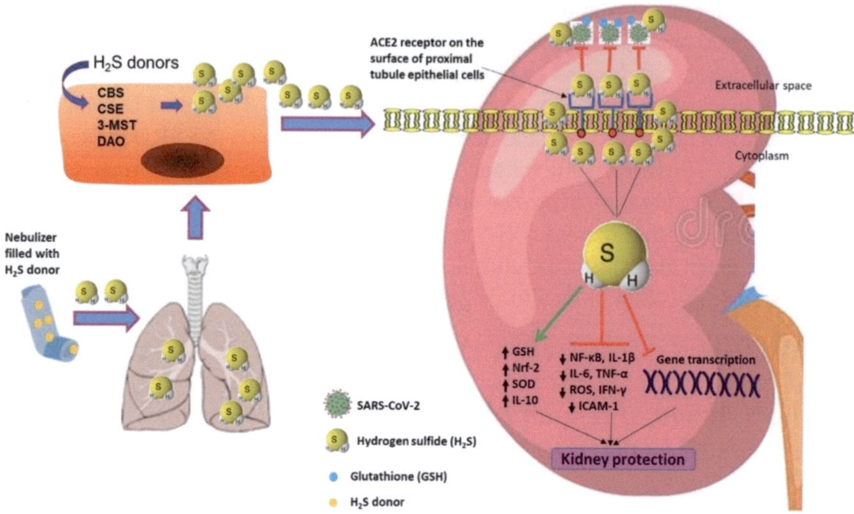

Fig. 6.2 Possible mechanism of action of H_2S against SARS-CoV-2. Administration of H_2S donors may increase endogenous production of H_2S by cystathionine β-synthase (CBS), cystathionine γ-lyase (CSE), 3-mercaptopyruvate sulfurtransferase (3-MST), and D-amino acid oxidase (DAO) and may also activate nonenzymatic pathway. H_2S interacts with angiotensin-converting enzyme 2 (ACE2) and TMPRSS2 (not shown) and may block the binding of SARS-CoV-2 to these host cell proteins, thereby inhibiting the entry of the virus into the host cell. H_2S may also alter SARS-CoV-2 membrane and inhibits its gene transcription including inhibiting the activation of nuclear factor-kappaB (NF-κB). In addition, H_2S may activate antioxidant pathway, leading to increased levels of antioxidant enzymes such as glutathione (GSH), nuclear factor-erythroid factor 2-related factor 2 (Nrf2), and superoxide dismutase (SOD) and suppressing overproduction of reactive oxygen species (ROS). Furthermore, H_2S may inhibit pro-inflammatory pathway, resulting in reduced production of pro-inflammatory mediators such as interleukin-1-beta (IL-1β), IL-6, tumor necrosis factor-alpha (TNF-α), interferon-gamma (IFN-γ), and intercellular adhesion molecule-1 (ICAM-1) while activating anti-inflammatory pathway, which increases the production of IL-10

contradictory findings could be attributed to the different context of H_2S application, as the former study used human respiratory epithelial cells and lung tissue samples from patients undergoing segmental/lobar pulmonary resections, whose pharmacological response to H_2S donors may be different from that of the mice carotid artery endothelial cells used in the latter study. Moreover, while two H_2S donors (NaHS and GYY4137) were administered in the former study, only one H_2S donor (NaHS) was used in the latter study, which could suggest that increased H_2S level in the former study may have accounted for the decreased expression of the TMPRSS2 (and possibly ACE2) proteins while a decreased H_2S level could result in increased expression of these host proteins in the latter study. A recent molecular dynamics simulation study showed that reduction of disulfides in ACE2 and S protein of SARS-CoV-2 into sulfhydryl groups impairs the binding of the S protein of SARS-CoV-2 to ACE2 [103]. Interestingly, administration of *N*-acetylcysteine (NAC, an antioxidant H_2S donor and a source of cysteine for endogenous GSH production) disrupted the disulfides, leading to inhibition of SARS-CoV-2 entry into the host cell [104]. This could also partly explain why the antiviral action of H_2S is suggested to be linked to its antioxidant property through increased GSH production. Moreover, NAC is a known mucolytic agent that breaks disulfide bonds in mucus, making it less viscous and easier to be expelled by other mucoactive agents (expectorants and mucokinetics) together with the action of the ciliary apparatus of the respiratory system. Thus, H_2S facilitates elimination of potentially harmful viruses such as SARS-CoV-2, suggesting its antiviral action in COVID-19.

Thirdly, the antiviral action of H_2S involves Toll-like receptors (TLRs), a class of pattern recognition receptors (PRRs) that initiate innate immune response for early immune recognition of a pathogen. Following the release of viral RNA (i.e., pathogen-associated molecular pattern) into host cells, it is recognized by PRRs such as TLRs in the host immune cells, which activates production and secretion of large amounts of pro-inflammatory cytokines and chemokines responsible for cytokine storm and organ damage as seen in the various kidney conditions discussed in previous sections [105]. Chen and colleagues [106] recently reported that deficiency in endogenous H_2S level contributes to sepsis-induced myocardial dysfunction (SIMD) in humans and mice via increased expression of TLRs. However, administration of NaHS in SIMD mice inhibited TLR pathway and prevented TLR-mediated inflammation. Although this study was not in relation to viruses, it is likely that antiviral action of H_2S involves the same mechanism. Besides, H_2S has been reported to inhibit activation and nuclear translocation of nuclear factor-kappaB (NF-κB, an inflammatory-related transcription factor), thereby suppressing the transcription of pro-inflammatory genes, leading to inhibition of the secretion of virus-induced chemokines and cytokines [91]. Fourthly, postmortem examination of transplanted kidney, lungs, and heart of COVID-19 deceased patients revealed endotheliitis and accumulation of apoptotic bodies [107], suggesting that inflammation of the endothelium (an important gatekeeper of cardiovascular health and homeostasis) and apoptotic cell death contributed to dysfunction or malfunction of these organs in the COVID-19 patients, which resulted in death of these patients. As a potential therapy for COVID-19 patients, there are studies showing the ameliorative effect of H_2S endothelial dysfunction in cardiovascular disorders such as hypertension, atherosclerosis, hyperhomocysteinemia, as well as diabetes [108, 109]. Besides, overactivation of the sympathetic nervous system has recently been implicated in COVID-19 patients with preexisting chronic lung diseases, kidney diseases, cardiovascular pathologies, obesity, and diabetes mellitus through factors including ACE2 imbalance, which contributes to organ damage in these patients [110]. Interestingly, H_2S donors such as NaHS are well known to suppress sympathetic activation [85, 111–113], and therefore inhibition of sympathetic outflow could be a potential therapeutic mechanism by H_2S donors for COVID-19 patients.

Another mechanism underlying the antiviral action of H_2S in relation to COVID-19 involves interaction with endoplasmic reticulum (ER) stress-related proteins. A recent preliminary virtual screening study in patients with COVID-19 pneumonia revealed higher gene expression and serum concentrations of glucose-regulated protein 78 (GRP78, an ER stress protein and the host cell surface protein to which the Spike protein of SARS-CoV-2 binds as revealed by molecular docking) compared to pneumonia patients without COVID-19 [114]. There are studies showing the inhibitory action of H_2S donors on GRP78 and other ER stress-related proteins in experimental models of human diseases. Yi et al. [115] reported that administration of NaHS downregulated the expression of GRP78 and other ER stress-related proteins, inhibited uranium-induced apoptosis of rat renal proximal tubular epithelial cells, and mitigated ER stress via activation of Akt/GSK-3β/Fyn-Nrf2 pathway, a protective molecular pathway. This in vitro result supports a previous result by Wei et al. [116] who observed attenuation of hyperhomocysteinemia-induced cardiomyocyte injury following H_2S administration in rats. Administration of NaHS also markedly inhibited cigarette smoke-induced overexpression of GRP78 and other markers of ER stress-mediated apoptosis and prevented lung tissue damage [117]. These pieces of experimental evidence suggest that H_2S donors could be potential antiviral agents that serve to treat COVID-19 patients by preventing the entry of SARS-CoV-2 into host cells via inhibition or downregulation of the expression of GRP78 and other ER stress-related proteins, thereby preventing apoptosis and organ damage. In addition to all these mechanisms, we also reported that H_2S decreases renal expression of kidney injury molecule (KIM-1, a biomarker of human renal proximal tubular injury) [83, 118], which has recently been found to be associated with COVID-19 nephropathy and potential receptor for SARS-CoV-2 entry into renal and lung cells [119]. Renal and lung epithelial cells of humans and mice co-expressed KIM-1 and SARS-CoV-2 spike protein [120], suggesting that KIM-1 could directly bind to SARS-CoV-2 spike protein following its induction by AKI or other pathological conditions involving the kidney, as this interaction was inhibited by anti-KIM-1 antibodies and the KIM-1 inhibitor, TW-37 [120]. Yang et al. [121] also implicated KIM-1 and ACE2 in a synergistic interaction, which mediated the invasion of SARS-CoV-2 in kidney cells and worsened COVID-19 infection in the kidney. We recently showed that activation of endogenous H_2S production by dopamine administration increases renal expression of H_2S-producing enzymes (CBS, CSE, and 3-MST) and serum H_2S level and decreases renal KIM-1 expression, leading to increased kidney protection in a rat model of deep hypothermia/rewarming-induced AKI [83]. We also observed decreased expression of KIM-1 in renal tubules and preservation of renal structures following administration of 5′-adenosine monophosphate, which correlated with increased renal H_2S-producing enzymes and serum H_2S level in a hamster model of therapeutic hypothermia [118]. These observations together with other potential mechanisms that decrease KIM-1 expression in kidney and lung tissues suggest that H_2S may offer a new therapy for COVID-19-associated nephropathy and pneumopathy. Other mechanisms underlying the antiviral action of H_2S or H_2S donors include inhibition of gene transcription along with antiviral immunosuppressive effect, as was reported in human cytomegalovirus [122] and alterations of the viral membrane, as XM-01 (an H_2S donor) inhibited the activities of enveloped viruses but had no effect on non-enveloped viruses [123]. The findings from all these studies strongly suggest that H_2S donors could serve a therapeutic purpose in COVID-19 and its complications including COVID-19-associated nephropathy (Fig. 6.2).

H_2S as a Potential Biomarker in Determining Final Outcome of COVID-19 Infection

Although there are currently no studies on the effect of H_2S on COVID-19-associated nephropathy, recent clinical study in a cohort of patients with COVID-19 pneumonia showed that circulating H_2S level was significantly higher along with increased lymphocyte count and reduced serum interleukin-6 (IL-6, an inflammatory marker) in survivors of the disease compared to healthy controls and those who died of the disease [124]. This observation suggests that H_2S could be a potential biomarker to determine the final outcome of pneumonia caused by COVID-19. It is important to note that IL-6 is considered a major pro-inflammatory mediator in the cytokine storm syndrome that causes respiratory failure and COVID-19-associated mortality [125]. There are studies including ours showing that H_2S is a potent inhibitor of pro-inflammatory pathway by inhibiting pulmonary and renal IL-6 and several other pro-inflammatory mediators such as IL-2, tumor necrosis factor-alpha (TNF-α), interferon-gamma (IFN-γ), intercellular adhesion molecule-1 (ICAM-1), and NF-κB while simultaneously increasing the levels of anti-inflammatory cytokines [126, 127]. Therefore, the findings by Renieris et al. [124] may suggest that the increased serum H_2S level in the COVID-19 survivors could be due to increased endogenous H_2S production from the lungs and perhaps the kidneys and other tissues to suppress the production of IL-6 and other pro-inflammatory mediators which are yet to be investigated. This is in agreement with the study by Li and colleagues [91] who observed reduced endogenous H_2S production and downregulation of CSE mRNA and protein expression (H_2S-producing enzyme) in airway epithelial cells infected with respiratory syncytial virus, the virus commonly associated with upper and lower respiratory tract infections in children of which there is no vaccine or effective treatment. Further evidence of the involvement of H_2S in virus-induced respiratory condition was reported when increased viral replication and airway inflammation were observed in CSE knockout mice infected with respiratory syncytial virus compared to wild-type mice [92]. Interestingly, treatment with the H_2S donor, GYY4137, markedly reduced the viral replication of not only respiratory syncytial virus but also human metapneumovirus and Nipah virus, which correlated with decreased production of pro-inflammatory mediators and improvement in airway dysfunction [92]. These findings provide strong evidence of the antiviral property of H_2S, which could be a potential therapeutic agent against COVID-19. In addition, administration of NAC to ten patients with severe COVID-19 significantly improved clinical and biochemical parameters [128] as well as clinical improvement in a critically ill COVID-19 patient with multisystem organ dysfunction, who was treated with intravenous administration of NAC (75 mg/kg over 4 h, then 35 mg/kg over 16 h, followed by 17 mg/kg over 24 h on day 2) along with low-dose hydroxychloroquine [129]. This finding is supported by another case of a severely ill COVID-19 patient who was cured and discharged following administration of NAC inhalation solution [130]. However, in a recent double-blind, randomized controlled trial, intravenous administration of NAC (14 g/kg in the first 4 h and 7 g/kg in the next 16 h) to severe COVID-19 patients in late stage of the disease showed no clinical benefits compared to placebo group [131]. This contradictory result could be attributable to differences in the dose of NAC and treatment regimen, synergistic effect with hydroxychloroquine, and timing of NAC administration, as the latter study administered NAC later than 7–10 days after the onset of COVID-19 symptoms compared to the former study. It further suggests that the aforementioned factors are crucial in the treatment of COVID-19 patients with NAC or other H_2S donors and should be matched with concurrent medical treatments. These clinical outcomes have led to conduction of several clinical trials with NAC to determine the most appropriate timing of administration in various stages of COVID-19. In the face of the potential positive role of H_2S in COVID-19 cases, Dominic et al. [132] recently refuted the report of Renieris et al. [124] by showing low circulating H_2S levels in Caucasian and African American COVID-19 patients compared to healthy controls and fatal cases. This conflicting finding could be due to important determinants such as age, race, sex, comorbidities (e.g., diabetes and hypertension), and stage of COVID-19 infection, which were not reported in the former study. Another important factor for consideration is the differences in the method of serum H_2S measurement, as H_2S decay was so fast in the latter study and may not have been very accurate. Besides, the authors of the latter study did not include high-performance liquid chromatography (a new method of H_2S quantification in biological systems) in their serum H_2S measurement, which their counterparts in the former study did, although both studies used the common monobromobimane method of H_2S measurement. This discrepancy in the two studies requires additional investigations and should take into consideration all important determining factors of H_2S, to establish the exact role of H_2S in determining the final outcome of COVID-19 infection.

The pathological characteristics of COVID-19 also include coagulopathy, during which there is progression of thrombosis and generation of DIC with increased platelet-leukocyte aggregates, which promote coagulation and vascular inflammation in the glomeruli of critically ill patients and partly account for COVID-19-related mortality [133]. Hence, inhibiting platelet-leukocyte aggregates is a therapeutic interest in COVID-19 patients, especially those with kidney conditions. Emerging evidence using animal and human whole blood shows that H_2S donors such as NaHS and GYY4137 inhibit the coagulation system by preventing DIC formation and platelet-leukocyte aggregation and facilitate thrombolysis, leading to impairment in thrombus stability [134, 135]. Therefore, these findings about the thrombolytic or antithrombotic property of H_2S could advance its potential clinical utility by COVID-19 patients.

Conclusion

Symptomatic COVID-19 patients develop renal complications, and patients with preexisting renal conditions also have a high chance of disease progression and mortality. Currently, there are no approved drugs that offer renal protection in COVID-19 patients although ritonavir-boosted nirmatrelvir and remdesivir and a number of vaccines have been approved by the US FDA for emergency use. With a new viral pandemic which has significant renal involvement, there is a need for future studies to determine the risk factors of kidney disease among COVID-19 patients. It is important to also determine the link between genetic polymorphisms and the risk of developing kidney diseases among certain races of people including those of African ancestry, who have genetic polymorphisms to kidney diseases, and to know whether there is an association between APOL1 high-risk carriers and risk of developing COVID-19-associated nephropathy. As the search for pharmacological agents for effective treatment of COVID-19 is underway, there are studies that are suggesting the potential clinical use of H_2S donors, as these agents fall under all three classifications of COVID-19 treatment—antiviral treatment, cytokine storm treatment, and thrombosis treatment. A growing body of scientific evidence shows that H_2S donors interact with ACE2, TMPRSS2, and other potential SARS-CoV-2 receptors on the host cell surface and alter SARS-CoV-2 membrane, thereby inhibiting the entry of the virus into the host cell and consequently preventing its replication (assembly and release). This mechanism is thought to suppress SARS-CoV-2-induced inflammatory pathway, leading to organ protection (Fig. 6.2). Other studies also suggest inhibition of gene transcription by H_2S donors along with antiviral immunosuppressive effect. In the light of these mechanisms of the antiviral action of H_2S donors, more experimental and clinical studies with H_2S donors, especially those that are already FDA approved and are in human clinical trials such as STS, NAC, ATB-346, and zofenopril, should be considered for preventive treatment or effective therapy against COVID-19 infection and should include their use in nebulizer for aerosol inhalation into the lungs and dissemination to extrapulmonary organs such as the kidney.Conflict of InterestNone.

References

1. Douglas M, Katikireddi SV, Taulbut M, et al. Mitigating the wider health effects of Covid-19 pandemic response. BMJ. 2020;369:m1557.
2. Velavan TP, Meyer CG. The COVID-19 epidemic. Trop Med Int Health. 2020;25(3):278–80.
3. Carriazo S, Kanbay M, Ortiz A. Kidney disease and electrolytes in COVID-19: more than meets the eye. Clin Kidney J. 2020;13(3):274–80.
4. Kudose S, Batal I, Santoriello D, et al. Kidney biopsy findings in patients with COVID-19. J Am Soc Nephrol. 2020;31(9):1959–68.
5. Pei G, Zhang Z, Peng J, et al. Renal involvement and early prognosis in patients with COVID-19 pneumonia. J Am Soc Nephrol. 2020;31(6):1157–65.

6. Wald R, Bagshaw SM. COVID-19-associated acute kidney injury: learning from the first wave. J Am Soc Nephrol. 2020;32(1):4–6.

7. Kuba K, Imai Y, Rao S, et al. A crucial role of angiotensin converting enzyme 2 (ACE2) in SARS coronavirus-induced lung injury. Nat Med. 2005;11(8):875–9.

8. Alhenc-Gelas F, Drueke TB. Blockade of SARS-CoV-2 infection by recombinant soluble ACE2. Kidney Int. 2020;97(6):1091–3.

9. He Q, Mok TN, Yun L, He C, Li J, Pan J. Single cell RNA sequencing analysis of human kidney reveals the presence of ACE2 receptor: a potential pathway of COVID-19 infection. Mol Genet Genom Med. 2020;8(10):e1442.

10. Pan XW, Xu D, Zhang H, Wang Z, Wang LH, Cui XG. Identification of a potential mechanism of acute kidney injury during the COVID-19 outbreak: a study based on single-cell transcriptome analysis. Intensive Care Med. 2020;31:1–3.

11. Wu J, Deng W, Li S, et al. Advances in research on ACE2 as a receptor for 2019-nCoV. Cell Mol Life Sci. 2021;78(2):531–44.

12. Cheng Y, Luo R, Wang K, et al. Kidney disease is associated with in-hospital death of patients with COVID-19. Kidney Int. 2020;97(5):829–38.

13. Hisashi K, Mamiko K. Interactions of coronaviruses with ACE2, angiotensin II, and RAS inhibitors—lessons from available evidence and insights into COVID-19. Hypertens Res. 2020;43:648–54.

14. Patel VB, Zhong JC, Grant MB, Oudit GY. Role of the ACE2/angiotensin 1–7 axis of the renin–angiotensin system in heart failure. Circ Res. 2016;118(8):1313–26.

15. Santos RAS, Sampaio WO, Alzamora AC, Motta-Santos D, Alenina N, Bader M, Campagnole-Santos MJ. The ACE2/angiotensin-(1–7)/MAS axis of the renin–angiotensin system: focus on angiotensin-(1–7). Physiol Rev. 2018;98(1):505–53.

16. Ng JH, Bijol V, Sparks MA, et al. Pathophysiology and pathology of acute kidney injury in patients with COVID-19. Adv Chronic Kidney Dis. 2020;27(5):365–76.

17. Robbins-Juarez SY, Qian L, King KL, et al. Outcomes for patients with COVID-19 and acute kidney injury: a systematic review and meta-analysis. Kidney Int Rep. 2020;5(8):1149–60.

18. Azam TU, Shadid HR, Blakely P, O'Hayer P, Berlin H, Pan M, Zhao P, et al. Soluble urokinase receptor (SuPAR) in COVID-19-related AKI. J Am Soc Nephrol. 2020;31(11):2725–35.

19. Perico L, Benigni A, Remuzzi G. Should COVID-19 concern nephrologists? Why and to what extent? The emerging impasse of angiotensin blockade. Nephron. 2020;144(5):213–21.

20. Benedetti C, Waldman M, Zaza G, et al. COVID-19 and the kidneys: an update. Front Med. 2020;7(423):1–13.

21. Cheruiyot I, Kipkorir V, Ngure B, et al. Acute kidney injury is associated with worse prognosis in COVID-19 patients: a systematic review and meta-analysis. Acta Biomed. 2020;91(3):1–12.

22. Su H, Yang M, Wan C, et al. Renal histopathological analysis of 26 postmortem findings of patients with COVID-19 in China. Kidney Int. 2020;98(1):219–27.

23. Swai J. Mortality rate of acute kidney injury in SARS, MERS, and COVID-19 infection: a systematic review and meta-analysis. Crit Care. 2020;24(1):555.

24. Izzedine H, Jhaveri KD. Acute kidney injury in patients with COVID-19: an update on the pathophysiology. Nephrol Dial Transplant. 2021;36(2):224–6.

25. Taher A, Alalwan AA, Naser N, Alsegai O, Alaradi A. Acute kidney injury in COVID-19 pneumonia: a single-center experience in Bahrain. Cureus. 2020;12:e9693.

26. Diao B, Wang C, Wang R, et al. Human kidney is a target for novel severe acute respiratory syndrome coronavirus 2 (SARS-CoV-2) infection. Nat Commun. 2021;12(1):2506.

27. Henry BM, Lippi G. Chronic kidney disease is associated with severe coronavirus disease 2019 (COVID-19) infection. Int Urol Nephrol. 2020;52(6):1193–4.

28. Yang L, Liu S, Liu J, et al. COVID-19: immunopathogenesis and immunotherapeutics. Signal Transduct Target Ther. 2020;5(1):128.

29. Qian JY, Wang B, Liu BC. Acute kidney injury in the 2019 novel coronavirus disease. Kidney Dis. 2020;6(5):318–23.

30. Ahmadian E, Hosseiniyan Khatibi SM, Razi Soofiyani S, Abediazar S, Shoja MM, Ardalan M, Zununi VS. Covid-19 and kidney injury: pathophysiology and molecular mechanisms. Rev Med Virol. 2021;31(3):e2176.
31. Portolés J, Marques M, López-Sánchez P, et al. Chronic kidney disease and acute kidney injury in the COVID-19 Spanish outbreak. Nephrol Dial Transplant. 2020;35(8):1353–61.
32. D'Marco L, Puchades MJ, Romero-Parra M, et al. Diabetic kidney disease and COVID-19: the crash of two pandemics. Front Med. 2020;7(199):6–8.
33. Apicella M, Campopiano MC, Mantuano M, et al. Review COVID-19 in people with diabetes: understanding the reasons for worse outcomes. Lancet Diabetes Endocrinol. 2020;8(9):782–92.
34. Gilbert RE, Caldwell L, Misra PS, Chan K, Burns KD, Wrana JL, Yuen DA. Overexpression of the severe acute respiratory syndrome Coronavirus-2 receptor, angiotensin-converting enzyme 2, in diabetic kidney disease: implications for kidney injury in novel coronavirus disease 2019. Can J Diabetes. 2021;45(2):162–166.e1.
35. Menon R, Otto EA, Sealfon R, Nair V, Wong AK, Theesfeld CL, et al. SARS-CoV-2 receptor networks in diabetic and COVID-19-associated kidney disease. Kidney Int. 2020;98(6):1502–18.
36. Ofori-Asenso R, Ogundipe O, Adom Agyeman A, et al. Cancer is associated with severe disease in COVID-19 patients: a systematic review and meta-analysis. Ecancermedicalscience. 2020;14:1–10.
37. Mihalopoulos M, Dogra N, Mohamed N, et al. COVID-19 and kidney disease: molecular determinants and clinical implications in renal cancer. Eur Urol Focus. 2020;6(5):1086–96.
38. Wallis CJD, Novara G, Marandino L, et al. Risks from deferring treatment for genitourinary cancers: a collaborative review to aid triage and management during the COVID-19 pandemic. Eur Urol. 2020;78(1):29–42.
39. Tripathi SC, Deshmukh V, Creighton CJ, et al. Renal carcinoma is associated with increased risk of coronavirus infections. Front Mol Biosci. 2020;7:579422.
40. Al-Quteimat OM, Amer AM. The impact of the COVID-19 pandemic on cancer patients. Am J Clin Oncol. 2020;43(6):452–5.
41. Ged Y, Markowski MC, Pierorazio PM. Advanced renal cell carcinoma and COVID-19—a personal perspective. Nat Rev Urol. 2020;17(8):425–7.
42. Srivastava A, Patel HV, Kim S, et al. Delaying surgery for clinical T1b-T2bN0M0 renal cell carcinoma: oncologic implications in the COVID-19 era and beyond. J Clin Oncol. 2021;39(6):283.
43. Bandyopadhyay D, Akhtar T, Hajra A, et al. COVID-19 pandemic: cardiovascular complications and future implications. Am J Cardiovasc Drugs. 2020;20(4):311–24.
44. Dobesh PP, Trujillo TC. Coagulopathy, venous thromboembolism, and anticoagulation in patients with COVID-19. Pharmacotherapy. 2020;40(11):1130–51.
45. Rapkiewicz AV, Mai X, Carsons SE, et al. Megakaryocytes and platelet-fibrin thrombi characterize multi-organ thrombosis at autopsy in COVID-19: a case series. EClinicalMedicine. 2020;24:100434.
46. Iba T, Levy JH, Connors JM, et al. The unique characteristics of COVID-19 coagulopathy. Crit Care. 2020;24(1):360.
47. Post A, den Deurwaarder ESG, Bakker SJL, et al. Kidney infarction in patients with COVID-19. Am J Kidney Dis. 2020;76(3):431–5.
48. Goshua G, Pine AB, Meizlish ML, et al. Endotheliopathy in COVID-19-associated coagulopathy: evidence from a single-centre, cross-sectional study. Lancet Haematol. 2020;7(8):e575–82.
49. Mukherjee A, Ghosh R, Furment MM. Case report: COVID-19 associated renal infarction and ascending aortic thrombosis. Am J Trop Med Hyg. 2020;103(5):1989–92.
50. Fu D, Yan B, Xu J, et al. COVID-19 infection in a patient with end-stage kidney disease. Nephron. 2020;144(5):245–7.

51. Kunutsor SK, Laukkanen JA. Renal complications in COVID-19: a systematic review and meta-analysis. Ann Med. 2020;52(7):345–53.
52. Ng JH, Hirsch JS, Wanchoo R, et al. Outcomes of patients with end-stage kidney disease hospitalized with COVID-19. Kidney Int. 2020;98(6):1530–9.
53. Kamel MH, Mahmoud H, Zhen A, et al. End-stage kidney disease and COVID-19 in an urban safety-net hospital in Boston, Massachusetts. PLoS One. 2021;16(6):e0252679.
54. Naaraayan A, Nimkar A, Hasan A, et al. End-stage renal disease patients on chronic hemodialysis fare better with COVID-19: a retrospective cohort study from the New York Metropolitan Region. Cureus. 2020;12(9):e10373.
55. La Milia V, Bacchini G, Bigi MC, et al. COVID-19 outbreak in a large hemodialysis center in Lombardy, Italy. Kidney Int. 2020;5(7):1095–9.
56. Ahmed W, Al Obaidli AAK, Joseph P, et al. Outcomes of patients with end stage kidney disease on dialysis with COVID-19 in Abu Dhabi, United Arab Emirates; from PCR to antibody. BMC Nephrol. 2021;22(1):198.
57. Peluso G, Campanile S, Scotti A, Tammaro V, Jamshidi A, Pelosio L, Caggiano M, et al. COVID-19 and living donor kidney transplantation in Naples during the pandemic. Biomed Res Int. 2020;2020:5703963.
58. González J, Ciancio G. Early experience with COVID-19 in kidney transplantation recipients: update and review. Int Braz J Urol. 2020;46(Suppl 1):145–55.
59. Abu Jawdeh BG. COVID-19 in kidney transplantation: outcomes, immunosuppression management, and operational challenges. Adv Chronic Kidney Dis. 2020;27(5):383–9.
60. Fisher DA, Carson G. Back to basics: the outbreak response pillars. Lancet. 2020;396:597–8.
61. Cravedi P, Mothi SS, Azzi Y, Haverly M, Farouk SS, Pérez-Sáez MJ, Redondo-Pachón MD, et al. COVID-19 and kidney transplantation: results from the TANGO International Transplant Consortium. Am J Transplant. 2020;20(11):3140–8.
62. Akalin E, Azzi Y, Bartash R, Seethamraju H, Parides M, Hemmige V, et al. Covid-19 and kidney transplantation. N Engl J Med. 2020;382(25):2475–7.
63. Hilbrands LB, Duivenvoorden R, Vart P, Franssen CFM, Hemmelder MH, Jager KJ, et al. COVID-19-related mortality in kidney transplant and dialysis patients: results of the ERACODA collaboration. Nephrol Dial Transplant. 2020;35(11):1973–83.
64. Genovese G, Friedman DJ, Ross MD, Lecordier L, Uzureau P, Freedman BI, et al. Association of trypanolytic ApoL1 variants with kidney disease in African-Americans. Science. 2010;329:841–5.
65. Kopp JB, Nelson GW, Sampath K, Johnson RC, Genovese G, An P, et al. APOL1 genetic variants in focal segmental glomerulosclerosis and HIV-associated nephropathy. J Am Soc Nephrol. 2011;22(11):2129–37.
66. Tayo BO, Kramer H, Salako BL, Gottesman O, McKenzie CA, Ogunniyi A, et al. Genetic variation in APOL1 and MYH9 genes is associated with chronic kidney disease among Nigerians. Int Urol Nephrol. 2013;45(2):485–94.
67. Ulasi II, Tzur S, Wasser WG, Shemer R, Kruzel E, Feigin E, et al. High population frequencies of APOL1 risk variants are associated with increased prevalence of non-diabetic chronic kidney disease in the Igbo people from South-Eastern Nigeria. Nephron Clin Pract. 2013;123(1–2):123–8.
68. Kissling S, Rotman S, Gerber C, Halfon M, Lamoth F, Comte D, et al. Collapsing glomerulopathy in a COVID-19 patient. Kidney Int. 2020;98(1):228–31.
69. Larsen CP, Bourne TD, Wilson JD, Saqqa O, Sharshir MA. Collapsing glomerulopathy in a patient with Coronavirus Disease 2019 (COVID-19). Kidney Int Rep. 2020;5(6):935–9.
70. Mohamed MMB, Lukitsch I, Torres-Ortiz AE, Walker JB, Varghese V, Hernandez-Arroyo CF, et al. Acute kidney injury associated with Coronavirus Disease 2019 in Urban New Orleans. Kidney360. 2020;1(7):614–22.
71. Peleg Y, Kudose S, D'Agati V, Siddall E, Ahmad S, Kisselev S, et al. Acute kidney injury due to collapsing glomerulopathy following COVID-19 infection. Kidney Int Rep. 2020;5(6):940–5.

72. Dummer PD, Limou S, Rosenberg AZ, Heymann J, Nelson G, Winkler CA, et al. APOL1 kidney disease risk variants: an evolving landscape. Semin Nephrol. 2015;35(3):222–36.
73. Kasembeli AN, Duarte R, Ramsay M, Mosiane P, Dickens C, Dix-Peek T, et al. APOL1 risk variants are strongly associated with HIV-associated nephropathy in black South Africans. J Am Soc Nephrol. 2015;26(11):2882–90.
74. Hirsch JS, Ng JH, Ross DW, Sharma P, Shah HH, Barnett RL, et al. Acute kidney injury in patients hospitalized with COVID-19. Kidney Int. 2020;98(1):209–18.
75. Nichols B, Jog P, Lee JH, Blackler D, Wilmot M, D'Agati V, et al. Innate immunity pathways regulate the nephropathy gene apolipoprotein L1. Kidney Int. 2015;87:332–42.
76. Wang M, Cao R, Zhang L, et al. Remdesivir and chloroquine effectively inhibit the recently emerged novel coronavirus (2019-nCoV) in vitro. Cell Res. 2020;30(3):269–71.
77. Wang R. Two's company, three's a crowd: can H_2S be the third endogenous gaseous transmitter? FASEB J. 2002;16(13):1792–8.
78. Xia M, Chen L, Muh RW, Li PL, Li N. Production and action of hydrogen sulfide, a novel gaseous bioactive substance in the kidneys. J Pharmacol Exp Ther. 2009;329:1056–62.
79. Mikami Y, Shinuya N, Kimura Y, Nagahara N, Ogasawara Y, Kimura H. Thioredoxin and dihydrolipoic acid are required for 3-mercaptopyruvate sulfurtransferase to produce hydrogen sulfide. Biochem J. 2011;439:479–85.
80. Modis K, Coletta C, Erdelyi K, Papapetropoulos A, Szabo C. Intramitochondrial hydrogen sulfide production by 3-mercaptopyruvate sulfurtransferase maintains mitochondrial electron transport flow and supports cellular biogenesis. FASEB J. 2013;27:601–11.
81. Shibuya N, Koike S, Tanaka M, et al. A novel pathway for the production of hydrogen sulfide from D-cysteine in mammalian cells. Nat Commun. 2013;4:1366.
82. Yamamoto J, Sato W, Kosugi T, Yamamoto T, Kimura T, Taniguchi S, et al. Distribution of hydrogen sulfide (H_2S)-producing enzymes and the roles of the H_2S donor sodium hydrosulfide in diabetic nephropathy. Clin Exp Nephrol. 2013;17(1):32–40.
83. Dugbartey GJ, Talaei F, Houwertjes MC, Goris M, Epema AH, Bouma HR, Henning RH. Dopamine treatment attenuates acute kidney injury in a rat model of deep hypothermia and rewarming—the role of renal H_2S-producing enzymes. Eur J Pharmacol. 2015a;769:225–33.
84. Tomita M, Nagahara N, Ito T. Expression of 3-mercaptopyruvate sulfurtransferase in the mouse. Molecules. 2016;21(12):1707.
85. Kulkarni KH, Monjok EM, Zeyssig R, Kouamou G, Bongmba ON, Opere CA, Njie YF, Ohia SE. Effect of hydrogen sulfide on sympathetic neurotransmission and catecholamine levels in isolated porcine iris-ciliary body. Neurochem Res. 2009;34(3):400–6.
86. Li L, Whiteman M, Guan YY, Neo KL, Cheng Y, Lee SW, et al. Characterization of a novel, water-soluble hydrogen sulfide-releasing molecule (GYY4137): new insights into the biology of hydrogen sulfide. Circulation. 2008;117:2351–60.
87. Gerő D, Torregrossa R, Perry A, Waters A, Le-Trionnaire S, Whatmore JL, Wood M, Whiteman M. The novel mitochondria-targeted hydrogen sulfide (H_2S) donors AP123 and AP39 protect against hyperglycemic injury in microvascular endothelial cells in vitro. Pharmacol Res. 2016;113(Pt A):186–98.
88. Powell CR, Dillon KM, Matson JB. A review of hydrogen sulfide (H_2S) donors: chemistry and potential therapeutic applications. Biochem Pharmacol. 2018;149:110–23.
89. Zhang H, Bai Z, Zhu L, Liang Y, Fan X, Li J, Wen H, Shi T, Zhao Q, Wang Z. Hydrogen sulfide donors: therapeutic potential in anti-atherosclerosis. Eur J Med Chem. 2020;205:112665.
90. Strazzula L, Nigwekar SU, Steele D, et al. Intralesional sodium thiosulfate for the treatment of calciphylaxis. JAMA Dermatol. 2013;149(8):946–9.
91. Li H, Ma Y, Escaffre O, Ivanciuc T, Komaravelli N, Kelley JP, Coletta C, Szabo C, Rockx B, Garofalo RP, Casola A. Role of hydrogen sulfide in paramyxovirus infections. J Virol. 2015;89(10):5557–68.
92. Ivanciuc T, Sbrana E, Ansar M, Bazhanov N, Szabo C, Casola A, Garofalo RP. Hydrogen sulfide is an antiviral and anti-inflammatory endogenous gasotransmitter in the airways. Role in respiratory syncytial virus infection. Am J Respir Cell Mol Biol. 2016;55(5):684–96.

93. Bazhanov N, Escaffre O, Freiberg AN, Garofalo RP, Casola A. Broad-range antiviral activity of hydrogen sulfide against highly pathogenic RNA viruses. Sci Rep. 2017;7:41029.
94. Bazhanov N, Ivanciuc T, Wu H, Garofalo M, Kang J, Xian M, Casola A. Thiol-activated hydrogen sulfide donors antiviral and anti-inflammatory activity in respiratory syncytial virus infection. Viruses. 2018;10(5):249.
95. Fang F, Li H, Cui W, Dong Y. Treatment of hepatitis caused by cytomegalovirus with allitridin injection—an experimental study. J Tongji Med Univ. 1999;19(4):271–4.
96. Martelli A, Citi V, Testai L, Brogi S, Calderone V. Organic isothiocyanates as hydrogen sulfide donors. Antioxid Redox Signal. 2020;32(2):110–44.
97. Lin CW, Tsai FJ, Tsai CH, Lai CC, Wan L, Ho TY, Hsieh CC, Chao PD. Anti-SARS coronavirus 3C-like protease effects of *Isatis indigotica* root and plant-derived phenolic compounds. Antiviral Res. 2005;68(1):36–42.
98. Palamara AT, Perno CF, Ciriolo MR, Dini L, Balestra E, D'Agostini C, Di Francesco P, Favalli C, Rotilio G, Garaci E. Evidence for antiviral activity of glutathione: in vitro inhibition of herpes simplex virus type 1 replication. Antiviral Res. 1995;27(3):237–53.
99. Kim J, Zhang J, Cha Y, Kolitz S, Funt J, Escalante Chong R, Barrett S, Kusko R, Zeskind B, Kaufman H. Advanced bioinformatics rapidly identifies existing therapeutics for patients with Coronavirus Disease-2019 (COVID-19). J Transl Med. 2020;18(1):257.
100. Horoz M, Bolukbas C, Bolukbas FF, Aslan M, Koylu AO, Selek S, Erel O. Oxidative stress in hepatitis C infected end-stage renal disease subjects. BMC Infect Dis. 2006;6:114.
101. Pozzi G, Masselli E, Gobbi G, Mirandola P, Taborda-Barata L, Ampollini L, Carbognani P, Micheloni C, Corazza F, Galli D, Carubbi C, Vitale M. Hydrogen sulfide inhibits TMPRSS2 in human airway epithelial cells: implications for SARS-CoV-2 infection. Biomedicine. 2021;9(9):1273.
102. Lin Y, Zeng H, Gao L, Gu T, Wang C, Zhang H. Hydrogen sulfide attenuates atherosclerosis in a partially ligated carotid artery mouse model via regulating angiotensin converting enzyme 2 expression. Front Physiol. 2017;8:782.
103. Hati S, Bhattacharyya S. Impact of thiol-disulfide balance on the binding of Covid-19 spike protein with angiotensin-converting enzyme 2 receptor. ACS Omega. 2020;5(26):16292–8.
104. Manček-Keber M, Hafner-Bratkovič I, Lainšček D, et al. Disruption of disulfides within RBD of SARS-CoV-2 spike protein prevents fusion and represents a target for viral entry inhibition by registered drugs. FASEB J. 2021;35(6):e21651.
105. Sallenave JM, Guillot L. Innate immune signaling and proteolytic pathways in the resolution or exacerbation of SARS-CoV-2 in Covid-19: key therapeutic targets? Front Immunol. 2020;11:1229.
106. Chen YH, Teng X, Hu ZJ, Tian DY, Jin S, Wu YM. Hydrogen sulfide attenuated sepsis-induced myocardial dysfunction through TLR4 pathway and endoplasmic reticulum stress. Front Physiol. 2021;12:653601.
107. Varga Z, Flammer AJ, Steiger P, et al. Endothelial cell infection and endotheliitis in COVID-19. Lancet. 2020;395(10234):1417–8.
108. Citi V, Martelli A, Gorica E, Brogi S, Testai L, Calderone V. Role of hydrogen sulfide in endothelial dysfunction: pathophysiology and therapeutic approaches. J Adv Res. 2020;27:99–113.
109. Sun HJ, Wu ZY, Nie XW, Bian JS. Role of endothelial dysfunction in cardiovascular diseases: the link between inflammation and hydrogen sulfide. Front Pharmacol. 2020;10:1568.
110. Porzionato A, Emmi A, Barbon S, et al. Sympathetic activation: a potential link between comorbidities and COVID-19. FEBS J. 2020;287(17):3681–8.
111. Guo Q, Jin S, Wang XL, Wang R, Xiao L, He RR, Wu YM. Hydrogen sulfide in the rostral ventrolateral medulla inhibits sympathetic vasomotor tone through ATP-sensitive K^+ channels. J Pharmacol Exp Ther. 2011;338(2):458–65.
112. Duan XC, Guo R, Liu SY, Xiao L, Xue HM, Guo Q, Jin S, Wu YM. Gene transfer of cystathionine beta-synthase into RVLM increases hydrogen sulfide-mediated suppression of sympathetic outflow via KATP channel in normotensive rats. Am J Physiol Heart Circ Physiol. 2015;308(6):H603–11.

113. Salvi A, Bankhele P, Jamil JM, Kulkarni-Chitnis M, Njie-Mbye YF, Ohia SE, Opere CA. Pharmacological actions of hydrogen sulfide donors on sympathetic neurotransmission in the bovine anterior uvea, in vitro. Neurochem Res. 2016;41(5):1020–8.
114. Palmeira A, Sousa E, Köseler A, et al. Preliminary virtual screening studies to identify GRP78 inhibitors which may interfere with SARS-CoV-2 infection. Pharmaceuticals (Basel). 2020;13(6):132.
115. Yi J, Yuan Y, Zheng J, Hu N. Hydrogen sulfide alleviates uranium-induced kidney cell apoptosis mediated by ER stress via 20S proteasome involving in Akt/GSK-3β/Fyn-Nrf2 signaling. Free Radic Res. 2018;52(9):1020–9.
116. Wei H, Zhang R, Jin H, et al. Hydrogen sulfide attenuates hyperhomocysteinemia-induced cardiomyocytic endoplasmic reticulum stress in rats. Antioxid Redox Signal. 2010;12(9):1079–91.
117. Lin F, Liao C, Sun Y, et al. Hydrogen sulfide inhibits cigarette smoke-induced endoplasmic reticulum stress and apoptosis in bronchial epithelial cells. Front Pharmacol. 2017;8:675.
118. Dugbartey GJ, Bouma HR, Strijkstra AM, Boerema AS, Henning RH. Induction of a torpor-like state by 5′-AMP does not depend on H_2S production. PLoS One. 2015;10(8):e0136113.
119. Wan C, Zhang C. Kidney injury molecule-1: a novel entry factor for SARS-CoV-2. J Mol Cell Biol. 2021;13(3):159–60.
120. Ichimura T, Mori Y, Aschauer P, et al. KIM-1/TIM-1 is a receptor for SARS-CoV-2 in lung and kidney. medRxiv. 2020;2020:20190694. https://doi.org/10.1101/2020.09.16.20190694.
121. Yang C, Zhang Y, Zeng X, et al. Kidney injury molecule-1 is a potential receptor for SARS-CoV-2. J Mol Cell Biol. 2021;13(3):185–96.
122. Zhen H, Fang F, Ye DY, Shu SN, Zhou YF, Dong YS, Nie XC, Li G. Experimental study on the action of allitridin against human cytomegalovirus in vitro: inhibitory effects on immediate-early genes. Antiviral Res. 2006;72(1):68–74.
123. Pacheco A. Sulfur-containing compounds as hydrogen sulfide donors and broad-spectrum antiviral agents. Washington State University ProQuest Dissertations Publishing; 2017.
124. Renieris G, Katrini K, Damoulari C, Akinosoglou K, Psarrakis C, Kyriakopoulou M, Dimopoulos G, Lada M, Koufargyris P, Giamarellos-Bourboulis EJ. Serum hydrogen sulfide and outcome association in pneumonia by the SARS-CoV-2 coronavirus. Shock. 2020;54(5):633–7.
125. Gubernatorova EO, Gorshkova EA, Polinova AI, Drutskaya MS. IL-6: relevance for immunopathology of SARS-CoV-2. Cytokine Growth Factor Rev. 2020;53:13–24.
126. Lobb I, Zhu J, Liu W, Haig A, Lan Z, Sener A. Hydrogen sulfide treatment improves long-term renal dysfunction resulting from prolonged warm renal ischemia-reperfusion injury. Can Urol Assoc J. 2014;8(5–6):413.
127. Zhang HX, Liu SJ, Tang XL, Duan GL, Ni X, Zhu XY, Liu YJ, Wang CN. H_2S attenuates LPS-induced acute lung injury by reducing oxidative/nitrative stress and inflammation. Cell Physiol Biochem. 2016;40(6):1603–12.
128. Ibrahim H, Perl A, Smith D, Lewis T, Kon Z, Goldenberg R, Yarta K, Staniloae C, Williams M. Therapeutic blockade of inflammation in severe COVID-19 infection with intravenous N-acetylcysteine. Clin Immunol. 2020;219:108544.
129. Puyo C, Kreig D, Saddi V, Ansari E, Prince O. Case report: use of hydroxychloroquine and N-acetylcysteine for treatment of a COVID-19 positive patient. F1000Research. 2020;9:491.
130. Liu Y, Wang M, Luo G, et al. Experience of N-acetylcysteine airway management in the successful treatment of one case of critical condition with COVID-19: a case report. Medicine (Baltimore). 2020;99(42):e22577.
131. de Alencar JCG, Moreira CL, Müller AD, Chaves CE, Fukuhara MA, et al. Double-blind, randomized, placebo-controlled trial with N-acetylcysteine for treatment of severe acute respiratory syndrome caused by COVID-19. Clin Infect Dis. 2021;72(11):e736–41.
132. Dominic P, Ahmad J, Bhandari R, Pardue S, Solorzano J, Jaisingh K, Watts M, Bailey SR, Orr AW, Kevil CG, Kolluru GK. Decreased availability of nitric oxide and hydrogen sulfide is a hallmark of COVID-19. Redox Biol. 2021;43:101982.

133. Pfister F, Vonbrunn E, Ries T, Jäck HM, Überla K, Lochnit G, Sheriff A, Herrmann M, Büttner-Herold M, Amann K, Daniel C. Complement activation in kidneys of patients with COVID-19. Front Immunol. 2021;11:594849.
134. Lu X, Li W, Wang G, Wang Q, Jiang Y, Gao J, Zhao X, Xu L. Effect of hydrogen sulfide on tissue factor-induced disseminated intravascular coagulation in rabbits. Zhonghua Wei Zhong Bing Ji Jiu Yi Xue. 2015;27(2):92–6.
135. Grambow E, Leppin C, Leppin K, Kundt G, Klar E, Frank M, Vollmar B. The effects of hydrogen sulfide on platelet-leukocyte aggregation and microvascular thrombolysis. Platelets. 2017;28(5):509–17.

Chapter 7
Hydrogen Sulfide for Prevention of Obstructive Nephropathy

Shouzhe Lin, Smriti Juriasingani, George J. Dugbartey, and Alp Sener

This chapter is a modified version by the same authors in the publication titled Is Hydrogen Sulfide a Potential Novel Therapy to Prevent Renal Damage During Ureteral Obstruction? Nitric Oxide. 2018; 73:15–21.

S. Lin · S. Juriasingani
Department of Microbiology and Immunology, Schulich School of Medicine and Dentistry, University of Western Ontario, London, ON, Canada

Matthew Mailing Centre for Translational Transplant Studies, University Hospital, London Health Sciences Centre, London, ON, Canada
e-mail: slin223@uwo.ca

G. J. Dugbartey (⊠)
Matthew Mailing Centre for Translational Transplant Studies, University Hospital, London Health Sciences Centre, London, ON, Canada

Department of Surgery, Schulich School of Medicine and Dentistry, St. Joseph's Health Care London, London, ON, Canada

Department of Pharmacology and Toxicology, School of Pharmacy, College of Health Sciences, University of Ghana, Accra, Ghana

Department of Physiology and Pharmacology, Accra College of Medicine, Accra, Ghana
e-mail: gdugbart@uwo.ca

A. Sener
Department of Microbiology and Immunology, Schulich School of Medicine and Dentistry, University of Western Ontario, London, ON, Canada

Matthew Mailing Centre for Translational Transplant Studies, University Hospital, London Health Sciences Centre, London, ON, Canada

Department of Surgery, Schulich School of Medicine and Dentistry, St. Joseph's Health Care London, London, ON, Canada
e-mail: alp.sener@lhsc.on.ca

G. J. Dugbartey, A. Sener, *Hydrogen Sulfide in Kidney Diseases*,
https://doi.org/10.1007/978-3-031-44041-0_7

143

Obstructive Nephropathy

Obstructive nephropathy occurs due to abnormalities in the urinary tract that result in the blockage of urine flow. The prevalence and etiology of obstructive nephropathy vary with age. The highest rate of obstructive nephropathy occurs in children; these incidences are typically congenital defects that arise during embryonic development, resulting in anatomical abnormalities that obstruct the urinary tract. Congenital obstructive nephropathy is one of the leading causes of end-stage renal disease (ESRD) in children and accounts for 16.5% of all pediatric renal transplantations in North America [1]. In the young and middle-aged adult, urinary obstructions are typically caused due to obstructive calculi (kidney stones). Studies estimate that approximately 10–15% of Americans will develop obstructive stones in their lifetime, with 40% risk of recurrence at 5 years that increases to 75% at 20 years [2]. In elderly patients, urinary tract obstructions are more common in males and are typically caused by benign prostatic hyperplasia or prostate cancer [3]. Ureteral obstructions can be unilateral or bilateral and can be classified based on the degree (complete or partial obstruction) and duration (acute and chronic). In this chapter, we will focus on the outcomes, pathophysiology, and potential therapies for mitigating renal damage caused by chronic complete unilateral ureteral obstruction (UUO).

Pathogenesis of Obstructive Nephropathy

Urinary tract obstruction is one of the many causes of acute kidney injury (AKI) and chronic kidney disease (CKD). A possible treatment for AKI is dialysis, a process that can take days to weeks. While the mortality rate attributed to AKI is approximately 50%, death from CKD-related injury or the need for dialysis and renal transplantation is generally the ultimate outcome of chronic ureteral obstruction [4]. AKI and CKD share similar pathogenesis, including cellular injury, cell death, and inflammation. Additionally, tubulointerstitial fibrosis is often observed in CKD and can also be detected in severe cases of AKI. All these processes can contribute to the irreversible renal injury and dysfunction caused by UUO [4].

Hemodynamics and Functional Changes in Obstructive Nephropathy

Upon complete UUO, an initial increase in renal blood flow into the obstructed kidney is observed. This is a result of prostaglandin and prostacyclin production due to medullary compression. After a few hours with persisting obstruction, renal blood flow decreases due to increased vascular resistance and production of vaso-constrictors such as angiotensin II (Ang II) and thromboxane A2. Together, these events lead to reduced glomerular filtration rate (GFR). Correspondingly, an initial increase in intratubular pressure is observed. While this rise is observed in the first few hours, intratubular pressure decreases to pre-obstructive values within the first 24 h. This decline in pressure is caused by decreased GFR, increased sodium reab-sorption, and increased removal of tubular fluid through lymphatic drainage. Collectively, these actions decrease renal fluid volume [3]. Obstruction can also cause functional changes in renal tubular cells. Initially, there is an increase in sodium reabsorption in the renal tubules to maintain renal fluid volume. However, as the obstruction persists, sodium wasting occurs due to renal tubular injury and defects in the sodium/potassium ATPase enzymes. This disrupts the lumen poten-tial, which is necessary for hydrogen and potassium excretion. The resulting reten-tion of hydrogen leads to renal tubular acidosis. Furthermore, this prevents the distal nephrons from concentrating urine, which contributes to diuresis and an inability to acidify urine upon relief of obstruction [3]. In chronic obstructive nephropathy, the reduction of renal blood flow is maintained, which places the kidney in a state of ischemia. Consequently, reactive oxygen species (ROS) that are harmful to renal tubular cells are generated, resulting in tubular injury and activation of renin–angio-tensin–aldosterone system (RAAS), which increases the production of Ang II. Together, these factors cause the recruitment of inflammatory cells to the site of injury, ultimately leading to cell death and release of transforming growth factor-beta 1 (TGF-β1) [3].

Renal Tubular Injury and Cell Death in Obstructive Nephropathy

Renal tubular cell death occurs via apoptosis or necrosis and is a result of the mechanical and oxidative stress associated with ureteral obstruction. Apoptosis (cell suicide) is the main form of cell death observed in urinary obstruction and CKD [4]. Apoptosis is characterized by chromosome condensation and cellular blebbing, and this form of cell death is regulated by increased expression of intra-cellular lethal molecules and downregulation of pro-survival mediators. A large variety of factors associated with obstruction, such as ischemia, hypoxia, Ang II, ROS, tumor necrosis factor α (TNF-α), and mechanical stretching, can lead to mitochondrial destabilization and release of cytochrome C. This ultimately stimu-lates the caspase-mediated apoptotic pathway and contributes to tubular cell death [5]. These apoptotic cells are subsequently removed by infiltrating macrophages and neighboring native cells [5]. Necrosis, on the other hand, is characterized by loss of cell membrane integrity and uncontrolled release of intracellular contents.

Lethal stimuli released due to tissue injury and oxidative stress cause necrotic cell death, which results in the release of damage-associated molecular patterns (DAMPs) such as high-mobility group box 1. The release of DAMPs activates Toll-like receptors, which recruits leukocytes to the site of injury and subsequently initiates tissue inflammation [6]. Though prominent in the early stages of pathogenesis and inflammation, necrosis is not frequently observed in chronic renal injury [4].

Renal Tissue Inflammation in Obstructive Nephropathy

Renal interstitial inflammation is an early response to obstructive nephropathy, and it is characterized by infiltration of leukocytes that are attracted to cytokines, chemokines, and membrane adhesion molecules released by injured renal parenchymal and endothelial cells. Interstitial leukocyte population increases from 12 h up to 14 days post-obstruction and consists predominantly of macrophages [4]. Macrophages can be classically activated (M1) to produce cytokines and chemokines that induce inflammation, tubular apoptosis, and fibrosis or alternatively activated (M2) to attenuate inflammation. M1 macrophages generate ROS and TNF-α, which ultimately exacerbate the death of renal epithelial cells [7]. Additionally, interleukin (IL)-1β production can be observed. Together with TNF-α, IL-1β targets nuclear factor-kappaB (NF-κB) to increase the production of pro-inflammatory mediators such as monocyte chemoattractant protein-1 (MCP-1) and IL-1β [8], resulting in an amplified inflammatory response. M2 macrophages, on the other hand, appear in the later stages of inflammation. They play a critical role in the uptake of apoptotic cells, suppression of immune responses, and induction of tissue remodeling [7]. These macrophages release IL-4, IL-13, IL-10, and TGF-β1 to reduce tissue inflammation and induce tissue repair. Importantly, TGF-β1 plays a crucial role in the induction of fibrosis, which leads to tissue scarring and loss of function [6].

Tubulointerstitial Fibrosis in Obstructive Nephropathy

As the chronic inflammation associated with obstructive nephropathy persists, the fibrotic characteristics of CKD are eventually observed. Fibrosis is characterized by activation of fibroblasts that deposit extracellular matrix (ECM) components, such as fibronectin and collagen type I and III into the interstitial space [9]. These fibroblasts can be a result of proliferating resident fibroblasts or they can be derived from tubular epithelial cells undergoing epithelial-mesenchymal transition (EMT) [10]. TGF-β1 is a pro-fibrotic cytokine released during inflammation that plays a critical role in initiating the EMT response. Upon stimulation with TGF-β1, Smad 2 and Smad 3 proteins are phosphorylated to induce fibrosis. Meanwhile, Smad 7, an inhibitor of the fibrotic pathway, is degraded via ubiquitination. Under these circumstances, renal epithelial cells lose their adhesions to neighboring cells and the basement membrane. They also display increased expression of mesenchymal proteins (such as vimentin), decreased expression of epithelial proteins (such as E-cadherin), and migration into the interstitium [4, 11]. Propagation of tubulointerstitial fibrosis is commonly observed in CKD, and it can lead to irreversible renal injury and loss of renal function [12]. Due to its ability to stimulate TGF-β1 production, Ang II is also a key mediator in the initiation of renal fibrosis. Previous studies have demonstrated that administration of enalapril, an angiotensin-converting enzyme (ACE) inhibitor, decreases production of TGF-β1 mRNA [13], and treatment with losartan, an angiotensin AT1 receptor inhibitor, attenuates the progression of renal fibrosis [14]. Additionally, the synthesis of active TGF-β1 requires the conversion of latent pre-pro-TGF-β1 to TGF-β1, its biologically active form, and this process is promoted by RAS [15]. Taken together, these studies suggest that Ang II plays a critical role in the initiation of renal fibrosis by stimulating TGF-β1 production. The increase in TGF-β1 levels leads to the induction of EMT in renal epithelial cells and ultimately results in tubulointerstitial fibrosis characteristic of CKD [16]. In addition, Ang II also contributes to fibrosis indirectly by increasing the proliferation of renal fibroblasts. Ang II produced as a result of ureteral obstruction causes vasoconstriction, which leads to local ischemia and hypoxia. Tubular cells subsequently undergo atrophy and cell death due to restricted blood flow, reduced nutrients, and depleted oxygen supply. The remaining cells undergo hypermetabolism, resulting in increased oxygen consumption and ultimately, perpetuation and exacerbation of hypoxia in the interstitium. This causes fibroblasts to proliferate and induce ECM production by epithelial cells [12]. Furthermore, Ang II stimulates TNF-α production, which increases the formation of superoxide anions and perpetuates inflammation, thereby indirectly exacerbating the progression of fibrosis [12]. The complex mechanisms underlying the pathogenesis of obstructive uropathy are summarized in Fig. 7.1.

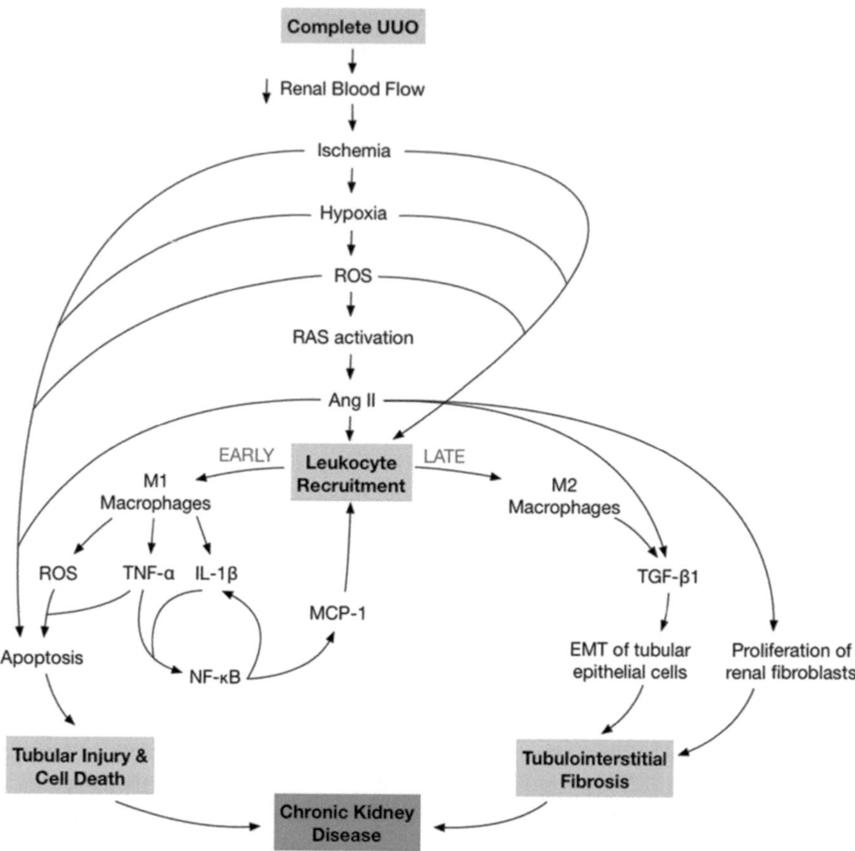

Fig. 7.1 The pathogenesis of obstructive nephropathy. Complete unilateral urinary obstruction (UUO) causes hemodynamic changes, inflammatory responses, and irreversible fibrosis that can ultimately lead to chronic kidney disease (CKD). Early hemodynamic changes and inflammatory responses (mediated by M1 macrophages) lead to tubular injury and cell death via apoptosis. As inflammation persists, TGF-β1 release by M2 macrophages causes epithelial-mesenchymal transition (EMT) of tubular epithelial cells. Additionally, persisting Ang II release due to decreased renal blood flow leads to proliferation of renal fibroblasts. Both of these mechanisms contribute to the fibrosis that is associated with CKD. Together, tubulointerstitial fibrosis along with tubular injury and cell death causes the pathophysiology associated with CKD

Recovery Upon Relief of Ureteral Obstruction

While surgical removal of UUO removes the source of injury, recovery of renal function is dependent on the duration of the obstruction, and it is important to note that renal function may not return to pre-obstruction levels [17]. Studies demonstrate that relief after 48 h of obstruction in neonatal rats was not able to recover the 40% loss of nephrons and did not improve tubular proliferation [18]. In addition, relief of obstruction was not able to fully return TGF-β1 and vimentin expression to normal levels, suggesting that tubular injury continues to persist [18]. Similarly, Chaabane et al. observed a 40% reduction in GFR and a 50% reduction of glomerulotubular integrity after a 30-day recovery following a 7-day obstruction in rats. Furthermore, albuminuria was also observed, implicating residual glomerular injury [19]. Therefore, while relief of UUO attenuates obstructive nephropathy, complete recovery of renal function is unlikely. Thus, prevention of renal injury during obstruction may be a potential treatment option to improve post-obstructive renal function [18].

Animal Models of Obstructive Nephropathy

One of the most widely used experimental models of obstructive nephropathy is the UUO model. Male rodents are typically used in this experimental model, as female sex organs increase the technical difficulty of the procedure. After placing the animal, usually a male rat, under general anesthesia, a midline incision is made in the abdomen and the left ureter is found. Two sutures, one proximal and one distal to the kidney, are made in the ureter to permanently ligate the ureter. This procedure inflicts renal injury upon the obstructed kidney while allowing the contralateral kidney to compensate for the unilateral loss of function [4]. There are several advantages of this model: it is a relatively simple procedure, it does not involve the use of an exogenous toxin, and it does not create a uremic environment [20]. Additionally, this model can be used to explore both acute and chronic renal injury, as the initial insult can result in AKI and persistence of obstruction can produce histological indices of CKD, particularly fibrosis, after a few weeks [4]. While renal injury in the UUO model can be histologically evaluated, functional changes of the obstructed kidney cannot be determined as the contralateral kidney compensates for the loss of renal function. Tapmeier et al. developed the unilateral ureteral obstruction and reimplantation (UUO-R) model, in which the obstructed ureter is reimplanted into the bladder, thus emulating relief of obstruction. The contralateral kidney is subsequently removed, which causes the animal to depend solely on the previously obstructed kidney and allows for both histological and functional evaluation of the obstructed kidney [21].

Pharmacological Interventions in Obstructive Nephropathy

To complement surgical relief of obstruction, pharmacological treatments may be used to prevent the recurrence of stones, treat existing stones, or manage symptoms associated with obstruction. Diuretics, such as thiazide diuretics and indapamide, can decrease calcium excretion and therefore reduce the risk of calcium stone formation. While beneficial, these drugs may cause hypocitraturia, hypokalemia, hyponatremia, dizziness, weakness, and gastrointestinal upset [22]. Potassium citrate and sodium citrate are two common urinary alkalinizers used to prevent crystallization. However, like diuretics, they may also cause gastrointestinal distress. Additionally, a common side effect of potassium-containing therapeutics is hyperkalemia, which can potentially be dangerous in patients with renal failure [22]. To treat uric acid stones, xanthine oxidase inhibitors are often used, as they decrease urinary acid excretion. However, they are often associated with hepatotoxicity, skin rashes, and gastrointestinal distress [22]. Due to poor intestinal or renal tubular transport of cystine, high urinary cystine levels may cause cystine stone formation. As such, tiopronin and D-penicillamine are typically used to form disulfides to decrease cystine excretion and reduce the risk of cystine stone formation [22]. Furthermore, severe flank pain is a common symptom among patients with urinary obstruction. As a result, acetaminophen, cyclooxygenase inhibitors, nonsteroidal anti-inflammatory drugs (NSAIDs), and opioids are typically prescribed to manage pain. However, these drugs can have mild-to-severe side effects, including gastrointestinal distress, hepatotoxicity, respiratory depression, and addiction [22]. Additionally, several pharmacological interventions are available to induce the expulsion of urinary stones. For instance, alpha-blockers may improve the expulsion of urinary stones by inducing ureter relaxation; however, these drugs may cause nausea and nasal congestion [22]. While effective, these drugs are not able to mitigate the accumulation of renal injury during obstruction. If prolonged, obstruction can cause irreversible renal injury and lead to permanent loss of renal function [23]. Furthermore, studies have shown that relief of obstruction can only mitigate, but not reverse, renal injury [24]. Therefore, preemptive therapies administered during obstruction may help improve renal function following the relief of obstruction.

Endogenous Gasotransmitters and Their Potential Roles in the Treatment of Obstructive Nephropathy

Recent evidence suggests that gasotransmitters can exhibit anti-inflammatory and antioxidant effects in various models of tissue injury [25]. Gasotransmitters are small, endogenously produced gaseous molecules that have specific cellular and molecular targets, can freely permeate membranes, and have physiological functions [26]. Currently, nitric oxide, carbon monoxide, and hydrogen sulfide are identified as gasotransmitters. Nitric oxide (NO) is produced endogenously from L-arginine by nitric oxide synthases (NOS). It leads to the activation of protein kinases and mediates various physiological responses [26]. In inflammatory processes, NO can act as a "double-edged sword" depending on its concentration. Pro-inflammatory cytokines lead to excessive production of NO that can cause phagocyte recruitment to the site of inflammation and lead to sepsis due to positive feedback that generates supraphysiological concentrations of NO [27, 28]. However, at low concentrations, NO plays an anti-inflammatory role by reducing the expression of endothelial cell adhesion molecules, which inhibits leukocyte adhesion to the endothelium [28]. Furthermore, studies have shown that treatment with L-arginine ameliorates renal fibrosis, apoptosis, and inflammation following UUO, which suggests that NO is a potential therapeutic agent in obstructive uropathy [29]. Carbon monoxide (CO) is endogenously produced by heme oxygenase, and like NO, it can also mediate physiological responses [30]. Though toxic at high concentrations, CO can be therapeutic at low doses. For instance, like NO, CO also exhibits anti-inflammatory effects at low doses. It has been demonstrated that CO can mitigate the production of pro-inflammatory cytokines and increase the production of anti-inflammatory mediators [31]. In renal ischemia-reperfusion injury, CO has been shown to decrease oxidative stress, tubular apoptosis, and inflammation [32]. CO has also exhibited therapeutic effects in various other models of tissue injury [33–35]. Studies by Wang et al. have demonstrated that low-dose treatments with CO in UUO leads to decreased renal fibrosis. CO can mitigate ECM deposition in vivo and attenuate the TGF-β1-mediated fibrosis pathway in vitro [36]. As such, CO also shows potential as a therapeutic agent to ameliorate renal injury caused by urinary obstruction.

Hydrogen Sulfide in Obstructive Nephropathy

Along with NO and CO, hydrogen sulfide (H_2S) was recently identified as the third gasotransmitter. Using L-cysteine, H_2S is endogenously produced by cystathionine β-synthase (CBS), cystathionine γ-lyase (CSE), and 3-mercaptopyruvate sulfurtransferase (3-MST). These enzymes are expressed in a majority of human cell types, and they produce H_2S in the nanomolar to micromolar range [35]. By acting on adenosine triphosphate-sensitive potassium (K_{ATP}) channels, H_2S exerts physiological effects on the cardiovascular system such as mediating smooth muscle cell relaxation and vasodilation [25]. Additionally, H_2S can regulate metabolism, scavenge ROS, mitigate apoptosis, and reduce inflammation [25, 36]. Due to its broad variety of functions, disruption of H_2S production has been implicated in diseases such as hypertension, cancer, CKD, and diabetes [35]. In the kidney, CSE, CBS, and 3-MST are primarily found in the proximal tubules [37]. These enzymes play a major role in regulating renal hemodynamics by altering blood flow, GFR, and urine excretion due to the vasodilatory properties of H_2S [38]. In addition, H_2S may play a role in regulating RAS via modulation of cAMP and ROS production [39]. Due to its multifaceted effects on renal physiology, dysregulation of H_2S production has been implicated in CKD and other renal pathologies [36].

In obstructive nephropathy, H_2S has been shown to mitigate tubulointerstitial fibrosis, oxidative stress, and inflammation. Tubulointerstitial fibrosis has been associated with decreased expression of CBS and CSE and therefore decreased H_2S concentration [40]. Interestingly, Jung et al. have demonstrated that exogenous treatment with sodium hydrosulfide (NaHS, an H_2S donor compound) can remediate the decrease in CBS and CSE expression [40]. Furthermore, after 7 days of treatment, NaHS reduced renal fibrosis and mitigated the increase in renal TGF-β1,

Smad3, and NF-κB expression, which suggests that the H_2S production pathway may be a potential target for reducing renal fibrosis associated with obstructive nephropathy [40]. The induction of renal fibrosis is exacerbated by oxidative stress, as ROS have been reported to increase the expression of Ang II and TGF-β1 [41]. Therefore, mitigating ROS production may potentially be a way to alleviate tubulointerstitial fibrosis. Studies have shown that H_2S can act as an ROS scavenger in neuroblastoma cells, hepatic cells, and kidney cells and thus may ultimately attenuate the progression of tissue injury [39, 42, 43]. A study by Jiang et al. demonstrated that intraperitoneal treatment with NaHS prior to and during obstructive nephropathy significantly alleviated oxidative stress associated with UUO after 10 days of treatment [44]. When compared to control, UUO animals treated with NaHS demonstrated decreased expression of malondialdehyde (MDA, a marker for increased lipid peroxidation associated with ROS accumulation) and increased expression of superoxide dismutase (SOD, a free radical scavenging enzyme) [44]. Correspondingly, NaHS significantly attenuated renal fibrosis associated with obstructive nephropathy [44]. Therefore, due to its antioxidant properties, H_2S may be able to reduce obstructive nephropathy.

Increasingly, H_2S is being recognized as a key regulator of tissue inflammation. As demonstrated in the lung, liver, and kidney and following ischemic injury, H_2S has the ability to attenuate leukocyte adhesion and downregulate the expression of NF-κB, IL-1β, and TNF-α [36, 45–47], thereby attenuating inflammation. This effect was similarly observed in the context of UUO. Following UUO, various studies observed an increase in macrophage accumulation and TNF-α expression in the kidney, which was significantly ameliorated upon treatment with NaHS [44, 48]. Similarly, a study by Song et al. demonstrated in a rat model of obstructive nephropathy that H_2S treatment mitigated renal inflammation and fibrosis [49]. After treating obstructive nephropathy animals with NaHS for 7 days, significantly decreased infiltration of macrophages and reduced renal expression of IL-1β, TNF-α, and MCP-1 mRNA were observed when compared to control animals [49]. As inflammation plays a critical role in the initiation and propagation of fibrosis [50], H_2S may indirectly attenuate the progression of renal fibrosis by mediating renal inflammatory response.

The role of H_2S in tissue fibrosis is well established. Studies have shown that H_2S can be protective in pulmonary, hepatic, cardiac, and renal fibrosis [51–53]. Renal fibrosis can be a detrimental outcome of long-term obstructive nephropathy. However, studies have demonstrated that supplementation with NaHS can attenuate the progression of renal fibrosis by reducing collagen deposition in renal interstitium [44, 49]. Similarly, using a slow-releasing H_2S donor GYY4137, Lin et al. also observed a reduction in renal fibrosis following 30-day UUO [54]. This suggests that H_2S may be a promising therapeutic agent against fibrotic diseases. The mechanism by which H_2S mitigates renal fibrosis associated with UUO has been explored extensively. A proposed mechanism postulates that H_2S attenuates renal fibrosis by preventing renal fibroblasts from differentiating into myofibroblasts, and as a result, decreasing the expression of α-smooth muscle actin and fibronectin [49]. Furthermore, H_2S may mitigate renal fibrosis by attenuating EMT. Using a scratch wound assay, Lin et al. demonstrated that H_2S attenuated cell migration in TGF-β1-induced EMT [54], while other studies demonstrated that H_2S inhibits the EMT pathway through Smad-dependent, ERK-dependent, and Wnt/catenin-dependent pathways [49, 55]. Collectively, these studies suggest that the anti-fibrotic effects of H_2S may be due to its ability to regulate its production, scavenge ROS, and attenuate inflammation. H_2S may directly mitigate renal fibrosis by inhibiting various fibrotic pathways. Taken together, these findings suggest that exogenous H_2S may be a potential therapy against obstructive nephropathy.

GYY4137, a Slow-Releasing H_2S Donor

The use of H_2S in the literature has largely been limited to sulfide salts such as NaHS. These molecules release supraphysiological amounts of H_2S instantaneously in solution and are therefore unlikely to emulate the slow and sustained release of H_2S in biological systems. GYY4137 is a novel water-soluble H_2S donor that releases H_2S over a sustained period of time (from hours to days) [56]. Studies have shown that exposing vascular smooth muscle cells to low concentrations of GYY4137 leads to sustained vasorelaxation, as opposed to the transient effects of NaHS [56]. To evaluate the effects of GYY4137 on inflammation, Li et al. induced inflammation in mice by administering lipopolysaccharide. Upon treatment with GYY4137, they observed reduced macrophage infiltration, along with decreased expression of TNF-α and IL-1β, confirming that GYY4137 retains the anti-inflammatory properties of H_2S [57]. Additionally, Lin et al. have recently demonstrated the anti-inflammatory and anti-fibrotic effects of GYY4137 in a rat model of chronic obstructive nephropathy. Mirroring the downregulation of EMT markers in renal tissue, administration of GYY4137 also attenuated the progression of EMT in vitro [54]. To summarize, these studies conclude that GYY4137 is a slow-releasing H_2S donor molecule with anti-inflammatory and anti-fibrotic properties and can exhibit protective effects in various models of tissue injury, including obstructive nephropathy.

Development of Clinically Viable H_2S-Releasing Therapeutics

Due to the promise that H_2S holds, there has been a surge in research and development of clinically viable H_2S donors. These include garlic-derived compounds including allyl disulfide, and more recently, H_2S-releasing drugs, such as sodium polysulthionate (SG-1002), intravenous sodium sulfide (IK-1001), zofenopril, and ATB-346 [58, 59]. SG-1002 has been shown to restore plasma H_2S and NO levels in patients with congestive heart failure and has recently been approved for phase 2 of clinical trials [58]. IK-1001 showed efficacy in myocardial infarction, and it was approved for phase 2 of clinical trials. However, the sponsor company halted drug development and terminated phase 2 trials for IK-1001 for undisclosed reasons [59]. Zofenopril is an ACE inhibitor prodrug that metabolizes to zofenoprilat, a sulfhydryl-containing metabolite. It exhibits cardioprotective and vasculoprotective properties and, due to its sulfhydryl moiety, also exhibits antioxidant effects [58]. Although NSAIDs are commonly used to manage pain and inflammation, they often carry the risk of gastrointestinal distress, bleeding, and ulceration. Antibe therapeutics recently developed ATB-346, a naproxen-based drug linked to an H_2S donor, with the aim of using the gastroprotective effects of H_2S to help minimize the side effects associated with NSAIDs. ATB-346 has recently successfully completed phase 2 of clinical trials in patients with osteoarthritis, which is a chronic inflammatory disease [58].

Cross Talk Between H_2S and the Other Gasotransmitters

An emerging body of evidence is uncovering diverse interactions between gasotransmitters and cellular processes they are involved in. Cross talk between H_2S and NO has been studied primarily in the context of the myocardium and the endothelium. It is known that NO and H_2S can activate each other's catalyzing enzymes [60]. In addition to its direct vasorelaxant effects, H_2S can activate endothelial NOS (eNOS) and promote the production of NO. NO-dependent mechanisms have been implicated in H_2S-induced endothelial proliferation and angiogenesis [60, 61]. These interactions have important implications for chronic diseases such as congestive heart failure (CHF). SG-1002, the H_2S-releasing therapeutic that is being clinically tested in CHF patients, takes advantage of the cross talk between H_2S and NO by upregulating eNOS through H_2S release to restore plasma H_2S and NO levels [58]. Increased TGF-β1 production in the atria, which indicates the presence of fibrosis, has also been observed in dogs after development of CHF [62]. Preclinical studies in mice have shown reduced myocardial fibrosis upon treatment with SG-1002 [63]. However, its effects on TGF-β1 production and fibrosis have not yet been studied explicitly in human CHF patients. While cross talk between H_2S and NO has also been studied in the context of several other diseases, cross talk between H_2S and CO has been studied to a much lesser extent. To our knowledge, cross talk between H_2S and other gasotransmitters has not been studied specifically in the context of obstructive uropathy. However, cross talk between H_2S and NO has recently been discovered to play a role in ameliorating high glucose-induced kidney cell injury in the context of type 2 diabetes mellitus [64]. Administration of NaHS has been shown to inhibit diabetes-induced oxidative stress, TGF-β1 production, and deposition of ECM components, which indicates that H_2S mitigates renal fibrosis in diabetic kidney injury [65]. Further investigation into the protective effects of H_2S in glucose-induced kidney injury by Feliers et al. showed that H_2S causes increased expression of inducible NOS (iNOS), which produces NO in kidney proximal tubular epithelial cells. They hypothesized that H_2S-mediated NO production is important for the antioxidant effects of H_2S in glucose-induced kidney injury. Upon silencing iNOS, they observed that the protective effects of H_2S were abolished which supports their hypothesis and suggests a high degree of interaction between H_2S and NO in ameliorating glucose-induced tubular injury [64]. Considering the chronic nature of type 2 diabetes mellitus and the discovery of cross talk between H_2S and NO in kidney tubular epithelial cells, which are key sites of injury in obstructive nephropathy, it is possible that similar cross talk mechanisms are involved in the H_2S-mediated amelioration observed in the previously discussed obstructive nephropathy studies. For example, treatment with L-arginine, the precursor to NO, has been shown to ameliorate renal fibrosis, apoptosis, and inflammation following UUO [29]. Taking into consideration the finding that H_2S causes increased expression of iNOS, which leads to NO production by kidney tubular epithelial cells [64], it is likely that NO-mediated protective effects factor into the improved renal outcomes observed in obstructive nephropathy studies upon treatment with H_2S. It is evident that further investigation into the role and mechanisms of cross talk between H_2S, NO, and CO, specifically in the context of obstructive nephropathy, is needed to thoroughly understand the effects of using H_2S-releasing therapeutics in obstructive nephropathy.

Conclusions and Future Therapeutic Implications

Prolonged ureteral obstruction can lead to chronic obstructive nephropathy, ultimately resulting in loss of renal function. While surgical relief of obstruction removes the source of insult, renal function and renal injury cannot be fully reversed, and this residual injury can lead to renal dysfunction in later life. H_2S possesses several protective properties, and it has been shown to mitigate chronic obstructive nephropathy. This suggests that, in the future, H_2S-based therapeutics may potentially be used in clinical practice to improve post-obstructive renal function and clinical outcomes. Though still in the early stages of development, H_2S-releasing drugs show considerable promise. If administered throughout the duration of UUO, H_2S-releasing drugs may be a potential solution to attenuate obstructive nephropathy and improve renal function following relief of urinary obstruction.

Conflict of Interest None.

References

1. Roth KS, Koo HP, Spottswood SE, Chan JCM. Obstructive uropathy: an important cause chronic renal failure in children. Clin Pediatr (Phila). 2002;41:309–14.
2. Spernat D, Kourambas J. Urolithiasis—medical therapies. BJU Int. 2011;108:9–13.
3. Klahr S. Obstructive nephropathy. Intern Med. 2000;39(5):355–61.

4. Ucero AC, Benito-Martin A, Izquierdo MC, Sanchez-Niño MD, Sanz AB, Ramos AM, et al. Unilateral ureteral obstruction: beyond obstruction. Int Urol Nephrol. 2014;46(4):765–76.
5. Truong LD, Choi J-J, Tsao CC, Ayala G, Sheikh-Hamad D, Nassar G, et al. Renal cell apoptosis in chronic obstructive uropathy: the roles of caspases. Kidney Int. 2001;60:924–34.
6. Lech M, Anders H-J. Macrophages and fibrosis: how resident and infiltrating mononuclear phagocytes orchestrate all phases of tissue injury and repair. Biochim Biophys Acta. 2013;1832(7):989–97.
7. Kluth DC, Erwig L-P, Rees AJ. Multiple facets of macrophages in renal injury. Kidney Int. 2004;66:542–57.
8. Sakurai H, Hisada Y, Ueno M, Sugiura M, Kawashima K, Sugita T. Activation of transcription factor NF-kB in experimental glomerulonephritis in rats. Biochim Biophys Acta. 1996;1316:132–8.
9. Eddy AA, López-Guisa JM, Okamura DM, Yamaguchi I. Investigating mechanisms of chronic kidney disease in mouse models. Pediatr Nephrol. 2012;27(8):1233–47.
10. Samarakoon R, Overstreet JM, Higgins SP, Higgins PJ. TGF-β1 → SMAD/p53/USF2 → PAI-1 transcriptional axis in ureteral obstruction-induced renal fibrosis. Cell Tissue Res. 2012;347(1):117–28.
11. Chevalier RL. Pathogenesis of renal injury in obstructive uropathy. Curr Opin Pediatr. 2006;18(2):153–60.
12. Iwano M, Neilson EG. Mechanisms of tubulointerstitial fibrosis. Curr Opin Nephrol Hypertens. 2004;13:279–84.
13. Kaneto H, Morrissey J, Klahr S. Increased expression of TGF-β1 mRNA in the obstructed kidney of rats with unilateral ureteral ligation. Kidney Int. 1993;44(2):313–21.
14. Manucha W, Oliverros L, Carrizo L, Seltzer A, Valles P. Losartan modulation on NOS isoforms and COX-2 expression in early renal fibrogenesis in unilateral obstruction. Kidney Int. 2004;65:2091–107.
15. Gibbons GH, Pratt RE, Dzau VJ. Vascular smooth muscle cell hypertrophy vs. hyperplasia autocrine transforming growth factor beta 1, expression determines growth response to angiotensin II. J Clin Invest. 1992;90:456–61.
16. Xu J, Lamouille S, Derynck R. TGF-beta-induced epithelial to mesenchymal transition. Cell Res. 2009;19(2):156–72.
17. Vaughan ED Jr, Gillenwater JY. Recovery following complete chronic unilateral ureteral occlusion: functional, radiographic and pathologic alterations. J Urol. 1971;106:27–35.
18. Chevalier RL, Kim A, Thornhill BA, Wolstenholme JT. Recovery following relief of unilateral ureteral obstruction in the neonatal rat. Kidney Int. 1999;55:793–807.
19. Chaabane W, Praddaude F, Buleon M, Jaafar A, Vallet M, Rischmann P, et al. Renal functional decline and glomerulotubular injury are arrested but not restored by release of unilateral ureteral obstruction (UUO). Am J Physiol Ren Physiol. 2013;304(4):F432–9.
20. Chevalier RL, Forbes MS, Thornhill BA. Ureteral obstruction as a model of renal interstitial fibrosis and obstructive nephropathy. Kidney Int. 2009;75(11):1145–52.
21. Tapmeier TT, Brown KL, Tang Z, Sacks SH, Sheerin NS, Wong W. Reimplantation of the ureter after unilateral ureteral obstruction provides a model that allows functional evaluation. Kidney Int. 2008;73(7):885–9.
22. York NE, Borofsky MS, Lingeman JE. Risks associated with drug treatments for kidney stones. Expert Opin Drug Saf. 2015;14:1865–77.
23. Kerr WS Jr. Effects of complete ureteral obstruction in dogs on kidney function. Am J Phys. 1956;184:521–6.
24. Wu AK, Tran TC, Sorensen MD, Durack JC, Stoller ML. Relative renal function does not improve after relieving chronic renal obstruction. BJU Int. 2012;109(10):1540–4.
25. Wang R. Two's company, three's a crowd: can H2S be the third endogenous gaseous transmitter? FASEB J. 2002;16(13):1792–8.
26. Qian Y, Matson JB. Gasotransmitter delivery via self-assembling peptides: treating diseases with natural signaling gases. Adv Drug Deliv Rev. 2017;110:137–56.

27. Sharma JN, Al-Omran A, Parvathy SS. Role of nitric oxide in inflammatory diseases. Inflammopharmacology. 2007;15(6):252–9.
28. Lefer AM, Lefer DJ. Nitric oxide. II. Nitric oxide protects in intestinal inflammation. Am J Phys. 1999;276(3 Pt 1):G572–5.
29. Sun D, Wang Y, Liu C, Zhou X, Li X, Xiao A. Effects of nitric oxide on renal interstitial fibrosis in rats with unilateral ureteral obstruction. Life Sci. 2012;90(23–24):900–9.
30. Gibbons SJ, Farrugia G. The role of carbon monoxide in the gastrointestinal tract. J Physiol. 2004;556(Pt 2):325–36.
31. Motterlini R, Foresti R. Heme oxygenase-1 as a target for drug discovery. Antioxid Redox Signal. 2013;20(11):1810–26.
32. Abe T, Fujino M, Yazawa K, Imamura R, Hatayama N, Kakuta Y, Tsutahara K, Okumi M, Ichimaru N, Kaimori JY, Isaka Y, Seki K, Takahara S, Li X-K, Nonomura N. High-pressure carbon monoxide preserves rat kidney grafts from apoptosis and inflammation. Lab Investig. 2017;97:468–77.
33. Bauer I, Pannen BHJ. Bench-to-bedside review: carbon monoxide—from mitochondrial poisoning to therapeutic use. Crit Care. 2009;13(4):1–10.
34. Wallace JL, Ianaro A, Flannigan KL, Cirino G. Gaseous mediators in resolution of inflammation. Semin Immunol. 2015;27(3):227–33.
35. Whiteman M, Le Trionnaire S, Chopra M, Fox B, Whatmore J. Emerging role of hydrogen sulfide in health and disease: critical appraisal of biomarkers and pharmacological tools. Clin Sci. 2011;121(11):459–88.
36. Lobb I, Sonke E, Aboalsamh G, Sener A. Hydrogen sulphide and the kidney: important roles in renal physiology and pathogenesis and treatment of kidney injury and disease. Nitric Oxide. 2014;46(2015):55–65.
37. Yamamoto J, Sato W, Kosugi T, Yamamoto T, Kimura T, Taniguchi S, et al. Distribution of hydrogen sulfide (H_2S)-producing enzymes and the roles of the H_2S donor sodium hydrosulfide in diabetic nephropathy. Clin Exp Nephrol. 2013;17(1):32–40.
38. Xia M, Chen L, Muh RW, Li P, Li N. Production and actions of hydrogen sulfide, a novel gaseous bioactive substance, in the kidneys. J Pharmacol Exp Ther. 2006;329(3):1056–62.
39. Xue H, Yuan P, Ni J, Li C, Shao D, Liu J, et al. H_2S inhibits hyperglycemia-induced intrarenal renin–angiotensin system activation via attenuation of reactive oxygen species generation. PLoS One. 2013;8(9):e74366.
40. Jung K-J, Jang H-S, Kim JI, Han SJ, Park J-W, Park KM. Involvement of hydrogen sulfide and homocysteine transsulfuration pathway in the progression of kidney fibrosis after ureteral obstruction. Biochim Biophys Acta. 2013;1832(12):1989–97.
41. Song K, Li Q, Yin X-Y, Lu Y, Liu C-F, Hu L-F. Hydrogen sulfide: a therapeutic candidate for fibrotic disease? Oxid Med Cell Longev. 2015;2015:458720.
42. Whiteman M, Armstrong JS, Chu SH, Jia-Ling S, Wong BS, Cheung NS, et al. The novel neuromodulator hydrogen sulfide: an endogenous peroxynitrite "scavenger"? J Neurochem. 2004;90(3):765–8.
43. Deng Y. Protective effects of hydrogen sulfide on oxidative stress and fibrosis in hepatic stellate cells. Mol Med Rep. 2012;7:247–53.
44. Jiang D, Zhang Y, Yang M, Wang S, Jiang Z, Li Z. Exogenous hydrogen sulfide prevents kidney damage following unilateral ureteral obstruction. Neurourol Urodyn. 2014;33:538–43.
45. Cao H, Zhou X, Zhang J, Huang X, Zhai Y, Zhang X, et al. Hydrogen sulfide protects against bleomycin-induced pulmonary fibrosis in rats by inhibiting NF-κB expression and regulating Th1/Th2 balance. Toxicol Lett. 2014;224(3):387–94.
46. Szabó C. Hydrogen sulphide and its therapeutic potential. Nat Rev Drug Discov. 2007;6(11):917–35.
47. Lobb I, Mok A, Lan Z, Liu W, Garcia B, Sener A. Supplemental hydrogen sulphide protects transplant kidney function and prolongs recipient survival after prolonged cold ischemia-reperfusion injury by mitigating renal graft apoptosis and inflammation. BJU Int. 2012;110(11 Pt C):E1187–95.

48. Dursun M, Alper O, Emin O, Suleyman S, Huseyin B, Ozgur DO, Cekmen Mustafa NO, Somay A. Protective effect of hydrogen sulfide on protective effect of hydrogen sulfide on renal injury in the experimental unilateral ureteral obstruction-induced renal injury. Int Braz J Urol. 2015;41:1185–93.
49. Song K, Wang F, Li Q, Shi Y-B, Zheng H-F, Peng H, et al. Hydrogen sulfide inhibits the renal fibrosis of obstructive nephropathy. Kidney Int. 2014;85(6):1318–29.
50. Meng X-M, Nikolic-Paterson DJ, Lan HY. Inflammatory processes in renal fibrosis. Nat Rev Nephrol. 2014;10(9):493–503.
51. Zhang S, Pan C, Zhou F, Yuan Z, Wang H, Cui W, et al. Hydrogen sulfide as a potential therapeutic target in fibrosis. Oxid Med Cell Longev. 2015;2015:593407.
52. Fang L-P, Lin Q, Tang C-S, Liu X-M. Hydrogen sulfide attenuates epithelial-mesenchymal transition of human alveolar epithelial cells. Pharmacol Res. 2010;61(4):298–305.
53. Zheng D, Dong S, Li T, Yang F, Yu X, Wu J, et al. Exogenous hydrogen sulfide attenuates cardiac fibrosis through reactive oxygen species signal pathways in experimental diabetes mellitus models. Cell Physiol Biochem. 2015;36(3):917–29.
54. Lin S, Visram F, Liu W, Haig A, Jiang J, Mok A, et al. GYY4137, a slow-releasing hydrogen sulfide donor, ameliorates renal damage associated with chronic obstructive uropathy. J Urol. 2016;196:1778–87.
55. Guo L, Peng W, Tao J, Lan Z, Hei H, Tian L, et al. Hydrogen sulfide inhibits transforming growth factor-β1-induced EMT via Wnt/catenin pathway. PLoS One. 2016;11(1):e01470181.
56. Li L, Whiteman M, Guan YY, Neo KL, Cheng Y, Lee SW, et al. Characterization of a novel, water-soluble hydrogen sulfide-releasing molecule (GYY4137): new insights into the biology of hydrogen sulfide. Circulation. 2008;117(18):2351–60.
57. Li L, Fox B, Keeble J, Salto-Tellez M, Winyard PG, Wood ME, et al. The complex effects of the slow-releasing hydrogen sulfide donor GYY4137 in a model of acute joint inflammation and in human cartilage cells. J Cell Mol Med. 2013;17(3):365–76.
58. Wallace JL, Vaughan D, Dicay M, MacNaughton WK, DeNucci G. Hydrogen sulfide-releasing therapeutics: translation to the clinic. Antioxid Redox Signal. 2018;28(16):1533–40.
59. Szabo C, Papapetropoulos A. International union of basic and clinical pharmacology. CII: pharmacological modulation of H_2S levels: H_2S donors and H_2S biosynthesis inhibitors. Pharmacol Rev. 2017;69(4):497–564.
60. Zhao W, Zhang J, Lu Y, Wang R. The vasorelaxant effect of H_2S as a novel endogenous gaseous KATP channel opener. EMBO J. 2001;20(21):6008–16.
61. Altaany Z, Yang G, Wang R. Crosstalk between hydrogen sulfide and nitric oxide in endothelial cells. J Cell Mol Med. 2013;17(7):879–88.
62. Hanna N, Cardin S, Leung TK, Nattel S. Differences in atrial versus ventricular remodeling in dogs with ventricular tachypacing-induced congestive heart failure. Cardiovasc Res. 2004;63(2):236–44.
63. Kondo K, Bhushan S, King A, Prabhu S, Hamid T, Koenig S, et al. H_2S protects against pressure overload induced heart failure via upregulation of endothelial nitric oxide synthase (eNOS). Circulation. 2014;127(10):1116–27.
64. Feliers D, Lee HJHJ, Kasinath BSBS. Hydrogen sulfide in renal physiology and disease. Antioxid Redox Signal. 2016;25(13):720–31.
65. Zhou X, Feng Y, Zhan Z, Chen J. Hydrogen sulfide alleviates diabetic nephropathy in a streptozotocin-induced diabetic rat model. J Biol Chem. 2014;289(42):28827–34.

Chapter 8
Hydrogen Sulfide Therapy as the Future of Renal Graft Preservation

George J. Dugbartey, Hjalmar R. Bouma, Manujendra N. Saha, Ian Lobb, Robert H. Henning, and Alp Sener

This chapter is a modified version by the same authors in the publication titled A Hibernation-Like State for Transplantable Organs: Is Hydrogen Sulfide Therapy the Future of Organ Preservation? Antioxid Redox Signal. 2018; 28(16):1503–1515.

G. J. Dugbartey (✉)
Department of Surgery, Division of Urology, London Health Sciences Center, Western University, London, ON, Canada

Multi-Organ Transplant Program, London Health Sciences Center, Western University, London, ON, Canada

Matthew Mailing Center for Translational Transplant Studies, London Health Sciences Center, Western University, London, ON, Canada

Department of Pharmacology and Toxicology, School of Pharmacy, College of Health Sciences, University of Ghana, Accra, Ghana

Department of Physiology and Pharmacology, Accra College of Medicine, Accra, Ghana
e-mail: gdugbart@uwo.ca

H. R. Bouma · R. H. Henning
Department of Clinical Pharmacy and Pharmacology, University of Groningen, University Medical Center Groningen, Groningen, The Netherlands
e-mail: h.r.bouma@umcg.nl; r.h.henning@umcg.nl

M. N. Saha
Department of Surgery, Division of Urology, London Health Sciences Center, Western University, London, ON, Canada

Matthew Mailing Center for Translational Transplant Studies, London Health Sciences Center, Western University, London, ON, Canada

I. Lobb
Matthew Mailing Center for Translational Transplant Studies, London Health Sciences Center, Western University, London, ON, Canada

Department of Microbiology and Immunology, London Health Sciences Center, Western University, London, ON, Canada

159

G. J. Dugbartey, A. Sener, *Hydrogen Sulfide in Kidney Diseases*,
https://doi.org/10.1007/978-3-031-44041-0_8

A. Sener
Department of Surgery, Division of Urology, London Health Sciences Center, Western
University, London, ON, Canada

Multi-Organ Transplant Program, London Health Sciences Center, Western University,
London, ON, Canada

Matthew Mailing Center for Translational Transplant Studies, London Health Sciences
Center, Western University, London, ON, Canada

Department of Microbiology and Immunology, London Health Sciences Center, Western
University, London, ON, Canada
e-mail: alp.sener@lhsc.on.ca

Cold Preservation of Renal Grafts for Transplantation

Kidney transplantation is the preferred therapeutic option for end-stage renal disease. Compared to dialysis, kidney transplantation offers the best long-term outcomes in terms of survival, quality of life, and cost-effectiveness [1]. Renal grafts
may be derived from living donors or deceased (i.e., brain dead or non-heart beat-
ing) donors and are routinely flushed with and stored in cold preservation solutions
such as the University of Wisconsin (UW) solution at 4 °C to decrease energy
demand during this storage period. Hypothermic kidney storage prior to transplantation results in ischemic kidney damage due to restriction of blood flow to the
kidney. The final stage of ischemic injury occurs during reperfusion, the effector
phase of ischemic injury, which develops when blood flow is restored in the graft.
The whole process is defined as ischemia/reperfusion injury (IRI). Cold storage
preserves graft quality, thus allowing time for transportation and recipient selection,
as compared to warm IRI [2]. However, the beneficial effects of cold storage of
donor kidneys are limited. While short-term cold storage reduces cellular oxygen
demand and thereby prevents tissue injury, prolonged cold storage leads to renal
injury. The ensuing cold ischemic injury is characterized by tubular injury and epithelial cell death, thereby increasing the incidence of delayed graft function (DGF)
and lowering graft survival [3]. It has been reported that every 6-h increase in cold
storage increases the risk of DGF by 23% [4]. Furthermore, prolonged cold storage
is associated with worse long-term graft survival [5]. Thus, cold IRI is unavoidable
but remains the major contributor to early and late graft dysfunction following kidney transplantation.

The mechanisms underlying cold IRI are complex and not fully elucidated. Some
studies have reported that such events include mitochondrial injury evidenced by
depletion of mitochondrial adenosine triphosphate (ATP) leading to loss of cellular
homeostasis, thereby affecting several cellular pathways involved in tissue regen-
eration and repair [5, 6]. Further, excess production of free radicals in the mitochondria seems to play a key role in cold-induced mitochondrial injury [7] and may lead
to inflammation and apoptosis of glomerular and tubular cells of cold-stored kidneys [8]. The restoration of blood supply and temperature in the renal graft during

reperfusion results in excessive reactive oxygen species (ROS) generation [8, 9], which initiates a cascade of events including activation of inflammatory and apoptotic pathways, leading to tissue injury [10]. Unfortunately, the search for therapeutic strategies to mitigate cold IRI has met little success so far. Thus, the quest for safe reduction of metabolism in transplant organs continues.

It is of interest to note that mammalian hibernators are able to survive periods of low metabolic rate and body temperature without signs of renal injury in contrast to nonhibernating species. Hibernators alternate their body temperature between 4 and 37 °C without cold IRI challenge. Recently, hydrogen sulfide (H_2S), a gas with a distinctive smell of rotten eggs, and the third member of the gasotransmitter family, has been implicated in organ protection in deep hibernation [11] and also seems to confer cytoprotection by lowering metabolism, increasing preservation time, and overall increasing renal graft survival after transplantation [12–15]. H_2S is produced enzymatically in all mammalian species including humans [16]. Two of these enzymatic pathways are cytosolically catalyzed by cystathionine β-synthase (CBS) and cystathionine γ-lyase (CSE). The third enzymatic pathway requires the mitochondrial enzyme, 3-mercaptopyruvate sulfurtransferase (3-MST), while the fourth pathway involves the peroxisomal enzyme, D-amino acid oxidase (DAO) [17, 18]. Apart from being produced endogenously, there are various forms of exogenous H_2S, which have been used experimentally in the form of donor molecules. The classic form of inhalation is seriously hampered by toxic effects to bystanders, while sulfide salts (NaHS and Na_2S) are short-lasting and may not always reach their target sites, particularly the mitochondria [19]. Fortunately, slow-releasing H_2S donors such as GYY4137 [20] and mitochondria-targeting slow-releasing H_2S donors (AP39 and AP123) have been developed [21–23] and may enable translation of fundamental findings on H_2S in modulating renal IRI into human kidney preservation.

In this chapter, we first discuss mammalian hibernation as a unique natural model of how nature deals with cold IRI with reference to the kidney as a typical organ highly vulnerable to cold IRI. We also highlight the protective role of H_2S during hibernation. Next, we present recent findings on H_2S as a gasotransmitter that confers cytoprotection during cold IRI in kidney transplantation, suggesting that it may become a novel method of preservation to help improve graft quality and increase the long-term success of kidney transplantation in the future.

Lessons Learned from Mammalian Hibernation

Mammalian hibernation may offer a great clinical promise to safely cold-store and reperfuse donor organs. Hibernation is an evolved strategy that conserves energy mainly seasonally and confers a significant survival advantage to individuals among select but diverse mammalian lineages [24]. To save energy demand during winter, mammalian hibernators undergo repetitive cycles of "torpor" and "arousal" [25, 26] (Fig. 8.1). Torpor is a state of reduced metabolism and body temperature usually

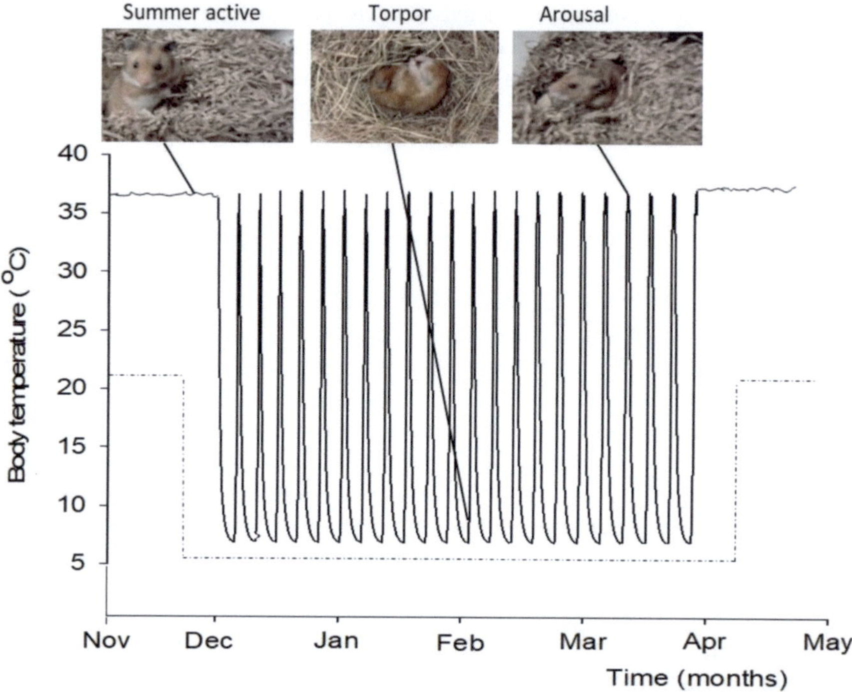

Fig. 8.1 Torpor-arousal cycle of a Syrian golden hamster with respect to appearance and core body temperature (Tb). The graph shows a simulation of Tb tracings (solid line) of a Syrian hamster (*Mesocricetus auratus*) inside a climate-controlled chamber. The dashed line represents the ambient temperature, which is lowered from 21 to 5 °C to induce hibernation and back to 21 °C to end the torpor-arousal cycle. Tb dropped from ~37 to ~7 °C as ambient temperature was lowered. Periodic arousals between each torpor bout are associated with restoration of euthermic temperature of ~37 °C despite constant ambient temperature. Photographs of hamsters at three different time points during the hibernation are shown above the graph

between 4 and 10 °C, depending on the species [27], and can be viewed as the natural equivalent of cold storage of donor organs. As illustrated in Fig. 8.1, torpor phase lasting days to weeks is intermittently interrupted by brief periods of arousal during which metabolism and body temperature return to euthermic levels [28]. Hence, arousal phase may represent a natural equivalent of reperfusion after cold storage.

While body temperature of smaller mammalian hibernators falls drastically during torpor and lasts days to weeks followed by intermittent arousals, larger hibernators such as bears remain in torpid state at 30–35 °C for 5–7 months in a year without eating, coupled with decreased metabolism, immobilization, and anuria due to complete reabsorption of the glomerular filtrate [29–31] (Fig. 8.2). A more extreme type of torpor is seen in hibernating arctic ground squirrels during which core body temperature measures −2.9 °C without freezing, and metabolism reduced to 1% of euthermic rate [27]. Interestingly, whereas torpor and arousal cause no

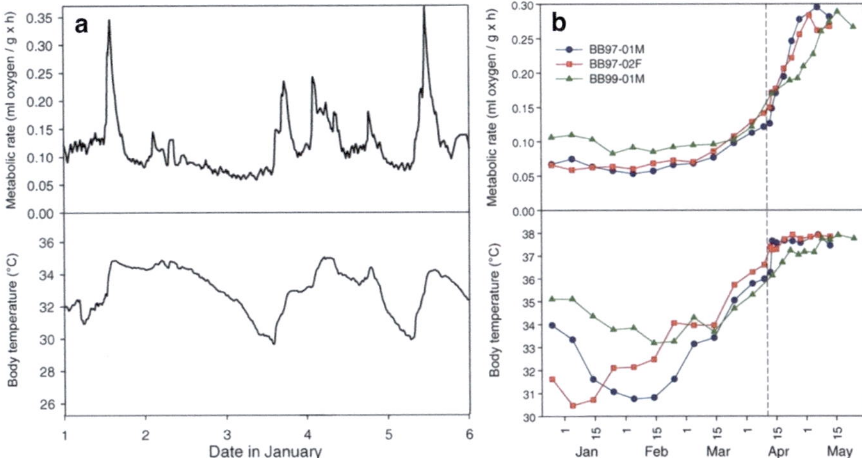

Fig. 8.2 Core body temperature and metabolic rate during torpor and arousal in bears. (**a**) Body temperature and oxygen consumption of a black bear (*Ursus americanus*) housed in an outside den during a 5-day period in January. (**b**) Body temperature and oxygen consumption of three bears during torpor and arousal. Vertical dashed line represents average time of emergence, which varied by ±2 days. (Data are adapted from Tøien et al., 2011 [8])

organ injury in all hibernating animals studied thus far [20, 32–35], cold storage and reperfusion result in extensive organ injury in nonhibernating species [12, 35] including humans. In the kidney, for example, the morphology of the renal cortex and medulla is not affected by hibernation in typical hibernating animals such as 13-lined ground squirrels and dormice, which are the most studied hibernating animals [33, 34, 36]. Moreover, the ultrastructure of the glomerular basement membrane, tubular brush border, and cytoskeleton are well preserved throughout torpor and arousal—a condition that would induce extensive damage in human deceased-donor kidneys [33, 34]. Renal protection in hibernating animals is such a strong intrinsic event that kidneys removed from hibernating 13-lined ground squirrels and stored in cold UW solution resisted apoptotic cell death as shown by reduced caspase-3 activity [33, 35].

The activation and suppression of mitochondrial metabolism and organ protection in hibernating animals seem tightly regulated, and the molecular mechanism of this regulation is not fully understood. Although it is yet to be identified which endogenous molecules are essential for entrance into torpor and/or arousal, H_2S has so far proven important in torpor-arousal cycle, as its level is markedly increased in the lung during torpor and reduced in arousal state in Syrian hamsters [11]. This finding suggests that H_2S may influence temperature-controlling neurotransmitters such as histamine, serotonin, and opioids, which have been proposed to play key roles in the regulation of torpor pattern by the central nervous system [37–39] as well as phospholipids of liver cell nuclei [40]. Additionally, organ protection in hibernation has been attributed to increased production of endogenous H_2S, which can also induce a torpor-like state in small nonhibernating mammals with effects on mitochondrial metabolism [11, 41, 42] and endogenous antioxidants such as glutathione and ascorbic acid [43] as well as upregulation of anti-apoptotic genes such as Bcl-2 and phospho-Akt [35, 44]. Renoprotective effect of H_2S was also observed in rats (nonhibernating animals) in which dopamine treatment upregulated renal expressions of CBS, CSE, and 3-MST and stimulated endogenous H_2S production, leading to protection against cold renal IRI [12]. Dopamine or serotonin treatment of rat smooth muscle aortic cells as well as rat kidney and other tissues prior to cold storage also protected against hypothermia/rewarming-induced apoptosis and subsequent hypothermic injury by strongly increasing endogenous H_2S level [45]. In addition, our group demonstrated that endogenous H_2S production protects kidneys of hamsters (natural hibernators) subjected to 5′-AMP-induced torpor-like state at 7 °C body temperature [46] (Figs. 8.3 and 8.4). Further, Blackstone and Roth demonstrated that pretreatment with inhaled H_2S for only 20 min markedly prolonged survival without any apparent detrimental effects in mice exposed to otherwise lethal hypoxia (5% oxygen) [41]. It appears that kidneys and tissues of mammalian hibernators are well protected from the damaging effects of hypothermia and reperfusion through upregulated antioxidant pathways and maintenance of mitochondrial homeostasis. These findings suggest that H_2S plays an important role in modulating cytoprotective pathways that govern protection against cold IRI and allow maintenance of mitochondrial function throughout torpor and arousal.

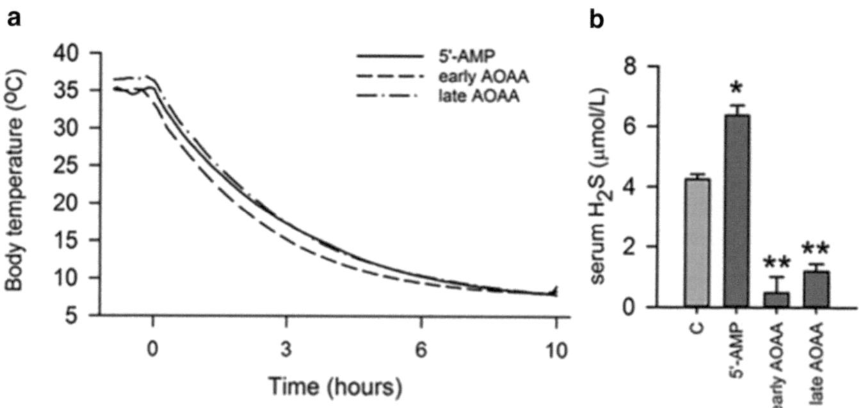

Fig. 8.3 5′-AMP induces torpor in natural hibernators and increases serum H_2S level. (**a**) 5′-AMP administration (at $t = 0$) resulted in a drop in body temperature from 37 to ~7 °C following 10 h of 5′-AMP injection, which was not affected by early or late administration of amino-oxyacetic acid (AOAA). (**b**) 5′-AMP administration markedly increased plasma H_2S level compared to control animals, while administration of AOAA before or 4 h after 5′-AMP injection reduced serum H_2S level. *C* control animals. */**$p < 0.05/0.01$ compared to control. Data are presented as mean ± SEM. (Data are adapted from Dugbartey et al., 2015 [46])

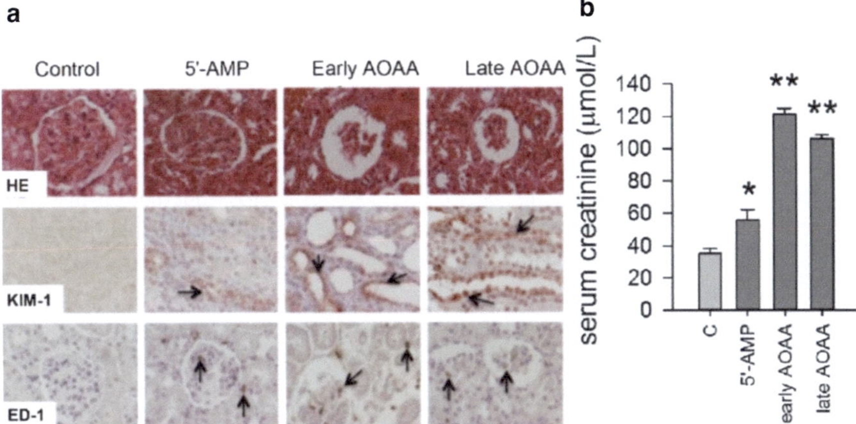

Fig. 8.4 Blocking endogenous H₂S production during 5′-AMP-induced torpor induces renal injury. (**a**) Representative photographs of kidney tissue from immuno(histochemical) staining (magnification ×400). Pharmacological inhibition of endogenous H₂S during 5′-AMP-induced torpor provokes kidney damage characterized by glomerular atrophy, tubular dilatation, atrophy of epithelial cells, and widening of tubular lumen. (**b**) Serum creatinine level showing the degree of renal functional derangement following pharmacological inhibition of endogenous H₂S in 5′-AMP-induced torpor. *HE* hematoxylin/eosin staining, *KIM-1* kidney injury molecule 1, *ED-1* antibody against CD68 specific for macrophages. Arrows point to positively stained areas (in brown), indicating tubular injury and inflammation. (Data are adapted from Dugbartey et al., 2015 [46])

Do Organs of Hibernators Suffer Ischemia During Torpor, or Is There an Element of Organ Preservation?

Since torpor is characterized by reduced metabolism and body temperature, a major question that immediately comes to mind is whether the profound reduction in cardiac output and oxygenation of the kidney and other tissues during hibernation results in renal ischemia during hibernation. The kidneys of nonhibernating animals in a healthy state receive about 20% of cardiac output, which mostly goes to the renal cortex, while the renal medulla receives only about 10% of the total renal perfusion [47], implying that the renal medulla is highly vulnerable to ischemia even at euthermic temperature. From a clinical point of view, ischemia occurs when there is an imbalance between blood oxygen demand and supply, which may result in cell death and tissue injury [48]. To date, there are no good data to strongly suggest whether "clinical" renal ischemia occurs during torpor and, if it occurs, whether it may serve as a primary stimulus for arousal from torpor. Likely, the profound lowering of metabolism during torpor runs parallel with the reduced perfusion, which ensures a balance between blood oxygen demand and supply and thereby prevents ischemia during torpor [49]. Despite the debate about whether torpor is associated with (renal) ischemia/reperfusion (I/R), the profound increase in metabolic rate upon rewarming after torpor likely results in high levels of oxidative stress and can potentially lead to cellular injury if not counterbalanced by protective mechanisms. Specific adaptations, consisting of upregulation of antioxidant enzymes and anti-apoptotic pathways, limit oxidative stress and protect against cell death throughout hibernation [50]. It should be noted that in contrast to hypothermic I/R, arousal from torpor may not be associated with a gross fluctuation in tissue oxygenation. In the brain of torpid Arctic ground squirrels, for example, there is a high arterial oxygen pressure and low expression of hypoxia-inducible factor-alpha, a marker of tissue hypoxia [51], suggesting that hibernators may not show signs of ischemia during torpor. In conclusion, it remains to be revealed whether hibernators suffer from renal ischemia from a clinical perspective during torpor and arousal.

H_2S Lowers Metabolic Rate at High Concentrations, but Stimulates ATP Production at Low Concentrations

At high concentration of 80 ppm, for example, H_2S can suppress metabolism through reversible inhibition of mitochondrial complex IV (cytochrome c oxidase) [42, 52]. Thus, it is not surprising that H_2S affects metabolism in animals. Inhibition of mitochondrial respiration was implicated in the induction of suspended animation in mice [52]. Inhalation of gaseous H_2S induces a hibernation-like state in non-hibernating mice by profoundly reducing metabolic rate and core body temperature and protecting against cold renal IRI [41, 42, 53]. Inhibition of oxidative phosphorylation by reversible antagonism at complex IV of the mitochondrial respiratory chain has been proposed to underlie the induction of such hypometabolic state by H_2S [42]. Whereas high dosages cause hypometabolism, low concentrations of H_2S (0.1–1 μM) enhance electron transport in the mitochondria by acting as an electron donor at the level of coenzyme Q—an electron carrier between complexes I and III in the mitochondrial electron transport chain (ETC). Such electron donation by H_2S stimulates cellular energy metabolism and adenosine triphosphate (ATP) production through oxidative phosphorylation [54, 55]. Recent studies also suggest that in the low-oxygen environment of ischemia/hypoxia, CBS and CSE enzymes translocate from the cytosol to the mitochondria to augment mitochondrial H_2S production by 3-MST through electron donation, thus protecting liver and heart mitochondria against ischemic injury [56, 57]. Perhaps, mitochondrial protection and preservation of ATP synthesis offered by H_2S at low concentrations explain why hibernators are protected from cold ischemic injury. In conclusion, H_2S at high concentration lowers metabolism but at low concentration acts as an electron donor and preserves mitochondrial function.

H_2S Protects and Prolongs Renal Graft Function During Cold Ischemia/Reperfusion and After Kidney Transplantation

Since the discovery of the therapeutic potential of H_2S, there has been more focus on the protective role of H_2S in warm IRI in the kidney compared to cold IRI in kidney transplantation. However, emerging evidence suggests that exogenous H_2S administration protects renal cells against cold I/R-induced apoptosis, vasoconstriction, oxidative stress, and inflammation and thus increases the survival rate of the renal graft after transplantation. For example, following 18 h of cold (4 °C) storage, NaHS treatment at 10 min before and after reperfusion has been shown to enhance renal blood flow (RBF) and increase renal graft function of porcine kidneys [58]. Studies by our own group have demonstrated that addition of NaHS to UW solution during preservation of rat donor kidneys significantly mitigates cold IRI and improves posttransplant renal graft function and survival following both moderate and severe periods of cold (4 °C) storage [8, 59]. Thus, H_2S protects and prolongs renal graft function during cold I/R and after kidney transplantation.

H_2S Scavenges ROS and Preserves Renal Function During Cold Ischemia/Reperfusion

It is well known that ROS is a chief mediator of cold IRI in human donor kidneys, and therefore the use of H_2S as an antioxidant has been suggested to mitigate oxidative stress during cold storage and reperfusion. Hosgood and Nicholson [58] observed a significant reduction of oxidative stress in porcine renal graft following treatment with NaHS before and during reperfusion. We also found that dopamine treatment preserved kidney function and integrity via maintenance (and upregulation) of renal CBS, CSE, and 3-MST and elevation of serum H_2S, resulting in a marked decrease in the levels of renal malondialdehyde (MDA, a product of lipid peroxidation in the cell and a marker of oxidative stress) in a rat model closely matching clinical whole-body deep cooling and rewarming [12]. Moreover, pharmacological inhibition of H_2S production with amino-oxyacetic acid (AOAA) in dopamine-treated hypothermic rats strongly reduced renal expression of CBS, CSE, and 3-MST and serum H_2S and significantly increased renal oxidative stress, resulting in severe renal injury [12]. This finding supports our previous study in which we showed that dopamine and serotonin doubled CBS expression via mammalian target of rapamycin, leading to increased endogenous H_2S production and reduced ROS levels in cultured smooth muscle cells [45]. This might also be the mechanism by which dopamine upregulates renal CSE and 3-MST under hypothermia/rewarming condition. Along the same train of thought, AOAA treatment also markedly reduced serum H_2S level (Fig. 8.3b) and creatinine clearance (Fig. 8.4b) in Syrian hamsters subjected to $5'$-AMP-induced torpor-like state at 7 °C body temperature (Fig. 8.3a) [46]. However, a major caveat in the use of AOAA (and other endogenous H_2S inhibitors) is its unspecificity to H_2S-producing enzymes, and therefore knockout/knockdown models are required to complement its use. The antioxidant effect of H_2S is also observed through therapeutic concentrations of the novel mitochondrial targeting molecule, AP39 [22], which significantly reduced ROS production and preserved mitochondrial membrane integrity in our novel in vitro model of cold hypoxia/hypercapnia and warm reoxygenation (H/R) injury [60] as well as in other in vitro models of hypoxia/oxidative stress injury in renal epithelial cells and in rat model of renal IRI [61], showing a direct mitochondrial effect of AP39. Mechanistically, H_2S regulates ROS production by enhancing the transport of homocysteine, which is reduced to cysteine, serving as a substrate for the synthesis of glutathione (the most abundant antioxidant in cells) and inhibiting the activity of nicotinamide adenine dinucleotide phosphate oxidase [NADPH oxidase (NOX), a major source of ROS in the kidney] [62]. Although the effect of H_2S on NOX expression and activity has not been described extensively in the context of kidney transplantation, Han et al. [63] recently reported that H_2S administration via NaHS increased total glutathione and other antioxidant levels and significantly decreased the expression of NOX4 and NOX1 (members of the NOX family), MDA production, and glutathione-to-oxidized glutathione ratio in a mouse model of warm renal IRI and in human vascular smooth muscle cells [64].

It is important to note that apart from functioning as an ROS scavenger, H_2S also boosts the endogenous antioxidant defense system by activating other antioxidant enzymes such as glutathione, catalase, superoxide dismutase, and nuclear factor erythroid 2-related factor 2 (Nrf-2) and by increasing levels of N-acetylcysteine [65, 66] (Fig. 8.5). However, considering the low concentration of endogenous H_2S in blood and tissues, its ability to directly scavenge ROS and its direct interaction with oxidants cannot completely account for its antioxidant effect. Studies suggest that H_2S interaction with NO and CO (members of the gasotransmitter family) in the mitochondrial respiratory chain could activate their individual antioxidant activities via activation and opening of adenosine triphosphate ATP-sensitive potassium (K^+_{ATP}) channels [67–69] and, therefore, could serve as a backup mechanism of the antioxidant activities of H_2S. In conclusion, H_2S treatment offers protection against cold IRI partly through its potent antioxidant action, which also includes recruitment and activation of other endogenous antioxidant pathways.

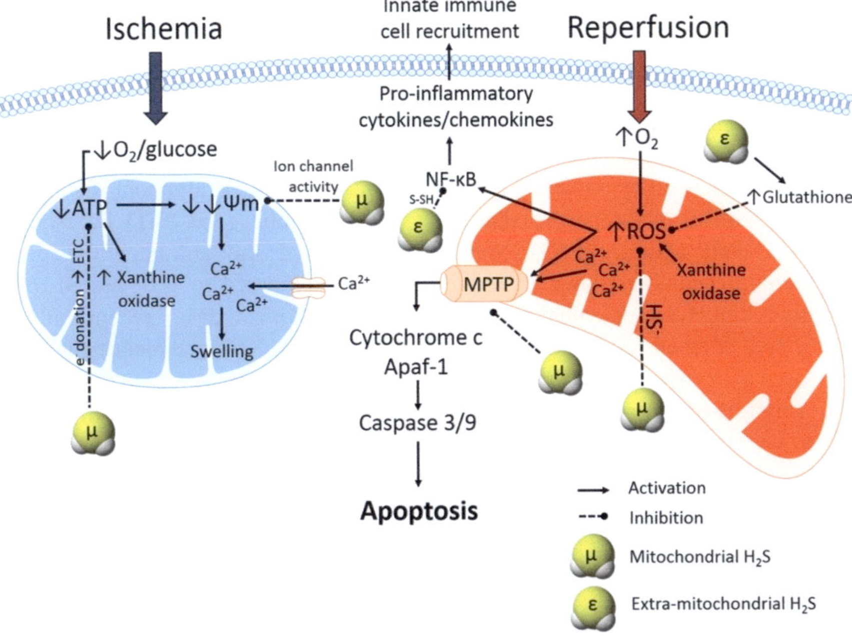

Fig. 8.5 Proposed mechanisms of H₂S-mediated protection of mitochondria during cold IRI. During ischemia, ATP depletion causes inhibition of mitochondrial Na⁺/K⁺ ion channels, resulting in decreased mitochondrial membrane potential (Ψm), influx of Ca^{2+} ions, and subsequent swelling of mitochondria. Prolonged periods of ischemia can permanently damage complexes in the electron transport chain (ETC), which produce a burst of reactive oxygen species (ROS) as oxygen floods cells upon reperfusion. ROS are also produced in mitochondria by conversion of xanthine dehydrogenase to xanthine oxidase during ischemia. Xanthine oxidase converts hypoxanthine to uric acid, producing superoxide as a by-product. High levels of mitochondrial ROS production combined with Ca^{2+}-induced mitochondrial swelling result in severe damage of mitochondrial membranes and formation of mitochondrial permeability transition pores (MPTP), releasing pro-apoptotic factors, cytochrome c, and apoptosis-inducing factor-1 (Apaf-1), which then activate the caspase 9/3 apoptotic signaling cascade, initiating cellular apoptosis. ROS-mediated mitochondrial damage also results in the activation of pro-inflammatory NF-κB signaling and ultimately innate immune cell recruitment. H₂S is proposed to directly mitigate the following mitochondrial mechanisms during IRI pathogenesis: (1) prevents loss of Ψm and subsequent Ca^{2+} influx through stimulation of ATP production via donation of electrons to the ETC and modulation of Ca^{2+} channel activity, (2) inhibits ROS production through direct inhibition (in HS⁻ form), and (3) directly inhibits MPTP formation via a cyclophilin D-independent mechanism. These mechanisms could be modulated through administration of external, mitochondrial targeted sources of H₂S, such as AP39. Additionally, external sources of extramitochondrial H₂S could indirectly blunt mitochondrial mechanisms of IRI pathogenesis via upregulation of the antioxidant glutathione and modulate pro-inflammatory NF-κB signaling via S-sulfhydration of the p65 subunit. The actions of mitochondrial (μ) and extramitochondrial (ε) sources of H₂S are, respectively, indicated in the figure

H_2S Maintains Mitochondrial Homeostasis and Inhibits Apoptosis During Cold Renal Ischemia/Reperfusion

We have previously shown that H_2S treatment protects donor kidneys against cold IRI at least partly by decreasing apoptosis in a rat model of kidney transplantation. This was evidenced by a marked reduction in rates of renal graft apoptosis in conjunction with decreased expression of the pro-apoptotic gene, BH3 interacting-domain death agonist (BID), and upregulation of the anti-apoptotic gene, extracellular signal-regulated kinase-1 (ERK-1), compared to UW-treated renal grafts without H_2S supplementation [8, 59]. Similar to our studies, a recent study by Meng et al. demonstrated that anti-apoptotic role of H_2S was associated with an increased expression of the anti-apoptotic protein, Bcl-2, and decreased expressions and activities of pro-apoptotic proteins (p38, Bax, and caspase-3) in both in vitro and in vivo models [70]. Considering both the increase in systemic H_2S levels and the importance of mitochondrial protection for preservation of renal function during mammalian hibernation, it has been increasingly suggested that H_2S may preserve mitochondrial integrity in a similar fashion during cold IRI. We have recently produced novel and exciting evidence that supports this potential protective mechanism of H_2S. In our study, we utilized AP39 to investigate whether targeting H_2S release to mitochondria improves the potency of its protective effects during cold renal IRI. Using an in vitro model of H/R injury, we demonstrated that the treatment of rat kidney cells with nanomolar concentrations of AP39 was at least 1000-fold more potent at preserving cellular viability following cold H/R injury compared to similar concentrations of the nonspecific H_2S donor, GYY4137 [60]. Treatment of renal grafts with AP39 during prolonged cold storage also resulted in improved posttransplant graft function and survival, suggesting that targeting of H_2S delivery to mitochondria could represent a viable and potent clinical strategy for minimizing the effect of IRI during transplantation [60]. Furthermore, AP39 stimulates mitochondrial respiration and generates mitochondrial sulfide and persulfide [22, 71], all of which act to maintain mitochondrial function during periods of hypoxia, thus making it an ideal candidate for organ preservation. Additionally, H_2S (NaHS and AP39) inhibited Ca^{2+}-mediated opening of mitochondrial permeability transition pore (MPTP) via a cyclophilin D-independent mechanism, preventing the release of pro-apoptotic factors from the mitochondria of hypertensive rat heart and also protecting rat myocardium against IRI [72–74]. Hence, as hypothermia stimulates Ca^{2+} influx and mitochondrial Ca^{2+} accumulation [75], it is highly possible that H_2S treatment of donor kidneys blocks Ca^{2+} influx and mitochondrial Ca^{2+} accumulation during cold storage by exerting a direct inhibitory effect on MPTP at a different site than cyclophilin D, thereby preventing the opening of MPTPs and preserving mitochondrial integrity (Fig. 8.5). Taken together, exogenous H_2S appears to exert an anti-apoptotic effect during cold renal IRI, which could be mediated by inhibitory actions against MPTP formation.

H_2S Induces Renal Vasodilation During Cold Ischemia/Reperfusion

Cold storage of donor organs induces vasoconstriction, which has been partially implicated in cold-induced organ injury during transplantation. Emerging reports indicate that H_2S induces vasodilation and thereby mitigates injurious effects of cold-induced vasoconstriction. Xia et al. [17] first demonstrated that infusion of NaHS in intrarenal arteries in rats increases RBF and glomerular filtration rate (GFR) by increasing vasodilation in pre- and post-glomerular arterioles and decreasing intrarenal vascular resistance, which would attenuate renal damage and improve oxygen and nutrient delivery to maintain functioning renal cells. This enhancement of RBF by H_2S may result from activation and opening of K^+_{ATP} channels and dilatation of blood vessels, as this appears to be the underlying mechanism of protection by H_2S in myocardial ischemia [76]. Following this initial demonstration of the effects of H_2S on renal hemodynamics, Hosgood and Nicholson used a porcine model of kidney transplantation to demonstrate that H_2S treatment significantly increases RBF in donor kidneys at 10 min before and after reperfusion compared to control group without H_2S supplementation [58]. We have also observed that NaHS administration improves RBF and reduces renal resistive index in a representative porcine model of donation-after-cardiac-death (DCD) kidney transplantation [13]. In addition, we subsequently developed a rat model of DCD kidney transplantation to show that treatment of DCD kidneys with H_2S during both warm and cold IRI results in decreased posttransplant graft injury and improved subsequent graft function and survival [77]. Thus, by improving resistive index and RBF, H_2S may improve perfusion parameters, which then may translate to improved renal function upon transplantation (Fig. 8.6). It is important to point out that cyclosporine, a widely used immunosuppressive drug after kidney transplantation, induces nephrotoxicity which begins with renal and systemic vasoconstriction leading to reduced glomerular filtration rate (GFR) and ultimately interstitial fibrosis and tubular atrophy [78]. Interestingly, a recent study has shown that H_2S infusion before and after reperfusion of cold-stored porcine kidneys reverses cyclosporine-induced vasoconstriction and glomerular atrophy by inducing vasodilation and increasing RBF, suggesting an additional protective role of H_2S-induced vasodilation during the transplant procedure [79]. Thus, the vasodilatory effects of H_2S appear to reduce renal resistance and increase RBF in donor kidneys following cold storage, resulting in improved reperfusion and function of renal grafts in the acute posttransplant period.

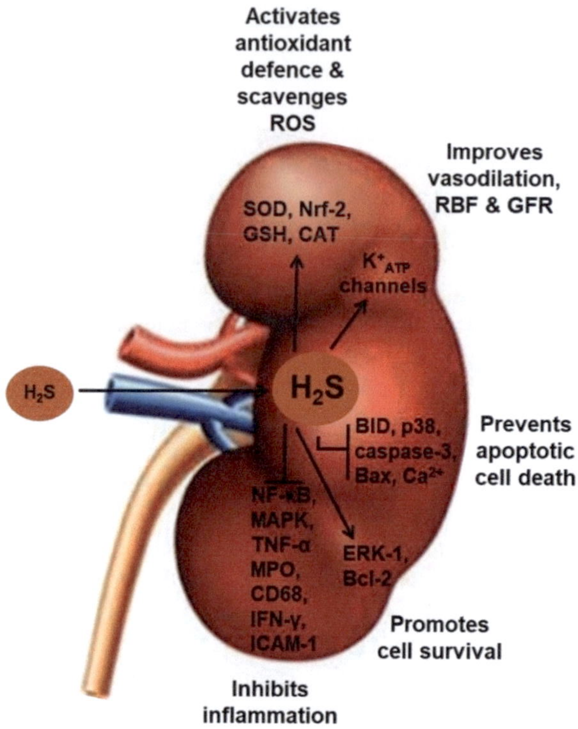

Fig. 8.6 Effects and mechanisms of H_2S against cold ischemia/reperfusion injury in kidney transplantation. Exogenous administration of hydrogen sulfide (H_2S) augments endogenous H_2S level, thereby stimulating the opening of adenosine triphosphate (ATP)-sensitive potassium (K^+_{ATP}) channels, causing vasodilation, and consequently increasing renal blood flow (RBF) and glomerular filtration rate (GFR). H_2S also inhibits the activation of apoptotic and inflammatory pathways, upregulates anti-apoptotic genes such as extracellular signal-regulated kinase-1 (ERK-1) and B-cell lymphoma-2 (Bcl-2), and thus promotes renal cell survival. Additionally, H_2S scavenges reactive oxygen species (ROS) and also activates endogenous antioxidants such as superoxide dismutase (SOD), glutathione (GSH), catalase (CAT), and nuclear factor erythroid 2-related factor 2 (Nrf-2), thereby bolstering the endogenous antioxidant defense system and thus reducing mitochondrial oxidative stress

H_2S Suppresses Renal Inflammation Induced by Cold Ischemia/Reperfusion

Apart from antioxidant, anti-apoptotic, and vasodilatory effects, the therapeutic properties of H_2S in kidney transplantation also include an anti-inflammatory component. For example, we have previously demonstrated that H_2S treatment of rat renal graft during cold storage significantly decreased infiltration of myeloperoxidase (MPO)-positive neutrophils, CD68-positive macrophages, and expression of the pro-inflammatory cytokines interferon-gamma (IFN-γ) and intercellular adhesion molecule-1 (ICAM-1) in the acute posttransplant period [8] (Fig. 8.5). Our finding was confirmed by a recent study in which H_2S administration suppressed the influx of myeloperoxidase (MPO)-positive neutrophils in the kidneys of rats subjected to warm IRI [61]. While the anti-inflammatory property of H_2S in kidney transplantation remains to be revealed, other studies have reported more potent anti-inflammatory effects and mechanisms of H_2S in various disease models [70]. The slow-releasing H_2S donor, GYY4137, inhibits nuclear factor-kappa B and mitogen-activated protein kinases (p38, ERK1/2 and JNK1/2) [80], two key mediators of inflammation. Such anti-inflammatory effect of H_2S was partially involved in myocardial protection through increased plasma H_2S concentration and CSE activity in a rat model of myocardial IRI [70]. H_2S inhibits the expression of leukocyte adhesion molecules, thereby preventing leukocyte "rolling" and attachment to the endothelium [81]. This inhibition was associated with the activation of K^+_{ATP} channels by H_2S, as K^+_{ATP} antagonist reversed the leukocyte inhibitory effect of H_2S and increased leukocyte adherence [81]. These mechanisms underlying the anti-inflammatory action of H_2S may thus partly account for the renal protection against cold IRI in transplantation.

Conclusion and Future Perspectives

To our knowledge, there are no therapeutic strategies that can successfully mitigate IRI associated with organ transplantation. Therefore, the therapeutic use of exogenous H_2S added to standard preservation solutions or inducing endogenous H_2S seems to be a promising approach to prolong renal graft preservation and mitigate the unavoidable cold IRI during transplantation of kidney and other solid organs (Fig. 8.7). Targeting exogenous H_2S administration to mitochondria increases the potency of its protective effects during IRI, implicating mitochondria as a primary site of action for H_2S-mediated renoprotection. Exogenous H_2S could potentially control mitochondrial mechanisms of IRI pathogenesis directly by driving ATP synthesis via donation of electrons to the ETC [54, 55], modulation of mitochondrial Ca^{2+} channels to prevent Ca^{2+} influx [82, 83], direct inhibition of mitochondrial ROS [84, 85], and prevention of MPTP formation [72] or indirectly via inhibition of pro-inflammatory NF-κB signaling [86] and upregulation of cellular antioxidant enzymes such as glutathione [87, 88]. Although extensive investigation in defining the molecular mechanisms behind IRI and the use of various therapeutic strategies have been proposed, ongoing clinical studies including those utilizing rPSGL-Ig (a p-selectin inhibitor) and mitoQ (an antioxidant) have provided some satisfying results in preventing renal IRI [89]. In all cases, more clinical trials with improved standardization of protocols are required in order to contribute to important advances in clinical therapy [90]. Apart from the involvement of H_2S in transplantation, additional lessons can be learned from dissecting mechanisms by which nature protects organs of hibernating animals from the damaging effects of cold exposure and

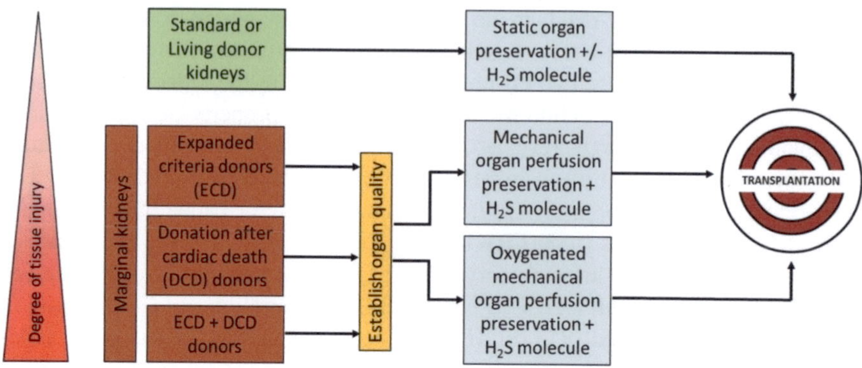

Fig. 8.7 Potential model of kidney preservation prior to transplantation. As donor organs become more marginal [expanded criteria donors (ECDs): age >60 or age >50 plus two of the following features—hypertension, terminal serum creatinine >1.5 mg/dL, or death from cerebrovascular accident; donation-after-cardiac-death (DCD) donors], better evaluative tools will need to be devised in order to better establish organ quality prior to transplantation. Once this has been carried out, transplant teams may decide whether the organ should be preserved in static or mechanical organ preservation in standard solutions. There is strong experimental evidence to suggest that supplementing these standard solutions with H₂S donor molecules may have a significant impact on both short- and long-term graft outcomes by modulating the deleterious effects of ischemia-reperfusion injury

reperfusion. Understanding such mechanisms will be beneficial for the development of more potent forms of the current therapeutics or novel therapeutic agents. In addition, future investigations should be aimed at developing new drugs or combination of current therapeutic agents that could afford a multi-target approach to minimizing IRI during transplantation. In this way, we may be able to take advantage of natural cytoprotective mechanisms utilized by hibernating mammals, such as H₂S-mediated mitochondrial preservation, to ultimately improve clinical outcomes and quality of life for renal transplant recipients.

Conflict of Interest None.

References

1. Cavallo MC, Sepe V, Conte F, Abelli M, Ticozzelli E, Bottazzi A, Geraci PM. Cost-effectiveness of kidney transplantation from DCD in Italy. Transplant Proc. 2014;46:3289–96.
2. Bon D, Chatauret N, Giraud S, Thuillier R, Favreau HT. New strategies to optimize kidney recovery and preservation in transplantation. Nat Rev Nephrol. 2012;8:339–47.
3. Debout A, Foucher Y, Trebern-Launay K, et al. Each additional hour of cold ischemic time significantly increases the risk of graft failure and mortality following renal transplantation. Kidney Int. 2015;87:343–9.
4. Ojo AO, Wolfe RA, Held PJ, Port FK, Schmouder RL. Delayed graft function: risk factors and implications for renal allograft survival. Transplantation. 1997;63:968.

5. Salahudeen AK, Haider N, May W. Cold ischemia and reduced long-term survival of cadaveric renal allografts. Kidney Int. 2004;65:713–8.
6. Stubenitsky BM, Booster MH, Kootstra G, Brasile L, Haisch C. Deleterious effect of prolonged cold ischemia on renal function. Transpl Int. 2001;14:256–60.
7. Mitchell T, Saba H, Laakman J, Parajuli N, Macmillan-Crow LA. Role of mitochondrial-derived oxidants in renal tubular cell cold-storage injury. Free Radic Biol Med. 2010;49:1273–82.
8. Lobb I, Mok A, Lan Z, Liu W, Garcia B, Sener A. Supplemental hydrogen sulfide protects transplant kidney function and prolongs recipient survival after prolonged cold ischemia-reperfusion injury by mitigating renal apoptosis and inflammation. BJU Int. 2012;110:E1187–95.
9. Carden DL, Granger DN. Pathophysiology of ischemia-reperfusion injury. J Pathol. 2000;190:255–66.
10. Malek M, Nematbakhsh M. Renal ischemia/reperfusion injury; from pathophysiology to treatment. J Renal Inj Prev. 2015;4:20–7.
11. Talaei F, Bouma HR, Hylkema MN, Strijkstra AM, Boereman AS, Schmidt M, Henning RH. The role of endogenous H$_2$S formation in reversible remodeling of lung tissue during hibernation in the Syrian hamster. J Exp Biol. 2012;15:2912–9.
12. Dugbartey GJ, Talaei F, Houwertjes MC, Goris M, Epema AH, Bouma HR, Henning RH. Dopamine treatment attenuates acute kidney injury in a rat model of deep hypothermia and rewarming—the role of renal H$_2$S-producing enzymes. Eur J Pharmacol. 2015;769:225–33.
13. Alabbassi A, Tran KC, Bloch M, Deng J, Mok A, Liu W, et al. The effects of CORM-3 and H$_2$S on renal protection during pulsatile perfusion. Am J Transplant. 2011;11:A1614.
14. George TJ, Arnaoutakis GJ, Beaty CA, Jandu SK, Santhanam L, Berkowitz DE, Shah AS. Inhaled hydrogen sulfide improves graft function in an experimental model of lung transplantation. J Surg Res. 2012;178:593–600.
15. George TJ, Arnaoutakis GJ, Beaty CA, Jandu SK, Santhanam L, Berkowitz DE, Shah AS. Hydrogen sulfide decreases reactive oxygen in a model of lung transplantation. J Surg Res. 2012;178:494–501.
16. Li Q, Lancaster JR Jr. Chemical foundations of hydrogen sulfide biology. Nitric Oxide. 2013;35:21–34.
17. Xia M, Chen L, Muh RW, Li PL, Li N. Production and actions of hydrogen sulfide, a novel gaseous bioactive substance, in the kidneys. J Pharmacol Exp Ther. 2009;329:1056–62.
18. Shibuya N, Koike S, Tanaka M, et al. A novel pathway for the production of hydrogen sulfide from D-cysteine in mammalian cells. Nat Commun. 2013;4:1366.
19. Kashfi K, Olson KR. Biology and therapeutic potential of hydrogen sulfide and hydrogen sulfide-releasing chimeras. Biochem Pharmacol. 2013;85:689–703.
20. Li I, Whiteman M, Guan YY, et al. Characterization of a novel, water-soluble hydrogen sulfide-releasing molecule (GYY4137): new insights into the biology of hydrogen sulfide. Circulation. 2008;117:2351–60.
21. Szczesny B, Modis K, Yanagi K, et al. AP39, a novel mitochondria-targeted hydrogen sulfide donor, stimulates cellular bioenergetics, exerts cytoprotective effects and protects against the loss of mitochondrial DNA integrity in oxidatively stressed endothelial cells in vitro. Nitric Oxide. 2014;41:120–30.
22. Le Trionairre S, Perry A, Bartosz S, et al. The synthesis and functional evaluation of a mitochondria-targeted hydrogen sulfide donor, (10-oxo-10-(4-(3-thioxo-3H-1,2-dithiol-5-yl)phenoxy)decyl)triphenyl phosphonium bromide (AP39). Med Chem Commun. 2014;5:728–36.
23. Gerő D, Torregrossa R, Perry A, Waters A, Le-Trionnaire S, Whatmore JL, Wood M, Whiteman M. The novel mitochondria-targeted hydrogen sulfide (H$_2$S) donors AP123 and AP39 protect against hyperglycemic injury in microvascular endothelial cells in vitro. Pharmacol Res. 2016;113(Pt A):186–98.
24. Quinones QJ, Ma Q, Zhang Z, Barnes BM, Podgoreanu MV. Organ protective mechanisms common to extremes of physiology: a window through hibernation biology. Integr Comp Biol. 2014;54:497–515.

25. de Vrij EL, Vogelaar PC, Goris M, et al. Platelet dynamics during natural and pharmacologically induced torpor and forced hypothermia. PLoS One. 2014;9(4):e93218.
26. Bouma HR, Dugbartey GJ, Boerema AS, Talaei F, Herwig A, Goris M, van Buiten A, Strijkstra AM, Carey HV, Henning RH, Kroese FGM. Reduction of body temperature governs neutrophil retention in hibernating and non-hibernating animals by margination. J Leukoc Biol. 2013;94(3):431–7.
27. Barnes BM. Freeze avoidance in a mammal: body temperatures below 0 °C in an Arctic hibernator. Science. 1989;244:1593–5.
28. Heldmaier G, Ortmann S, Elvert R. Natural hypometabolism during hibernation and daily torpor in mammals. Respir Physiol Neurobiol. 2004;141:317–29.
29. Stenvinkel P, Jani AH, Johnson RJ. Hibernating bears (Ursidae): metabolic magicians of definite interest for the nephrologist. Kidney Int. 2013;83(2):207–12.
30. Brown DC, Mulhausen RO, Andrew DJ, et al. Renal function in anesthetized dormant and active bears. Am J Phys. 1971;220:293–8.
31. Toien O, Blake J, Edgar DM, et al. Hibernation in black bears: independence of metabolic suppression from body temperature. Science. 2011;331:906–9.
32. Camici PG, Prasad SK, Rimoldi OE. Stunning, hibernation and assessment of myocardial viability. Circulation. 2008;117:103–14.
33. Jani A, Epperson E, Martin J, Pacic A, Ljubanovic D, Martin SL, Edelstein CL. Renal protection from prolonged cold ischemia and warm reperfusion in hibernating squirrels. Transplantation. 2011;92:1215–21.
34. Zancanaro C, Malatesta M, Mannello F, Vogel P, Fakan S. The kidney during hibernation and arousal from hibernation. A natural model of organ preservation during cold ischemia and reperfusion. Nephrol Dial Transplant. 1999;14:1982–90.
35. Jain S, Keys D, Martin S, Edelstein CL, Jani A. Protection from apoptotic cell death during cold storage followed by rewarming in 13-lined ground squirrel tubular tells: the role of prosurvival factors X-linked inhibitor of apoptosis and phospho-Akt. Transplantation. 2016;100(3):538–45.
36. Sandovici M, Henning RH, Hut RA, Strijkstra AM, Epema AH, van Goor H, Deelman LE. Differential regulation of glomerular and interstitial endothelial nitric oxide synthase expression in the kidney of hibernating ground squirrel. Nitric Oxide. 2004;11(2):194–200.
37. Haak LL, Mignot E, Kilduff TS, Dement WC, Heller HC. Regional changes in central monoamine and metabolic levels during the hibernation cycle in the golden-mantled ground squirrel. Brain Res. 1991;563:215–20.
38. Kramarova LI, Lee TF, Cui Y, Wang LC. State-dependent variation in the inhibitory effect of [D-Ala^2, D-Leu^5]-enkephalin on hippocampal serotonin release in ground squirrels. Life Sci. 1991;48:175–81.
39. Sallmen T, Beckman AL, Stanton TL, et al. Major changes in the brain histamine system of the ground squirrel *Citellus lateralis* during hibernation. J Neurosci. 1999;19:1824–35.
40. Lakhina AA, Markevich LN, Zakharova NM, Afanasyev VN, Kolomiytseva IK, Fesenko EE. Phospholipids of liver cell nuclei during hibernation of Yakutian ground squirrel. Dokl Biochem Biophys. 2016;469(1):235–8.
41. Blackstone E, Roth MB. Suspended animation-like state protects mice from lethal hypoxia. Shock. 2007;27:370–2.
42. Blackstone E, Morrison M, Roth MB. H_2S induces a suspended animation-like state in mice. Science. 2005;308:518.
43. Drew KL, Osborne PG, Frerichs KU, Hu Y, Koren RE, Hellenbeck JM, Rice ME. Ascorbate and glutathione regulation in hibernating ground squirrels. Brain Res. 1999;851:1–8.
44. Fleck CC, Carey HV. Modulation of apoptotic pathways in intestinal mucosa during hibernation. Am J Physiol Regul Integr Comp Physiol. 2005;289:R586–95.
45. Talaei F, Bouma HR, van der Graaf AC, Strijkstra AM, Schmidt M, Henning RH. Serotonin and dopamine protect from hypothermia/rewarming damage through the CBS/H_2S pathway. PLoS One. 2011;6:e22568.

46. Dugbartey GJ, Bouma HR, Strijkstra AM, Boerema AS, Henning RH. Induction of a torpor-like state by 5′-AMP does not depend on H_2S production. PLoS One. 2015;10(8):e0136113.
47. Beltowski J. Hypoxia in the renal medulla: implication for hydrogen sulfide signaling. J Pharmacol Exp Ther. 2010;334(2):358–63.
48. Braunwald E, Bonow RO. Braunwald's heart disease: a textbook of cardiovascular medicine. Philadelphia: Saunders; 2012. p. 44.
49. Carey HV, Andrews MT, Martin SI. Mammalian hibernation: cellular and molecular responses to depressed metabolism and low temperature. Physiol Rev. 2003;83(4):1153–81.
50. Bouma HR, Verhaag EM, Otis JP, Heldmaier G, Swoap SJ, Strijkstra AM, Henning RH, Carey HV. Induction of torpor: mimicking natural metabolic suppression for biomedical applications. J Cell Physiol. 2012;227(4):1285–90.
51. Ma YL, Zhu X, Rivera PM, Toien O, Barnes BM, LaManna JC, Smith MA, Drew KL. Absence of cellular stress in brain after hypoxia induced by arousal from hibernation in Arctic ground squirrels. Am J Physiol Regul Integr Comp Physiol. 2005;289:R1297–306.
52. Baumgart K, Radermacher P, Wagner F. Applying gases for microcirculatory and cellular oxygenation in sepsis: effects of nitric oxide, carbon monoxide, and hydrogen sulfide. Curr Opin Anesthesiol. 2009;22:168–76.
53. Bos EM, Leuvenink HG, Snijder PM, et al. Hydrogen sulfide-induced hypometabolism prevents renal ischemia/reperfusion injury. J Am Soc Nephrol. 2009;20:1901–5.
54. Modis K, Coletta C, Erdelyi K, Papapetropoulos A, Szabo C. Intramitochondrial hydrogen sulfide production by 3-mercaptopyruvate sulfurtransferase maintains mitochondrial electron flow and supports cellular bioenergetics. FASEB J. 2013;27:601–11.
55. Goubern M, Andriamihaja M, Nubel T, Blachier F, Bouillaud F. Sulfide, the first inorganic substrate for human cells. FASEB J. 2007;21:1699–706.
56. Fu M, Zhang W, Wu L, Yang G, Li H, Wang R. Hydrogen sulfide (H_2S) metabolism in mitochondria and its regulatory role in energy production. Proc Natl Acad Sci U S A. 2012;109(8):2943–8.
57. Teng H, Wu B, Zhao K, Yang G, Wu L, Wang R. Oxygen-sensitive mitochondria accumulation of cystathionine β synthase mediated by Lon protease. Proc Natl Acad Sci U S A. 2013;110(31):12679–84.
58. Hosgood SA, Nicholson ML. Hydrogen sulphide ameliorates ischaemia-reperfusion injury in an experimental model of non-heart-beating donor kidney transplantation. Br J Surg. 2010;97:202–9.
59. Lobb I, Davidson M, Carter D, Liu W, Haig A, Gunaratnam L, Sener A. Hydrogen sulfide treatment mitigates renal allograft ischemia-reperfusion injury during cold storage and improves early transplant kidney function and survival following allogeneic renal transplantation. J Urol. 2015;194:1806–15.
60. Lobb I, Jiang J, Lian D, et al. Hydrogen sulfide protects renal grafts against prolonged cold ischemia-reperfusion injury via specific mitochondrial actions. Am J Transplant. 2017;17(2):341–52.
61. Ahmad A, Olah G, Szczesny B, Wood ME, Whiteman M, Szabo C. AP39, a mitochondrially targeted hydrogen sulfide donor, exerts protective effects in renal epithelial cells subjected to oxidative stress in vitro and in acute renal injury in vivo. Shock. 2016;45(1):88–97.
62. Shan XQ, Aw TY, Jones DP. Glutathione-dependent protection against oxidative injury. Pharmacol Ther. 1990;47:61–71.
63. Han SJ, Kim JI, Park JW, Park KM. Hydrogen sulfide accelerates the recovery of kidney tubules after renal ischemia/reperfusion injury. Nephrol Dial Transplant. 2015;30:1497–506.
64. Muzaffar S, Shukla N, Bond M, Newby AC, Angelini GD, Sparatore A, Del Soldato P, Jeremy JY. Exogenous hydrogen sulfide inhibits superoxide formation, NOX-1 expression and Rac1 activity in human vascular smooth muscle cells. J Vasc Res. 2008;45(6):521–8.
65. Calvert JW, Jha S, Gundewar S, et al. Hydrogen sulfide mediates cardioprotection through Nrf2 signaling. Circ Res. 2009;105:365–74.

66. Shimada S, Fukai M, Wakayama K, et al. Hydrogen sulfide augments survival signals in warm ischemia and reperfusion of the mouse liver. Surg Today. 2015;45:892–903.
67. Murphy ME, Brayden JE. Nitric oxide hyperpolarizes rabbit mesenteric arteries via ATP-sensitive potassium channels. J Physiol. 1995;486(Pt 1):47–58.
68. Pareira de Avila MA, Giusti-Paiva A, de Oliveira G, Nascimento C. The peripheral antinociceptive effect induced by the heme oxygenase/carbon monoxide pathway is associated with ATP-sensitive K^+ channels. Eur J Pharmacol. 2014;726:41–8.
69. Zhao W, Zhang J, Lu Y, Wang R. The vasorelaxant effect of H_2S as a novel endogenous gaseous K(ATP) channel opener. EMBO J. 2001;20(21):6008–16.
70. Meng G, Wang J, Xiao Y, Bai W, Xie L, Shan L, Moore PK, Ji Y. GYY4137 protects against myocardial ischemia and reperfusion injury by attenuating oxidative stress and apoptosis in rats. J Biomed Res. 2015;29:203–13.
71. Wedmann R, Onderka C, Wei S, Szijártó IA, et al. Improved tag-switch method reveals that thioredoxin acts as depersulfidase and controls the intracellular levels of protein persulfidation. Chem Sci. 2016;7(5):3414–26.
72. Strutynska NA, Dorofeieva NO, Vavilova HL, Sahach VF. Hydrogen sulfide inhibits Ca^{2+}-induced mitochondrial transition pore opening in spontaneously hypertensive rats. Fiziol Zh. 2013;59:3–10.
73. Chatzianastasiou A, Bibli SI, Andreadou I, Efentakis P, Kaludercic N, Wood ME, Whiteman M, Di Lisa F, Daiber A, Manolopoulos VG, Szabó C, Papapetropoulos A. Cardioprotection by H_2S donors: nitric oxide-dependent and -independent mechanisms. J Pharmacol Exp Ther. 2016;358(3):431–40.
74. Karwi QG, Bornbaum J, Boengler K, Torregrossa R, Whiteman M, Wood ME, Schulz R, Baxter GF. AP39, a mitochondria-targeting hydrogen sulfide (H_2S) donor, protects against myocardial reperfusion injury independently of salvage kinase signalling. Br J Pharmacol. 2017;174(4):287–301.
75. Brinkkoetter PT, Song H, Lösel R, et al. Hypothermic injury: the mitochondrial calcium, ATP and ROS love–hate triangle out of balance. Cell Physiol Biochem. 2008;22:195–204.
76. Zhang Z, Huang H, Liu P, Tang C, Wang J. Hydrogen sulfide contributes to cardioprotection during ischemia-reperfusion injury by opening K ATP channels. Can J Physiol Pharmacol. 2007;85:1248–53.
77. Grewal J, Lobb I, Saha M, Haig A, Jiang J, Sener. MP29-16 hydrogen sulfide supplementation mitigates effects of ischemia reperfusion injury in a murine model of donation after cardiac death renal transplantation. J Urol. 2016;195(4):e386.
78. Senero J, Rodrigues-Santos P, Vala H, et al. Transition from cyclosporine-induced renal dysfunction to nephrotoxicity in an in vivo rat model. Int J Mol Sci. 2014;15:8979–97.
79. Lee G, Hosgood SA, Patel MS, Nicholson ML. Hydrogen sulphide as a novel therapy to ameliorate cyclosporine nephrotoxicity. J Surg Res. 2015;197:419–26.
80. Wu Z, Peng H, Lin W, Liu Y. GYY4137, a hydrogen sulfide-releasing molecule, inhibits the inflammatory response by suppressing the activation of nuclear factor-kappa B and mitogen-activated protein kinases in Coxsackie virus B3-infected rat cardiomyocytes. Mol Med Rep. 2015;11:1837–44.
81. Zanardo RC, Brancaleone V, Distrutti E, Fiorucci S, Cirino G, Wallace JL. Hydrogen sulfide is an endogenous modulator of leukocyte-mediated inflammation. FASEB J. 2006;20:2118–20.
82. Tomasova L, Pavlovicova M, Malekova L, Misak A, Kristek F, Grman M, et al. Effects of AP39, a novel triphenylphosphonium derivatised anethole dithiolethione hydrogen sulfide donor, on rat haemodynamic parameters and chloride and calcium Cav3 and RyR2 channels. Nitric Oxide. 2015;46:131–44.
83. Tang G, Wu L, Wang R. Interaction of hydrogen sulfide with ion channels. Clin Exp Pharmacol Physiol. 2010;37(7):753–63.
84. Carballal S, Trujillo M, Cuevasanta E, Bartesaghi S, Möller MN, Folkes LK, et al. Reactivity of hydrogen sulfide with peroxynitrite and other oxidants of biological interest. Free Radic Biol Med. 2011;50(1):196–205.

85. Nagy P, Winterbourn CC. Rapid reaction of hydrogen sulfide with the neutrophil oxidant hypochlorous acid to generate polysulfides. Chem Res Toxicol. 2010;23(10):1541–3.
86. Sen N, Paul BD, Gadalla MM, Mustafa AK, Sen T, Xu R, et al. Hydrogen sulfide- linked sulfhydration of NF-kappaB mediates its antiapoptotic actions. Mol Cell. 2012;45(1):13–24.
87. Kimura Y, Goto Y, Kimura H. Hydrogen sulfide increases glutathione production and suppresses oxidative stress in mitochondria. Antioxid Redox Signal. 2010;12(1):1–13.
88. Yang G, Zhao K, Ju Y, Mani S, Cao Q, Puukila S, et al. Hydrogen sulfide protects against cellular senescence via S-sulfhydration of Keap1 and activation of Nrf2. Antioxid Redox Signal. 2013;18(15):1906–19.
89. Dare AJ, Bolton EA, Pettigrew GJ, Bradley JA, Saeb-Parsy K, Murphy MP. Protection against renal ischemia-reperfusion injury in vivo by the mitochondria targeted antioxidant MitoQ. Redox Biol. 2015;5:163–8.
90. Pantazi E, Bejoui M, Folch-Puy E, Adam R, Rosello-Catafau J. Advances in treatment strategies for ischemia reperfusion injury. Expert Opin Pharmacother. 2016;17:169–79.

Chapter 9
Hydrogen Sulfide Against Ischemia-Reperfusion Injury in Transplantation of Kidney and Other Transplantable Solid Organs

George J. Dugbartey and Alp Sener

This chapter is a modified version by the same authors in the publication titled H2S donor molecules against cold ischemia-reperfusion injury in preclinical models of solid organ transplantation. Pharmacol Res. 2021 Oct; 172:105842.

G. J. Dugbartey (✉)
Division of Urology, Department of Surgery, London Health Sciences Center, Western University, London, ON, Canada

Multi-Organ Transplant Program, London Health Sciences Center, Western University, London, ON, Canada

Matthew Mailing Center for Translational Transplant Studies, London Health Sciences Center, Western University, London, ON, Canada

Department of Pharmacology and Toxicology, School of Pharmacy, College of Health Sciences, University of Ghana, Accra, Ghana

Department of Physiology and Pharmacology, Accra College of Medicine, Accra, Ghana
e-mail: gdugbart@uwo.ca

A. Sener
Division of Urology, Department of Surgery, London Health Sciences Center, Western University, London, ON, Canada

Multi-Organ Transplant Program, London Health Sciences Center, Western University, London, ON, Canada

Matthew Mailing Center for Translational Transplant Studies, London Health Sciences Center, Western University, London, ON, Canada

Department of Microbiology and Immunology, Schulich School of Medicine and Dentistry, University of Western Ontario, London, ON, Canada
e-mail: alp.sener@lhsc.on.ca

G. J. Dugbartey, A. Sener, *Hydrogen Sulfide in Kidney Diseases*,
https://doi.org/10.1007/978-3-031-44041-0_9

Ischemia-Reperfusion Injury in Kidney Transplantation

Transplantation of kidney and other solid organs is the ultimate therapeutic option that gives patients suffering from end-organ dysfunction a second chance to live with improved quality of life. However, the success of this life-saving intervention is severely hampered by a complicated, unavoidable, and unresolved clinical situation referred to as ischemia-reperfusion injury (IRI). Renal IRI is caused when blood supply to the renal tissue is temporarily stopped (ischemia) and then restored (reperfusion) after the ischemic period, which potentiates further renal tissue damage [1–3]. It represents a major factor that influences both short- and long-term survival rates of renal grafts—increasing acute tubular necrosis, decreasing graft survival, and delaying graft function—thereby complicating graft quality, posttransplant patient care, and kidney transplantation outcomes. In kidney transplantation, the donor kidney is temporarily cold-stored after procurement, inducing a period of cold ischemia before it is transplanted into the recipient patient (reperfusion). Thus, cold IRI, which is seen as the transplant surgeon's enemy, has been an inevitable and well-recognized clinical challenge since the inception of solid-organ transplantation in the mid-twentieth century. The pathophysiology of cold renal IRI is a complex cascade of interconnected events including vasoconstriction (microcirculatory disturbance and microvascular dysfunction), thrombogenesis, mitochondrial (free radical-mediated) injury, endoplasmic reticulum stress, vigorous inflammatory responses, cell damage and cell death, and many more. Therefore, prevention of cold IRI by pretreatment of renal grafts or modification of the cold preservation solution with protective pharmacological agents should begin before graft recovery. A novel pharmacological strategy to combat cold renal IRI and improve renal graft quality involves supplementation of standard preservation solution with hydrogen sulfide donor molecules during graft preservation or administration of hydrogen sulfide donor molecules to the kidney donor prior to donor kidney procurement and to the recipient at the start and during reperfusion after graft preservation. This chapter focuses on organ protection by hydrogen sulfide against cold IRI during transplantation of kidney and other transplantable solid organs. The chapter also discusses underlying molecular mechanisms of protection by hydrogen sulfide and how the translation of these promising findings from bench to bedside can lay the foundation for hydrogen sulfide donor drugs in clinical organ transplantation in the future.

Hydrogen Sulfide and Its Sources of Production

Hydrogen sulfide (H_2S) has been recently established as the third member of a class of endogenously produced gaseous signaling molecules collectively referred to as gasotransmitters, which include nitric oxide and carbon monoxide and regulate a myriad of physiological functions. Like other gasotransmitters, H_2S is an amphipathic compound, a property that makes it readily pass through lipid bilayer of cell membranes, resulting in quick and easy transport between cells and tissues without requiring specific transporters or receptors [4]. In addition to controlling physiological functions, this volatile intracellular messenger molecule has emerged as a potent cytoprotective mediator, possessing therapeutic properties such as vasodilatory, anti-apoptotic, anti-inflammatory, anti-fibrotic, and antioxidant properties that enable it to exhibit its intracellular signaling functions. Hence, alterations in its physiological levels and its synthesizing enzymes or defects in its signaling cascade have been associated with various pathological conditions of the organ systems including tissue injury that occurs due to cold IRI in organ transplantation. Emerging evidence shows that endogenous manipulation and/or exogenous administration of the levels of H_2S is cytoprotective against these pathological processes.

Endogenous Source of Hydrogen Sulfide in the Body

H_2S is commonly known as sewer gas or swamp gas. It is a colorless and flammable gas with high solubility in water and lipids. However, it has a pungent "rotten-egg" odor at low atmospheric concentration and is also denser than air [5, 6]. Until two decades ago, H_2S gained notoriety among industrial workers for its toxicity and death at high concentrations, which is attributable to its ability to reversibly inhibit the activity of the terminal enzyme, complex IV, of the mitochondrial electron transport chain (ETC) [7]. However, newer evidence from the past two decades suggests the development of a new paradigm that low concentrations of H_2S exhibit therapeutic potential, targeting a number of cellular and molecular pathways such as oxidative, inflammatory, fibrotic, and apoptotic pathways in various human diseases including IRI in organ transplantation and drug-induced toxicities [8–14].

Enzymatic Production of Hydrogen Sulfide in the Body

Endogenous H_2S is produced in all mammalian cells by enzymatic and nonenzymatic pathways [6]. The enzymatic pathway, which involves four main enzymes, is the major pathway of endogenous H_2S generation. The first two enzymes in the enzymatic pathway are cytosolic enzymes cystathionine β-synthase (CBS) and cystathionine γ-lyase (CSE), which participate in the so-called transsulfuration pathway that uses the sulfur-containing essential amino acid, L-cysteine, as substrate. The third enzymatic pathway involves the mitochondrial enzyme, 3-mercaptopyruvate sulfurtransferase (3-MST), in which L-cysteine is transaminated by cysteine aminotransferase to the intermediate product, 3-mercaptopyruvate, followed by its desulfhydration to pyruvate by the action of 3-MST. Finally, H_2S is also produced by the peroxisomal enzyme, D-amino acid oxidase (DAO), from D-cysteine, an optical isomer of cysteine [15–18]. After H_2S production by these enzymes, it is immediately released or stored in bound form or in acid-labile sulfur form in the cells [19]. Current evidence has provided a broader picture of the distribution of these H_2S-producing enzymes, suggesting that their expression is tissue specific. For example, CBS is abundantly expressed in regions of the brain such as the hippocampus, cerebellum, cerebral cortex, and brain stem [20]; in liver and pancreas; in glomerulus; in brush border and cytoplasm of the epithelial cells of the proximal tubule of the kidney [21–24]; and in cornea, conjunctiva, and iris of the eye [25]. CSE is also predominantly found in the cardiovascular system (aorta, mesenteric artery, portal vein, and other vascular tissue) [26–28] as well as in the endothelial cells, mesangial cells, podocytes, and brush border and cytoplasm of the epithelial cells of renal proximal tubules [9, 22]. In addition, 3-MST is expressed in neural and glial cells in the brain, bronchiolar cells in the lungs, pericentral hepatocytes in the liver, perinuclear area of myocardial cells of the heart, epithelial cells of renal proximal tubules, pancreatic islets, and blood vessels [24, 29–31], while DAO is expressed predominantly in the kidney and cerebellum [17].

Nonenzymatic Production of Hydrogen Sulfide in the Body

In addition to its enzymatic production, emerging evidence suggests that endogenous H_2S is also produced in a nonenzymatic manner from glucose, glutathione, elemental sulfur, and garlic-derived organic and inorganic polysulfides [32–35] although this pathway is poorly understood and less considered. It has been suggested that glucose could react with sulfur-containing amino acids such as methionine, cysteine, or homocysteine to generate H_2S and other gaseous sulfur compounds, while direct reduction of glutathione and elemental sulfur also produces H_2S [34, 35].

Exogenous Sources of Hydrogen Sulfide

Apart from its endogenous production, exogenous H_2S is currently being used in different experimental settings. Gaseous H_2S is the authentic source of exogenous H_2S. However, its application in experimental setting is less ideal due to difficulty to obtain precisely controlled concentration and possibility of toxic effect of excess H_2S [36]. Hence, exogenous H_2S in the form of inorganic sulfide salts such as sodium hydrosulfide (NaHS) and sodium sulfide (Na_2S) has been developed and functions as fast-releasing H_2S donors in various experimental models of human diseases including experimental models of organ transplantation [37, 38]. Nonetheless, a major drawback in the use of these inorganic sulfide salts is the fact that they offer a short-lasting H_2S release and do not sometimes reach their target sites, particularly the mitochondria. This makes them less ideal H_2S donors for therapeutic purpose. This limitation of the inorganic sulfide salts pushed forward the development of slow-releasing H_2S donors such as GYY4137 that offer a more sustained and longer lasting H_2S release than the inorganic sulfide salts [39]. More recently, the mitochondrially targeted slow-releasing H_2S donor, AP39, was developed by Prof. Whiteman's group and was shown to be more protective than NaHS and GYY4137 in animal models of organ transplantation and other disease models by augmenting mitochondrial H_2S production by 3-MST and offering a longer period of treating time [8, 40–42]. In addition, garlic-derived organic polysulfides such as diallyl sulfide (DAS), diallyl disulfide (DADS), and diallyl trisulfide (DATS) represent exogenous natural sources of H_2S, which are also currently being investigated experimentally in the context of organ transplantation and in the treatment of cardiovascular diseases [32, 33, 43–45]. Thiosulfate, a major metabolite of H_2S in the form of sodium thiosulfate, is another source of exogenous H_2S, which has also shown promise in warm IRI of kidney, heart, and brain [46–48] as well as in renovascular hypertension [49, 50]. Other H_2S donor molecules such as ATB-346 and zofenopril (whose H_2S generation is currently debatable) are currently in human clinical trials for cardiovascular and other disorders ([51], www.clinicaltrials.gov).

H_2S Protects Against Cold IRI in Kidney Transplantation

The current clinically approved method of renal graft preservation for transplantation is static cold storage (SCS) in various preservation solutions such as the University of Wisconsin (UW) solution or histidine–tryptophan–ketoglutarate (HTK) solution on ice at 4 °C, with the aim of mitigating cold IRI by slowing cellular activity and reducing production of toxic metabolites prior to transplantation [52–54]. However, SCS also contributes to cold IRI of the renal graft, with increased rates of acute tubular necrosis, decreased graft survival, and delayed graft function [55–58]. This suggests modification of the preservation solution with additives that could combat cold renal IRI and reduce the incidence of posttransplant complications. While limiting cold ischemic time is currently the only approach to minimize cold renal IRI, there is a growing interest to experimentally explore novel pharmacological strategies involving H_2S donor molecules as prophylaxis against cold IRI in kidney transplantation, which could increase the quality of the preserved renal graft for transplantation and perhaps safely extend the cold ischemic time with minimal injury.

Ever since Blackstone et al. [7] first demonstrated in 2005 that gaseous H_2S can induce a safe, reversible hypometabolism and hypothermia in mice through reversible inhibition of complex IV of the mitochondrial ETC, there have been several studies including those of our own group, exploiting this fascinating finding using various H_2S donor molecules to mitigate cold IRI in kidney transplantation. We have previously shown that supplementing cold UW solution with H_2S donor molecules such as NaHS (150 μM), and D-cysteine (2 mmol/kg), AP39 (200 nM) and varying doses of GYY147 protects rats and porcine donor kidneys from prolonged warm and cold IRI and improves graft function following transplantation [2, 3, 8, 59–61]. The mechanisms behind this protection include mitigating oxidative stress induced by increased production of reactive oxygen species (ROS, a natural by-product of cellular oxidative metabolism that is injurious to cells and tissues) by mitochondria; downregulating pro-apoptotic genes (e.g., BID) and upregulating anti-apoptotic genes (e.g., ERK-1); suppressing pro-inflammatory pathways through reduction of myeloperoxidase-positive neutrophils, CD68-positive macrophages, interferon gamma (IFN-γ), and intercellular adhesion molecule-1 (ICAM-1); and increasing renal blood flow with decreasing renal resistive index through vasodilation [2, 3, 8, 59–61] (Fig. 9.1). In terms of mitigating the deleterious effects of cold IRI in which mitochondrial dysfunction is a major contributing factor, AP39 demonstrates greater potential because it targets the mitochondria via its triphenylphosphonium motif, which facilitates H_2S entry into the mitochondria,

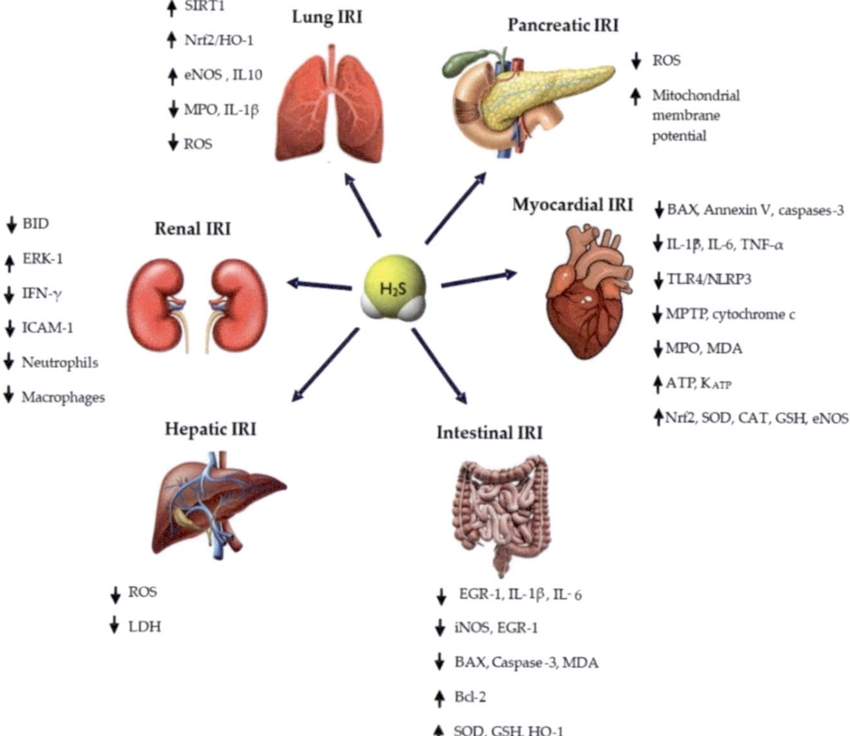

Fig. 9.1 Treatment with hydrogen sulfide (H_2S) attenuates cold ischemia-reperfusion injury (IRI) via modulation of several molecular mechanisms including inflammatory, apoptotic, antioxidant, and vascular mechanisms. *SIRT1* sirtuin 1, *Nrf2* nuclear factor erythroid 2-related factor 2, *HO-1* heme oxygenase-1, *eNOS* endothelial nitric oxide synthase, *ROS* reactive oxygen species, *BID* BH3-interacting domain death agonist, *ERK1* extracellular signal-regulated kinase 1, *MDA* malondialdehyde, *EGR-1* early growth response gene-1, *IL-1β* interleukin-1-beta, *IL-6* interleukin-6, *IL-10* interleukin-10, *BAX* Bcl-2-associated X protein, *Bcl-2* B-cell lymphoma-2, *SOD* superoxide dismutase, *GSH* glutathione, *CAT* catalase, *MPTP* mitochondrial permeability transition pore, *Caspase-3* cysteine-aspartic proteases-3, *TLR4* Toll-like receptor-4, *IFN-γ* interferon-gamma, *ICAM-1* intercellular adhesion molecule-1, *LDH* lactate dehydrogenase, *MPO* myeloperoxidase, *ATP* adenosine triphosphate, K_{ATP} adenosine triphosphate-sensitive potassium channel, and *NLRP3* nicotinamide-binding domain and leucine-rich repeat-containing protein-3

thereby restoring mitochondrial bioenergetics and preserving its integrity and function. It is worth mentioning that ROS production in the mitochondria under pathological conditions is primarily by mitochondrial ETC, which hyperpolarizes the mitochondria to create optimal condition for increased ROS production [62]. H_2S treatment with NaHS (100–300 μM) or overexpression of CSE (H_2S-producing enzyme) has been reported to normalize mitochondrial membrane potential in oxidatively stressed vascular endothelial cells by acting as an electron donor in the mitochondrial ETC, leading to suppression of mitochondrial ROS production [63]. Although this mechanism has not been investigated in transplantation of the kidney and other transplantable organs, it is possible that the inhibition of ROS-induced oxidative stress by H_2S donor molecules, especially the mitochondrially targeted AP39, in our kidney transplant models is via the same mechanism. This, however, needs to be investigated. We have also shown that prolonged SCS in cold UW solution supplemented with AP39 leads to improved graft function and reduced tissue injury following allogeneic kidney transplantation in rats [8]. In addition, Bos et al. [64] reported that mRNA expression of CSE in human kidney transplant biopsies at organ procurement (from brain-dead or living donors) was positively associated with renal function in the first 14 days following transplantation, as measured by glomerular filtration rate, and could lay the foundation for the use of H_2S donor molecules in clinical kidney transplantation in the future. Also, renal production of H_2S was significantly reduced in CSE knockout mice, which was associated with increased renal IRI and mortality compared to wild-type mice. These effects were reversed following intraperitoneal administration of 1 mg/kg NaHS and were found to be via reduced production of ROS [64]. This suggests that H_2S production from CSE is an important contributor to renal protection against IRI in kidney transplantation. While other important molecular mechanisms of renal protection by these H_2S donor molecules will provide a more comprehensive understanding of their mechanisms of action in the context of kidney transplantation, these empirical findings so far provide insights into the renoprotective mechanism of H_2S donor molecules in kidney transplantation. Hence, these data could push forward the potential clinical utility of H_2S donor molecules as pharmacological agents, especially those targeting the mitochondria in organ preservation solutions, as they appear to extend cold ischemic time with minimal injury and improve the quality of renal grafts after transplantation.

H_2S Against Cold IRI in Other Solid-Organ Grafts

H_2S Protects Against Cold IRI in Heart Transplantation

The protection of donor organs against cold IRI by H_2S donor molecules is also observed in the preservation of donor hearts before transplantation. In a collaborative study with our research team using in vitro and in vivo murine model of heart transplantation, preservation of donor hearts in AP39-supplemented UW solution protected donor heart function against prolonged period (24 h) of cold IRI measured by quantitative ultrasound scan, together with cardiac fibrosis [65]. In addition, AP39 (100 nM) treatment markedly increased viability of cardiomyocytes, while it significantly reduced apoptotic (BAX and annexin V) and expression of pro-inflammatory (IL-1β, IL-6, tumor necrosis factor-alpha [TNF-α]) genes, leading to preservation of mitochondrial function following cold hypoxia/reoxygenation in vitro [65] (Fig. 9.1). Our observations support those of Sun et al. [45], who exploited mesoporous silica nanoparticles (MSNs) as the carrier of diallyl trisulfide (DATS, an H_2S donor), a novel long-term slow and controlled-releasing H_2S system (DATS-MSN, 22.2 μM) that requires glutathione to release H_2S, in cold UW solution in a rat model of heart transplantation in comparison with UW solution supplemented with 25 μM NaHS and 26.5 μM GYY4137, whose H_2S generation depends on cysteine. Following 6 h of donor heart preservation and 1 h of reperfusion, the authors reported a significantly higher cardioprotection in donor hearts that were preserved in cold UW solution supplemented with DATS-MSN compared to those preserved in NaHS- and GYY4137-supplemented UW solution as well as control group preserved in UW solution without H_2S supplementation. The DATS-MSN-induced cardioprotection, resulting in higher graft performance than the other groups, was characterized by increased left ventricular developed pressure, decreased levels of plasma creatine kinase-MB and troponin I (cardiac damage markers), reduced myocardial inflammation (myeloperoxidase [MPO], IL-1β, TNF-α), increased activities of antioxidants (glutathione [GSH], catalase [CAT], and superoxide dismutase [SOD]), decreased cardiomyocyte apoptosis index (BAX, caspase-3), and preserved mitochondrial integrity as illustrated in Fig. 9.1. This culminated in long-term graft survival and function following 8 weeks of transplantation [45]. In addition, DATS-MSN treatment protected cardiomyocytes against hypoxic injury in vitro by inhibiting TLR4/NLRP3, an inflammatory pathway [45].

It is worth mentioning that the DATS-MSN used by Sun et al. [45] and the AP39 used in our collaborative study are slow-releasing H_2S donors that resulted in mitochondrial protection, although at very different concentrations due to their nature, characterized by preservation of mitochondrial integrity with inhibition of apoptosis and inflammation in both studies. Moreover, NaHS is a fast-releasing but short-lasting H_2S donor, while GYY4137 is a slow- and sustained-releasing but nonspecific H_2S donor whose actions do not sometimes reach the mitochondria. Hence, superior cardioprotection was observed in the DATS-MSN group over NaHS and GYY4137 groups. Cardioprotection by H_2S donor molecules through inhibition of apoptotic machinery is also seen in other experimental models of heart disease in relation to myocardial IRI. In hypertensive rats subjected to myocardial IRI, for example, treatment with varying concentrations of NaHS and AP39 protected the heart and rat myocardium in a dose-dependent manner against IRI via inhibition of Ca^{2+}-mediated opening of mitochondrial permeability transition pores (MPTPs) through a cyclophilin D-independent mechanism [66–68] and thus prevented mitochondrial release of pro-apoptotic factors. Although this mechanism has not been reported in the context of cold myocardial IRI in transplantation, it is very likely that H_2S inhibits Ca^{2+} influx and blocks mitochondrial Ca^{2+} accumulation during SCS since hypothermia is a known stimulator of Ca^{2+} influx and mitochondrial Ca^{2+} accumulation [69], thus preventing the opening of MPTP and thereby preserving mitochondrial function during SCS.

It is important to reiterate that DATS can be activated by glutathione (a potent endogenous antioxidant) to release H_2S in a controlled manner, while H_2S by itself activates glutathione and other antioxidants such as catalase, superoxide dismutase, and nuclear factor erythroid 2-related factor 2 (Nrf-2) [70, 71] and thus may partly account for the cardioprotection after transplantation. However, given that the concentration of H_2S in blood and tissue is usually very low, its interaction with other antioxidant enzymes and ROS scavenging property alone cannot completely explain its antioxidant effect in tissues. The results of some studies suggest an interplay between H_2S and the other two members of the gasotransmitter family (nitric oxide and carbon monoxide) in the mitochondrial ETC, and activation and opening of adenosine triphosphate-sensitive potassium (K_{ATP}) channels, leading to activation of their individual antioxidant activities [72–74] and partly contributing to the antioxidant effect of H_2S in tissues. In addition, Predmore et al. [33] reported that administration of 200 µg/kg of DATS prior to reperfusion restored myocardial H_2S level, significantly activated endothelial nitric oxide synthase (eNOS, nitric oxide-synthesizing enzyme predominantly in vascular endothelium and responsible for vasodilation and other biological effects), and increased nitric oxide metabolites as well as activation of Nrf2 antioxidant pathway, resulting in cardioprotection in a mouse model of myocardial IRI. The cardioprotection was characterized by marked reduction in infarct size per area at risk, per left ventricular area, and plasma troponin; improved myocardial contractile function; as well as improved mitochondrial respiration at the subcellular level compared to control mice [33]. In conclusion, supplementation of standard preservation solution with H_2S donor molecules is a simple, easy, and inexpensive pharmacological strategy to safely protect donor heart against cold IRI in transplantation through activation of antioxidant defense system and inhibition of inflammatory, apoptotic, and other potentially damaging pathways.

H₂S Protects Against Cold IRI in Lung Transplantation

Besides the kidney and heart, H_2S donor molecules have also proven to be protective in experimental models of lung transplantation. In a rat model of orthotopic lung transplantation, intraperitoneal administration of 14 µmol/kg NaHS in recipient rats after 3 h of SCS of grafts and 15 min before reperfusion improved lung function and protection after transplantation in comparison with control rats without NaHS treatment. The improvement in pulmonary function and protection was associated with markedly increased H_2S level and expression of CSE protein in the graft lung tissues with significantly decreased membrane lipid oxidation level, myeloperoxidase activity, and levels of IL-1β (a pro-inflammatory cytokine) while increasing the production of IL-10 (a potent anti-inflammatory cytokine) [75] (Fig. 9.1). In a separate experiment by the same authors, pharmacological inhibition of endogenous H_2S production by intraperitoneal administration of 37.5 mg/kg propargylglycine (CSE inhibitor) in recipient rats at 15 min prior to the start of lung transplantation aggravated lung injury and worsened pulmonary function in the graft tissues after transplantation [75]. This suggests that activation of CSE/H_2S pathway in the recipient prior to lung transplantation confers protection against cold IRI following lung transplantation partly through antioxidant and anti-inflammatory pathways. Moreover, the effect of propargylglycine on CSE expression and activity in such a short time may suggest that CSE-producing cells in the lungs are probably more sensitive to propargylglycine than those of other tissues, leading to death of CSE-producing cells within such a short period. It is also possible that the 37.5 mg/kg dose of propargylglycine used by the authors might be higher than what is used in other studies. Therefore, this needs to be further investigated. In another experiment of lung transplantation in which donor rabbits inhaled 150 ppm of gaseous H_2S for 2 h before 18 h of SCS followed by addition of a bolus of 100 µg/kg NaHS through the reperfusion circuit at the beginning of reperfusion and a continuous infusion of 1 mg/kg/h NaHS for the duration of reperfusion (2 h), the authors observed a significant decrease in mitochondrial ROS as well as a decrease in cold IRI with improved oxygenation, ventilation, lower pulmonary artery pressures, and better graft function after transplantation compared to control group without NaHS treatment [76, 77]. This highlights the ROS scavenging property of H_2S as discussed above.

Other potential protective mechanisms observed in other experimental models of lung diseases in relation to lung IRI might partly account for the antioxidant effect of H_2S against cold IRI in lung transplantation. In type 2 diabetic rats treated with GYY4137 and then subjected to a surgical model of lung IRI, for example, the authors observed significant activation of sirtuin 1 (SIRT1) signaling and attenuated lung IRI with improved lung functional recovery, reduced oxidative damage, inflammation, and apoptosis (Fig. 9.1) [78]. It is important to point out that SIRT1 is a nicotinamide adenine dinucleotide (NAD)-dependent histone deacetylase with multiple biological functions such as transcription and cell cycle regulation, anti-apoptosis, and activator of antioxidant enzymes [79–81]. Hence, the authors further reported that GYY4137 treatment activated SIRT1 signaling, which in turn upregulated antioxidant signaling pathways mediated by Nrf2/heme oxygenase-1 (HO-1) and eNOS, thereby reducing apoptosis and inflammation and ultimately preserving lung function under diabetic IRI condition. Therefore, this mechanism might apply in cold lung IRI during transplantation and could partly contribute to the antioxidant effect of H_2S donor molecules against cold IRI in lung transplantation. Taken together, administration of H_2S donor molecules to the donor prior to lung procurement and to the recipient at the start of and during reperfusion after SCS provides a novel means to pharmacologically protect graft lung tissue against cold IRI in transplantation.

H₂S Protects Against Cold IRI in Liver Transplantation

Ever since Abe and Kimura first reported the therapeutic potential of H_2S in 1996 [5], there has been more focus on its application in warm IRI in the liver compared to cold IRI in liver transplantation. However, emerging evidence from experimental models suggests that exogenous administration of H_2S donor molecules during graft preservation increases survival rates of liver grafts after transplantation. In a rat model of donation after cardiac death liver transplantation, preservation of donor rat liver in HTK solution at 4 °C for 24 h and supplemented with 10 µM sodium sulfide (Na_2S, an H_2S donor) at the beginning of SCS and followed by 90 min of ex vivo reperfusion resulted in hepatoprotection (improved liver microcirculation, morphology, and function), which was observed as markedly increased levels and activities of liver antioxidant enzymes with significant reduction in levels of lactate dehydrogenase, malondialdehyde (MDA, a by-product of lipid peroxidation and an indication of ROS production), and other liver damage markers during cold I/R compared to preservation in HTK solution without Na_2S supplementation [82] (Fig. 9.1). This finding supports a previous report by the same authors, in which 48 h of SCS of rat livers in UW solution at 4 °C supplemented with 3.4 mM of diallyl disulfide (DADS, an H_2S donor) improved parameters of liver function in an isolated perfused rat liver model [44]. This implies that addition of H_2S donor molecules during SCS of liver grafts could serve a pharmacological purpose of improving standard methods of liver preservation for transplantation.

H₂S Protects Against Cold IRI in Pancreas Transplantation

Pancreas transplantation is currently one of the preferred treatments in patients with unstable type 1 diabetes mellitus with the aim of restoring normoglycemia and avoiding the complications of diabetes. However, as with other solid organs, poor graft quality and high incidence of early graft loss due to cold IRI hamper a successful pancreas transplantation, with graft pancreatitis as a major complication following pancreas transplantation [83]. Hence, improvement or modification in the preservation technique could attenuate cold pancreatic IRI and avoid the complications during the postoperative period. In a porcine model of pancreas transplantation, supplementation of UW solution with 400 nM AP39 for 18 h followed by islet isolation produced significantly higher islet yields before and after purification with markedly reduced ROS production and significantly elevated mitochondrial membrane potential compared to control group as illustrated in Fig. 9.1 [84]. In a separate experiment by the same authors, preservation of pancreas in UW solution supplemented with AP39 mitigated cold IRI, improved the outcome of islet transplantation, and prevented graft pancreatitis in type 1 diabetic mice induced with streptozotocin (an anticancer drug that destroys insulin-producing pancreatic beta cells) [84]. This observation suggests that addition of H_2S donor molecules to preservation solution during SCS may be a novel pharmacological approach to improve islet transplantation outcomes through activation of antioxidant defense system and avoiding complications associated with pancreas transplantation.

H_2S Protects Against Cold IRI in Intestinal Transplantation

Intestinal transplantation remains the best treatment option for patients with intestinal failure—patients who have lost their ability to maintain normal nutritional support and permanently depend on parenteral nutrition [85, 86]. The gold standard of SCS of donor organs in UW or HTK solution at 4 °C was developed for kidney and other solid-organ preservation and is suboptimal for intestinal grafts, notwithstanding the good results for these organs [87–89]. As the intestine is extremely sensitive to cold ischemia, relatively long cold ischemic times in these less ideal preservation solutions exacerbate cold IRI and render the outcome of intestinal preservation for transplantation inferior to that of other solid organs [87, 89]. Hence, these preservation solutions and preservation techniques need improvement for optimal intestinal graft preservation and patient survival.

Whereas there is a substantial body of experimental evidence on the action of H_2S donor molecules against cold IRI in the transplantation of other solid organs, data on H_2S donor compounds against cold intestinal IRI is currently lacking. One study reported hydrogen gas, which can be produced industrially from H_2S [90], to protect against cold intestinal IRI, leading to preservation of graft function in a rat model of isogeneic intestinal transplantation [91]. In their study, SCS of intestinal graft in 100% hydrogen-bubbled UW solution for 6 h prior to transplantation preserved intestinal mucosal graft morphology and markedly decreased levels of MDA and expressions of pro-inflammatory elements such as early growth response gene-1 (EGR-1), IL-1β, IL-6, and inducible nitric oxide synthase during the early phase of cold IRI compared to control [91] (Fig. 9.1). In addition, the authors reported that the intestinal graft protection was partly due to significant upregulation of anti-apoptotic HO-1 in the grafts preserved in UW solution supplemented with 100% hydrogen gas compared to control group without hydrogen gas supplementation [91].

Although H_2S donor molecules have not been investigated in cold intestinal IRI, a number of studies have reported protective effect of H_2S donor molecules against warm intestinal IRI. In an experiment to determine whether pharmacologic postconditioning of intestinal tissue with H_2S protects against warm intestinal IRI, Henderson et al. [92] reported markedly reduced apoptotic index in enterocytes (epithelial cells that line the inner surface of the intestine and perform absorptive function) following treatment with 10 μM and 100 μM NaHS under hypoxic condition compared to control group without NaHS treatment. The result of this in vitro study was supported by that of an in vivo study by the same authors in which intravenous administration of NaHS at the same concentrations after 1–3 h of intestinal ischemia and 20 min before reperfusion in rats resulted in reduction in intestinal IRI characterized by significant quantitative preservation of villus height [92], an indication of a greater surface area for nutrient absorption than in control rats who received no NaHS. This observation is in agreement with the findings from a previous study in which 14 µmol/kg NaHS administration after 30 min of intestinal occlusion significantly decreased serum level and activity of MDA and markedly elevated serum and intestinal levels and activities of the antioxidant enzymes SOD and GSH [93], suggesting that intestinal protection by H_2S against IRI is partly due to its antioxidant property. Also, administration of low and high doses (40 mg/kg and 80 mg/kg, respectively) of GYY4137 reduced plasma levels of MDA and intestinal pro-apoptotic proteins (BAX and caspase-3) and increased expression of intestinal anti-apoptotic protein (Bcl-2) as well as plasma SOD, leading to preservation of intestinal integrity in a rat model of intestinal IRI [94]. It is worth noting that while the intestines of rats treated with low and high doses of GYY4137 were protected against IRI compared to the control group without GYY4137 treatment, high-dose-treated rats had a better intestinal protection than those treated with low-dose GYY4137. This implies that the degree of intestinal protection by GYY4137 against IRI is dose dependent. Recently, NaHS (2 nmol/kg and 2000 nmol/kg) and GYY4137 (50 mg/kg) were also found to improve postischemic recovery of mesenteric perfusion, mucosal integrity, and inflammation via eNOS-dependent pathways in a mouse model of intestinal IRI [95, 96]. Taken together, H_2S donor molecules protect against intestinal IRI by activating antioxidant, anti-inflammatory, anti-apoptotic, and vasodilatory pathways.

Translation from Bench to Bedside

Several lines of empirical evidence in the last few years have shown that various H_2S donor molecules minimize organ damage caused by cold IRI in solid-organ transplantation and improve graft survival and function during the posttransplant period. Among all the H_2S donor molecules experimentally investigated so far in this context, AP39 demonstrates a greater potential with improved graft function and reduced tissue injury following prolonged SCS in standard preservation solution and after organ transplantation. This is because AP39 specifically targets the mitochondria and facilitates H_2S entry. However, AP39 is not a clinically viable H_2S donor molecule. Bearing this limitation in mind, it is important to consider a clinically relevant H_2S donor which could help translate the fascinating findings of the effect of H_2S donor molecules in organ transplantation from bench to bedside. Along this train of thought, thiosulfate, an H_2S donor drug in the form of sodium thiosulfate, which is already approved by the US Food and Drug Administration (FDA) and currently being used to treat calciphylaxis in patients with end-stage kidney disease, acute cyanide poisoning, and cisplatin toxicities with cancer [97–100], can lay the foundation for H_2S donor drugs in clinical organ transplantation in the future. In addition, H_2S donor drugs such as ATB-346 (H_2S-generating naproxen molecule) are currently in clinical trials for gastric ulcer, osteoarthritis, and chronic pain (www.clinicaltrials.gov). Zofenopril, a specific FDA-approved antihypertensive drug whose chemical structure contains sulfur moiety and whose therapeutic actions have been reported to be associated with increased H_2S release [101], is also in human clinical trials for cardiovascular diseases and type 2 diabetes mellitus (www.clinicaltrials.gov), and its therapeutic benefits together with ATB-346 could be further investigated and expanded to include organ transplantation. In the light of this, our research team is currently exploring the potential clinical application of some of these clinically viable H_2S donor drugs in kidney transplantation [102]. Also, the finding that human renal CSE mRNA expression at the time of renal graft procurement from brain-dead or living donors was associated with a positive post-transplant outcome [64] is a positive indication of its potential beneficial effect in human kidney transplantation as also observed in animal models.

Limitations and the Way Forward

In the face of these promising findings, there are several limitations which may keep H_2S donor molecules decades away from clinical use. For example, all the H_2S donor molecules studied in these transplantable organs appear to modulate very limited molecular mechanisms and do not provide extensive molecular evidence in their mechanisms of action. Future studies will require a broader investigation into other very important molecular pathways such as soluble guanylate cyclase/cyclic guanosine monophosphate, mitogen-activated protein kinase, reperfusion injury salvage kinase pathway, hypoxia-inducible factor/vascular endothelial growth factor system, heat-shock protein family, autophagy pathway, H_2S relationship with the other two established gasotransmitters (nitric oxide and carbon monoxide), as well as the impact of these H_2S donor molecules in the mitochondrial ETC in the context of organ transplantation. These studies should also consider the effect of the H_2S donor molecules on the immune system after organ transplantation to know whether H_2S-induced protection after organ transplantation will require administration of immunosuppressive drugs to recipients prior to and after transplantation as is the case in clinical organ transplantation. Moreover, there is currently no data on the effect of H_2S donor molecules on cold IRI in intestinal transplantation. Future studies should address this gap in the literature, which will among other things add to the expanding body of literature that supports the cyto- and organ-protective effect of H_2S donor molecules against cold IRI in solid-organ transplantation. Also, SG-1002, which was previously thought to be an H_2S donor, is not an H_2S donor but rather a collection of salts which can generate H_2S in aqueous solution and barely increases blood sulfide level. Although it shows efficacy in rodent studies, it appears to be going nowhere in humans. In the same vein, GIC-1001 was in clinical development but it is no longer. AP39 also recently entered into human clinical trial in a study that compared two treatment strategies in patients with acute coronary syndrome without ST elevation. However, the study was terminated for undisclosed reason (www.clinicaltrials.gov). Another limitation is the lack of effective and quick method to measure H_2S concentration, especially in a noninvasive way in these transplant studies. The fact that these H_2S donor molecules generate H_2S is not enough to assume that all the effects attributed to them are because of H_2S. This implies that the relevance of the doses of these H_2S donor molecules to the effective dose of H_2S needs to be determined. Unfortunately, there are no techniques with the sensitivity, selectivity, and real-time capability to measure the effective dose of H_2S following administration of these H_2S donor molecules. A solution to this problem will also necessitate measurement of nitric oxide and carbon monoxide considering that the concentration of H_2S in blood and tissue is usually very low, and therefore an interplay between H_2S and other gasotransmitters could reinforce the protective action of H_2S in organ transplantation. Addressing all these limitations in future studies will very likely unravel several therapeutic feasibilities of this gaseous signaling molecule and will help move H_2S donor molecules closer towards human clinical trials.

Conclusion

Cold IRI is a well-recognized inevitable pathological condition that hampers the success of solid-organ transplantation, culminating in posttransplant complications including early loss of solid-organ graft. Modification of standard transplantation protocol to include addition of H_2S donor molecules to standard preservation solutions or administration of H_2S donor molecules to the organ donor prior to organ procurement and to the recipient at the start and during reperfusion after SCS is a novel pharmacological strategy that has been shown experimentally to mitigate cold IRI during transplantation of kidney and other transplantable solid organs through inhibition of a multitude of pathways involving ROS-induced oxidative stress, inflammation, microcirculatory disturbance and microvascular dysfunction, and apoptotic and other potential but unidentified pathways. From an optimistic perspective, H_2S donor molecules show a great clinical promise that could decrease acute and chronic organ rejection and thereby improve the quality of organ grafts. Translating these promising findings from bench to bedside can lay the foundation for H_2S donor drugs in clinical organ transplantation in the future. However, this will require more animal experiments and human clinical trials to determine important factors such as therapeutic doses, timing of treatment in the organ donor, preservation solution, and organ recipient, as well as evaluate adverse effects. Overall, pretreatment of donor organs and supplementation of preservation solutions with H_2S donor molecules or their administration to the organ recipient show significant therapeutic potential in terms of improving transplantation outcomes, and this approach merits further experimental and clinical investigations. In conclusion, the future of organ transplantation is bright with these exciting research findings that promise to overcome the unavoidable obstacle of cold IRI in organ transplantation.

Conflict of Interest   None.

References

1. Dorweiler B, Pruefer D, Andrasi TB, Maksan SM, Schmiedt W, Neufang A, Vahl CF. Ischemia-reperfusion injury. Eur J Trauma Emerg Surg. 2007;33(6):600–12.
2. Lobb I, Davison M, Carter D, Liu W, Haig A, Gunaratnam L, Sener A. Hydrogen sulfide treatment mitigates renal allograft ischemia-reperfusion injury during cold storage and improves early transplant kidney function and survival following allogeneic renal transplantation. J Urol. 2015;194(6):1806–15.
3. Grewal J, Lobb I, Saha M, Haig A, Jiang J, Sener A. Mp29-16 hydrogen sulfide supplementation mitigates effects of ischemia reperfusion injury in a murine model of donation after cardiac death renal transplantation. J Urol. 2016;195(4):e386.
4. Wang R. Gasotransmitters: growing pains and joys. Trends Biochem Sci. 2014;39(5):227–32.
5. Abe K, Kimura H. The possible role of hydrogen sulfide as an endogenous neuromodulator. J Neurosci. 1996;6(3):1066–71.
6. Polhemus DJ, Lefer DJ. Emergence of hydrogen sulfide as an endogenous gaseous signaling molecule in cardiovascular disease. Circ Res. 2014;114(4):730–7.
7. Blackstone E, Morrison M, Roth MB. H_2S induces a suspended animation-like state in mice. Science. 2005;308(5721):518.
8. Lobb I, Mok A, Lan Z, Liu W, Garcia B, Sener A. Supplemental hydrogen sulphide protects transplant kidney function and prolongs recipient survival after prolonged cold ischaemia-reperfusion injury by mitigating renal graft apoptosis and inflammation. Br J Urol Int. 2012;110(11c):E1187–95.
9. Yamamoto J, Sato W, Kosugi T, Yamamoto T, Kimura T, Taniguchi S, et al. Distribution of hydrogen sulfide (H_2S)-producing enzymes and the roles of the H_2S donor sodium hydrosulfide in diabetic nephropathy. Clin Exp Nephrol. 2013;17(1):32–40.
10. Dugbartey GJ, Bouma HR, Lobb I, Sener A. Hydrogen sulfide: a novel nephroprotectant against cisplatin-induced renal toxicity. Nitric Oxide. 2016;57:15–20.
11. Dugbartey GJ. Diabetic nephropathy: a potential savior with 'rotten-egg' smell. Pharmacol Rep. 2017;69:331–9.
12. Dugbartey GJ. H_2S as a possible therapeutic alternative for the treatment of hypertensive kidney injury. Nitric Oxide. 2017;64:52–60.
13. Dugbartey GJ. The smell of renal protection against chronic kidney disease: hydrogen sulfide offers a potential stinky remedy. Pharmacol Rep. 2018;70(2):196–205.
14. Dugbartey GJ, Bouma HR, Saha MN, Lobb I, Henning RH, Sener A. A hibernation-like state for transplantable organs: is hydrogen sulfide therapy the future of organ preservation? Antioxid Redox Signal. 2018;28(16):1503–15.
15. Xia M, Chen L, Muh RW, Li PL, Li N. Production and action of hydrogen sulfide, a novel gaseous bioactive substance in the kidneys. J Pharmacol Exp Ther. 2009;329:1056–62.
16. Mikami Y, Shinuya N, Kimura Y, Nagahara N, Ogasawara Y, Kimura H. Thioredoxin and dihydrolipoic acid are required for 3-mercaptopyruvate sulfurtransferase to produce hydrogen sulfide. Biochem J. 2011;439:479–85.
17. Shibuya N, Koike S, Tanaka M, et al. A novel pathway for the production of hydrogen sulfide from D-cysteine in mammalian cells. Nat Commun. 2013;4:1366.
18. Modis K, Coletta C, Erdelyi K, Papapetropoulos A, Szabo C. Intramitochondrial hydrogen sulfide production by 3-mercaptopyruvate sulfurtransferase maintains mitochondrial electron transport flow and supports cellular biogenesis. FASEB J. 2013;27:601–11.
19. Kimura H. Production and physiological effects of hydrogen sulfide. Antioxid Redox Signal. 2014;20(5):783–93.
20. Gong QH, Wang Q, Pan LL, Liu XH, Xin H, Zhu YZ. *S*-propargyl-cysteine, a novel hydrogen sulfide-modulated agent, attenuates lipopolysaccharide-induced spatial learning and memory impairment: involvement of TNF signaling and NF-kappaB pathway in rats. Brain Behav Immun. 2011;25:110–9.

21. Bao L, Vlcek C, Paces V, Kraus JP. Identification and tissue distribution of human cystathionine beta-synthase mRNA isoforms. Arch Biochem Biophys. 1998;350(1):95–103.
22. Lee HJ, Mariappan MM, Feliers D, Cavaglieri RC, Sataranatarajan K, Abboud HE, et al. Hydrogen sulfide inhibits high glucose-induced matrix protein synthesis by activating AMP-activated protein kinase in renal epithelial cells. J Biol Chem. 2012;387(7):4451–61.
23. Dugbartey GJ, Talaei F, Houwertjes MC, Goris M, Epema AH, Bouma HR, Henning RH. Dopamine treatment attenuates acute kidney injury in a rat model of deep hypothermia and rewarming—the role of renal H_2S-producing enzymes. Eur J Pharmacol. 2015;769:225–33.
24. Jin S, Pu S, Hou C, Ma F, Li N, Li X, Tan B, Tao B, Wang M, Zhu Y. Cardiac H_2S generation is reduced in ageing diabetic mice. Oxid Med Cell Longev. 2015;2015:758358.
25. Persa C, Osmotherly K, Kate C-W, Moon S, Lou MF. The distribution of cystathionine beta-synthase (CBS) in the eye: implication of the presence of a trans-sulfuration pathway for oxidative stress defense. Exp Eye Res. 2006;83(4):817–23.
26. Kawabata A, Ishiki T, Nagasawa K, Yoshida S, Maeda Y, Takahashi T, et al. Hydrogen sulfide as a novel nociceptive messenger. Pain. 2007;132:74–81.
27. Wang XB, Huang XM, Ochs T, Li XY, Jin HF, Tang CS, Du JB. Effect of sulfur dioxide preconditioning on rat myocardial ischemia/reperfusion injury by inducing endoplasmic reticulum stress. Basic Res Cardiol. 2011;106(5):865–78.
28. Bos EM, Wang R, Snijder PM, Boersema M, Damman J, Fu M, Moser J, Hillebrands JL, Ploeg RJ, Yang G, Leuvenink HG, van Goor H. Cystathionine γ-lyase protects against renal ischemia/reperfusion by modulating oxidative stress. J Am Soc Nephrol. 2013;24(5):759–70.
29. Nagahara N, Hirasawa T, Yoshii T, Niimura Y. Is novel signal transducer sulfur oxide involved in the redox cycle of persulfide at the catalytic site cysteine in a stable reaction intermediate of mecaptopyruvate sulfurtransferase? Antioxid Redox Signal. 2012;16:747–53.
30. Coletta C, Módis K, Szczesny B, Brunyánszki A, Oláh G, Rios EC, Yanagi K, Ahmad A, Papapetropoulos A, Szabo C. Regulation of vascular tone, angiogenesis and cellular bioenergetics by the 3-mercaptopyruvate sulfurtransferase/H_2S pathway: functional impairment by hyperglycemia and restoration by DL-α-lipoic acid. Mol Med. 2015;21(1):1–14.
31. Tomita M, Nagahara N, Ito T. Expression of 3-mercaptopyruvate sulfurtransferase in the mouse. Molecules. 2016;21(12):1707.
32. Benavides GA, Squadrito GL, Mills RW, Patel HD, Isbell TS, Patel RB, et al. Hydrogen sulfide mediates the vasoactivity of garlic. Proc Natl Acad Sci U S A. 2007;104:17977–82.
33. Predmore BL, Kondo K, Bhushan S, et al. The polysulfide diallyl trisulfide protects the ischemic myocardium by preservation of endogenous hydrogen sulfide and increasing nitric oxide bioavailability. Am J Physiol Heart Circ Physiol. 2012;302(11):H2410–8.
34. Kolluru GK, Shen X, Bir SC, Kevil CG. Hydrogen sulfide chemical biology: pathophysiological roles and detection. Nitric Oxide. 2013;35:5–20.
35. Li Q, Lancaster JR Jr. Chemical foundations of hydrogen sulfide biology. Nitric Oxide. 2013;35:21–34.
36. Zhao Y, Biggs TD, Xian M. Hydrogen sulfide (H_2S)-releasing agents: chemistry and biological applications. Chem Commun (Camb). 2014;50(80):11788–805.
37. Caliendo G, Cirino G, Santagada V, Wallace JL. Synthesis and biological effects of hydrogen sulfide (H_2S): development of H_2S-releasing drugs as pharmaceuticals. J Med Chem. 2010;53:6275–86.
38. Kashfi K, Olso KR. Biology and therapeutic potential of hydrogen sulfide and hydrogen sulfide-releasing chimeras. Biochem Pharmacol. 2013;85:689–703.
39. Li L, Whiteman M, Guan YY, Neo KL, Cheng Y, Lee SW, et al. Characterization of a novel, water-soluble hydrogen sulfide-releasing molecule (GYY4137): new insights into the biology of hydrogen sulfide. Circulation. 2008;117:2351–60.
40. Le Trionairre S, Perry A, Bartosz S, et al. The synthesis and functional evaluation of mitochondria-targeted hydrogen sulfide donor, (10-oxo-10-(4-(3-thioxo-3H-1,2-dithiol-5-yl)phenoxy)decyl)triphenyl phosphonium bromide (AP39). Med Chem Commun. 2014;5:728–36.

41. Ahmad A, Olah G, Szczesny B, Wood ME, Whiteman M, Szabo C. AP39, a mitochondrially-targeted hydrogen sulfide donor, exerts protective effects in renal epithelial cells subjected to oxidative stress in vitro and in acute renal injury, in vivo. Shock. 2016;45:88–97.

42. Zhao FL, Fang F, Qiao PF, Yan N, Gao D, Yan Y. AP39, a mitochondria-targeted hydrogen sulfide donor, supports cellular bioenergetics and protects against Alzheimer's disease by preserving mitochondrial function in APP/PS1 mice and neurons. Oxid Med Cell Longev. 2016;2016:8360738.

43. Ginter E, Simko V. Garlic (*Allium sativum* L.) and cardiovascular diseases. Bratisl Lek Listy. 2010;111:452–6.

44. Balaban CL, Rodriguez JV, Guibert EE. Delivery of the bioactive gas hydrogen sulfide during cold preservation of rat liver: effects on hepatic function in an ex vivo model. Artif Organs. 2011;35:508515.

45. Sun X, Wang W, Dai J, Huang J, Shi M, Chu X, Wang F, Guo C, Wang C, Pang L, Wang Y. Donor heart preservation with a novel long-term and slow-releasing hydrogen sulfide system. Nitric Oxide. 2018;81:1–10.

46. Marutani E, Yamada M, Ida T, et al. Thiosulfate mediates cytoprotective effects of hydrogen sulfide against neuronal ischemia. J Am Heart Assoc. 2015;4(11):e002125.

47. Mohan D, Balasubramanian ED, Ravindran S, Kurian GA. Renal mitochondria can withstand hypoxic/ischemic injury secondary to renal failure in uremic rats pretreated with sodium thiosulfate. Indian J Pharmacol. 2017;49(4):317–21.

48. Ravindran S, Boovarahan SR, Shanmugam K, Vedarathinam RC, Kurian GA. Sodium thiosulfate preconditioning ameliorates ischemia/reperfusion injury in rat hearts via reduction of oxidative stress and apoptosis. Cardiovasc Drugs Ther. 2017;31(5–6):511–24.

49. Snijder PM, Frenay AR, Koning AM, et al. Sodium thiosulfate attenuates angiotensin II-induced hypertension, proteinuria and renal damage. Nitric Oxide. 2014;42:87–98.

50. Bijarnia RK, Bachtler M, Chandak PG, van Goor H, Pasch A. Sodium thiosulfate ameliorates oxidative stress and pre-serves renal function in hyperoxaluric rats. PLoS One. 2015;10(4):e0124881.

51. Wallace JL, Vaughan D, Dicay M, MacNaughton WK, de Nucci G. Hydrogen sulfide-releasing therapeutics: translation to the clinic. Antioxid Redox Signal. 2018;28(16):1533–40.

52. Opelz G, Döhler B. Multicenter analysis of kidney preservation. Transplantation. 2007;83(3):247–53.

53. Morris PJ. Kidney transplantation, principles and practice. 6th ed. Saunders; 2008. p. 126–7.

54. Bond M, Pitt M, Akoh J, Moxham T, Hoyle M, Anderson R. The effectiveness and cost-effectiveness of methods of storing donated kidneys from deceased donors: a systematic review and economic model. Health Technol Assess. 2009;13(38):3–4.

55. Dragun D, Hoff U, Park JK, et al. Prolonged cold preservation augments vascular injury independent of renal transplant immunogenicity and function. Kidney Int. 2001;60(3):1173–81.

56. Salahudeen AK, Haider N, May W. Cold ischemia and the reduced long-term survival of cadaveric renal allo-grafts. Kidney Int. 2004;65(2):713–8.

57. Quiroga I, McShane P, Koo DD, et al. Major effects of delayed graft function and cold ischaemia time on renal allograft survival. Nephrol Dial Transplant. 2006;21(6):1689–96.

58. Kayler LK, Magliocca J, Zendejas I, Srinivas TR, Schold JD. Impact of cold ischemia time on graft survival among ECD transplant recipients: a paired kidney analysis. Am J Transplant. 2011;11(12):2647–56.

59. Hosgood SA, Nicholson ML. Hydrogen sulphide ameliorates ischaemia-reperfusion injury in an experimental model of non-heart-beating donor kidney transplantation. Br J Surg. 2010;97(2):202–9.

60. Lobb I, Zhu J, Liu W, Haig A, Lan Z, Sener A. Hydrogen sulfide treatment improves long-term renal dysfunction resulting from prolonged warm renal ischemia-reperfusion injury. Can Urol Assoc J. 2014;8(5–6):413.

61. Lobb I, Jiang J, Lian D, Liu W, Haig A, Saha MN, Torregrossa R, Wood ME, Whiteman M, Sener A. Hydrogen sulfide protects renal grafts against prolonged cold ischemia-reperfusion injury via specific mitochondrial actions. Am J Transplant. 2017;17(2):341–52.
62. Gero D, Szabo C. Glucocorticoids suppress mitochondrial oxidant production via upregulation of uncoupling protein 2 in hyperglycemic endothelial cells. PLoS One. 2016;11(4):e0144813.
63. Suzuki K, Olah G, Modis K, Colleta C, Kulp G, Gero D, et al. Hydrogen sulfide replacement therapy protects the vascular endothelium in hyperglycemia by preserving mitochondrial function. Proc Natl Acad Sci U S A. 2011;108(33):13829–34.
64. Bos EM, Wang R, Snijder PM, Boersema M, Damman J, Fu M, Moser J, Hillebrands JL, Ploeg RJ, Yang G, Leuvenink HG, van Goor H. Cystathionine gamma-lyase protects against renal ischemia/reperfusion by modulating oxidative stress. J Am Soc Nephrol. 2013;24(5):759–70.
65. Zhu C, Su Y, Juriasingani S, Zheng H, Veramkovich V, Jiang J, Sener A, Whiteman M, Lacefield J, Nagpal D, Alotaibi F, Liu K, Zheng X. Supplementing preservation solution with mitochondria-targeted H_2S donor AP39 protects cardiac grafts from prolonged cold ischemia-reperfusion injury in heart transplantation. Am J Transplant. 2019;19(11):3139–48.
66. Strutynska NA, Dorofeieva NO, Vavilova HL, Sahach VF. Hydrogen sulfide inhibits Ca^{2+}-induced mitochondrial transition pore opening in spontaneously hypertensive rats. Fiziol Zh. 2013;59:310.
67. Chatzianastasiou A, Bibli SI, Andreadou I, Efentakis P, Kaludercic N, Wood ME, Whiteman M, Di Lisa F, Daiber A, Manolopoulos VG, Szabó C, Papapetropoulos A. Cardioprotection by H_2S donors: nitric oxide-dependent- and independent mechanisms. J Pharmacol Exp Ther. 2016;358:43140.
68. Karwi QG, Bornbaum J, Boengler K, Torregrossa R, Whiteman M, Wood ME, Schulz R, Baxter GF. AP39, a mitochondria-targeting hydrogen sulfide (H_2S) donor, protects against myocardial reperfusion injury independently of salvage kinase signalling. Br J Pharmacol. 2017;174:287301.
69. Brinkkoetter PT, Song H, Lösel R, Schnetzke U, Gottmann U, Feng Y, Hanusch C, Beck GC, Schnuelle P, Wehling M, van der Woude FJ, Yard BA. Hypothermic injury: the mitochondrial calcium, ATP and ROS love–hate triangle out of balance. Cell Physiol Biochem. 2008;22:195204.
70. Calvert JW, Jha S, Gundewar S, et al. Hydrogen sulfide mediates cardioprotection through Nrf2 signaling. Circ Res. 2009;105:365–74.
71. Shimada S, Fukai M, Wakayama K, et al. Hydrogen sulfide augments survival signals in warm ischemia and reperfusion of the mouse liver. Surg Today. 2015;45:892–903.
72. Murphy ME, Brayden JE. Nitric oxide hyperpolarizes rabbit mesenteric arteries via ATP-sensitive potassium channels. J Physiol. 1995;486:47–58.
73. Zhao W, Zhang J, Lu Y, Wang R. The vasorelaxant effect of H_2S as a novel endogenous gaseous K(ATP) channel opener. EMBO J. 2001;20:6008–16.
74. Pareira de Avila MA, Giusti-Paiva A, de Oliveira G, Nascimento C. The peripheral antinociceptive effect induced by the heme oxygenase/carbon monoxide pathway is associated with ATP-sensitive K^+ channels. Eur J Pharmacol. 2014;726:41–8.
75. Wu J, Wei J, You X, Chen X, Zhu H, Zhu X, Liu Y, Xu M. Inhibition of hydrogen sulfide generation contributes to lung injury after experimental orthotopic lung transplantation. J Surg Res. 2013;182:e2533.
76. George TJ, Arnaoutakis GJ, Beaty CA, Jandu SK, Santhanam L, Berkowitz DE, Shah AS. Hydrogen sulfide decreases reactive oxygen in a model of lung transplantation. J Surg Res. 2012;178:494501.
77. George TJ, Arnaoutakis GJ, Beaty CA, Jandu SK, Santhanam L, Berkowitz DE, Shah AS. Inhaled hydrogen sulfide improves graft function in an experimental model of lung transplantation. J Surg Res. 2012;178:593600.
78. Jiang T, Yang W, Zhang H, Song Z, Liu T, Lv X. Hydrogen sulfide ameliorates lung ischemia-reperfusion injury through sirt1 signaling pathway in type 2 diabetic rats. Front Physiol. 2020;11:596.

79. Haigis MC, Guarente LP. Mammalian sirtuins-emerging roles in physiology, aging, and calorie restriction. Genes Dev. 2006;20:2913–21.
80. Verdin E, Hirschey MD, Finley LW, Haigis MC. Sirtuin regulation of mitochondria: energy production, apoptosis, and signaling. Trends Biochem Sci. 2010;35:669–75.
81. Zhang W, Huang Q, Zeng Z, Wu J, Zhang Y, Chen Z. Sirt1 inhibits oxidative stress in vascular endothelial cells. Oxidative Med Cell Longev. 2017;2017:7543973.
82. Balaban CL, Rodriguez JV, Tiribelli C, Guibert EE. The effect of a hydrogen sulfide releasing molecule (Na$_2$S) on the cold storage of livers from cardiac dead donor rats. A study in an ex vivo model. Cryobiology. 2015;71:2432.
83. Prudhomme T, Kervella D, Le Bas-Bernardet S, Cantarovich D, Karam G, Blancho G, Branchereau J. Ex situ perfusion of pancreas for whole-organ transplantation: is it safe and feasible? A systematic review. J Diabetes Sci Technol. 2020;14(1):120–34.
84. Nishime K, Miyagi-Shiohira C, Kuwae K, Tamaki Y, Yonaha T, Sakai-Yonaha M, Saitoh I, Watanabe M, Noguchi H. Preservation of pancreas in the University of Wisconsin solution supplemented with AP39 reduces reactive oxygen species production and improves islet graft function. Am J Transplant. 2021;21(8):2698–708.
85. Iyer KR, Kunecki M, Boullata JI, Fujioka K, Joly F, Gabe S, Pape UF, Schneider SM, Virgili Casas MN, Ziegler TR, Li B, Youssef NN, Jeppesen PB. Independence from parenteral nutrition and intravenous fluid support during treatment with teduglutide among patients with intestinal failure associated with short bowel syndrome. JPEN J Parent Enteral Nutr. 2017;41(6):946–51.
86. Celik N, Mazariegos GV, Soltys K, Rudolph JA, Shi Y, Bond GJ, Sindhi R, Ganoza A. Pediatric intestinal transplantation. Gastroenterol Clin N Am. 2018;47(2):355–68.
87. Guo M, Lu C, Gao Y, Zhang H, Chen D, Li Y. Lifor solution: an alternative preservation solution in small bowel transplantation. Gastroenterol Res Pract. 2016;2016:3925751.
88. Lautenschläger I, Pless-Petig G, Middel P, de Groot H, Rauen U, Stojanovic T. Cold storage injury to rat small-bowel transplants-beneficial effect of a modified HTK solution. Transplantation. 2018;102(10):1666–73.
89. Lysyy T, Finotti M, Maina RM, Morotti R, Munoz-Abraham AS, Bertacco A, Ibarra C, Barahona M, Agarwal R, D'Amico F, Rodriguez-Davalos MI, Mulligan D, Geibel J. Human small intestine transplantation: segmental susceptibility to ischemia using different preservation solutions and conditions. Transplant Proc. 2020;52(10):2934–40.
90. Zaman J, Chakma A. Production of hydrogen and sulfur from hydrogen sulfide. Fuel Process Technol. 1995;41(2):159–98.
91. Buchholz BM, Masutani K, Kawamura T, Peng X, Toyoda Y, Billiar TR, Bauer AJ, Nakao A. Hydrogen-enriched preservation protects the isogeneic intestinal graft and amends recipient gastric function during transplantation. Transplantation. 2011;92(9):985–92.
92. Henderson PW, Weinstein AL, Sohn AM, Jimenez N, Krijgh DD, Spector JA. Hydrogen sulfide attenuates intestinal ischemia-reperfusion injury when delivered in the post-ischemic period. J Gastroenterol Hepatol. 2010;25(10):1642–7.
93. Liu H, Bai X, Shi S, Cao Y. Hydrogen sulfide protects from intestinal ischaemia-reperfusion injury in rats. J Pharm Pharmacol. 2009;61(2):207–12.
94. Cui N, Luo H, Zhao Y. Protective effect of GYY4137, a water-soluble hydrogen sulfide-releasing molecule, on intestinal ischemia-reperfusion. Mol Med Rep. 2020;21(3):1633–9.
95. Jensen AR, Drucker NA, Khaneki S, Ferkowicz MJ, Markel TA. Hydrogen sulfide improves intestinal recovery following ischemia by endothelial nitric oxide-dependent mechanisms. Am J Physiol Gastrointest Liver Physiol. 2017;312(5):G450–6.
96. Drucker NA, Jensen AR, Te Winkel JP, Markel TA. Hydrogen sulfide donor GYY4137 acts through endothelial nitric oxide to protect intestine in murine models of necrotizing enterocolitis and intestinal ischemia. J Surg Res. 2019;234:294–302.
97. Pfeifle CE, Howell SB, Felthouse RD, Woliver TB, Andrews PA, Markman M, Murphy MP. High-dose cisplatin with sodium thiosulfate protection. J Clin Oncol. 1985;3(2):237–44.

98. Breen PH, Isserles SA, Westley J, Roizen MF, Taitelman UZ. Effect of oxygen and sodium thiosulfate during combined carbon monoxide and cyanide poisoning. Toxicol Appl Pharmacol. 1995;134(2):229–34.
99. Strazzula L, Nigwekar SU, Steele D, et al. Intralesional sodium thiosulfate for the treatment of calciphylaxis. JAMA Dermatol. 2013;149(8):946–9.
100. Freyer DR, Chen L, Krailo MD, et al. Effects of sodium thiosulfate versus observation on development of cisplatin-induced hearing loss in children with cancer (ACCL0431): a multicentre, randomised, controlled, open-label, phase 3 trial. Lancet Oncol. 2017;18(1):63–74.
101. Bucci M, Vellecco V, Cantalupo A, Brancaleone V, Zhou Z, Evangelista S, et al. Hydrogen sulfide accounts for the peripheral vascular effects of zofenopril independently of ACE inhibition. Cardiovasc Res. 2014;102:138–47.
102. Zhang MY, Dugbartey GJ, Juriasingani S, Akbari M, Liu W, Haig A, McLeod P, Arp J, Sener A. Sodium thiosulfate-supplemented UW solution protects renal grafts against prolonged cold ischemia-reperfusion injury in a murine model of syngeneic kidney transplantation. Biomed Pharmacother. 2022;145:112435.

Chapter 10
FDA-Approved Hydrogen Sulfide Donor Drug and Its Clinical Applications in Nephrology

George J. Dugbartey, Max Y. Zhang, and Alp Sener

This chapter is an expanded version by the same authors in the publication titled Hydrogen Sulfide Metabolite, Sodium Thiosulfate: Clinical Applications and Underlying Molecular Mechanisms. Int J Mol Sci. 2021; 22(12):6452.

G. J. Dugbartey (✉)
Matthew Mailing Center for Translational Transplant Studies, London Health Sciences Center, Western University, London, ON, Canada

Division of Urology, Department of Surgery, London Health Sciences Center, Western University, London, ON, Canada

Multi-Organ Transplant Program, London Health Sciences Center, Western University, London, ON, Canada

Department of Pharmacology and Toxicology, School of Pharmacy, College of Health Sciences, University of Ghana, Accra, Ghana

Department of Physiology and Pharmacology, Accra College of Medicine, Accra, Ghana
e-mail: gdugbart@uwo.ca

M. Y. Zhang
Matthew Mailing Center for Translational Transplant Studies, London Health Sciences Center, Western University, London, ON, Canada

Department of Microbiology and Immunology, Schulich School of Medicine and Dentistry, University of Western Ontario, London, ON, Canada
e-mail: yzha493@uwo.ca

A. Sener
Matthew Mailing Center for Translational Transplant Studies, London Health Sciences Center, Western University, London, ON, Canada

Division of Urology, Department of Surgery, London Health Sciences Center, Western University, London, ON, Canada

Multi-Organ Transplant Program, London Health Sciences Center, Western University, London, ON, Canada

Department of Microbiology and Immunology, Schulich School of Medicine and Dentistry, University of Western Ontario, London, ON, Canada
e-mail: alp.sener@lhsc.on.ca

Sodium Thiosulfate, an FDA-Approved H$_2$S Donor Drug

Sodium thiosulfate (STS) is an odorless, inorganic, and water-soluble compound with the chemical formula $Na_2S_2O_3$ and a molecular weight of 158.11 g/mol. It is a major oxidation production of hydrogen sulfide (H$_2$S) and is typically available as a white crystalline or powdered substance in the form of pentahydrate ($Na_2S_2O_3 \cdot 5H_2O$) [1]. Currently on the World Health Organization's list of essential medicines, STS has several other uses including as a common food preservative, a water dechlorinator, a photographic fixative, and a bleaching agent for paper pulp [2]. It possesses therapeutic properties such as antioxidant, anti-inflammatory, and antihypertensive properties [3–7]. It is approved by the Food and Drug Administration (FDA) and is currently clinically useful in the treatment of acute cyanide poisoning, carbon monoxide toxicity, cisplatin toxicities in cancer therapy, and calcific uremic arteriolopathy (calciphylaxis) in dialysis patients [8–11]. STS is administered intravenously or applied topically because it is rapidly degraded in the stomach. Emerging reports also suggest its potential application in ischemia-reperfusion injury (IRI) in solid-organ transplantation [12–14]. In this chapter, we present hydrogen sulfide (H$_2$S) as an endogenous signaling molecule and describe its biochemical and molecular pathways from which thiosulfate is generated. In addition, we also discuss the clinical usefulness and potential clinical applications of STS in renovascular hypertension, renal ischemia-reperfusion injury, chronic kidney disease, and uremic pruritus and its underlying molecular mechanisms. We also discuss future perspectives of STS on kidney transplantation.

Hydrogen Sulfide as a Gasotransmitter

H$_2$S is a colorless, flammable, and water-soluble gas with the characteristic smell of rotten eggs [15, 16]. For several centuries, H$_2$S was notoriously known for its toxic effects and death among agricultural and industrial workers at high concentrations. The mechanism underlying the toxic effect of H$_2$S involves reversible antagonism of cytochrome c oxidase (complex IV), the terminal complex of the mitochondrial electron transport chain [17]. In the past two decades, however, this obnoxious-smelling, membrane-permeable gas has risen above its negative public image and is now known to play several important functions in physiological processes at low concentrations. Additionally, it exhibits diverse therapeutic potential with the ability to target several molecular pathways in several diseases and drug-induced toxicities [18–22]. H$_2$S is also established among researchers as the third member of the family of gasotransmitters, endogenous gaseous signaling molecules, next to nitric oxide and carbon monoxide [15]. It has the ability to alter the activity of proteins from many cellular signaling pathways involved in apoptosis, angiogenesis, inflammation, metabolism, proliferation, and oxygen sensing. It can also play a detoxifying role during oxidative stress by increasing the development of glutathione [23–25], the most abundant naturally occurring antioxidant in the body, and by reacting directly with peroxynitrite (ONOO−) as a direct scavenging property of H_2S towards cellular ROS. H_2S is endogenously produced in all mammalian cells through metabolic pathways that use the sulfur-containing amino acid L-cysteine and 3-mercaptopyruvate via three enzymes: cystathionine β-synthase (CBS), cystathionine γ-lyase (CSE), and 3-mercaptopyruvate sulfurtransferase (3-MST) (Fig. 10.1). It has also been found that H_2S can be produced from D-cysteine using the peroxisomal enzyme, D-amino acid oxidase [26]. Besides its endogenous production, H_2S is also administered exogenously through a number of its donor compounds, including STS and GYY4137 [27–29].

Generation of STS from H_2S

At a physiological level, thiosulfate can be generated in tissues from the mitochondrial sulfide oxidation pathway, using H_2S as the substrate. This process involves three mitochondrial enzymes: quinone oxidoreductase, sulfur dioxygenase, and

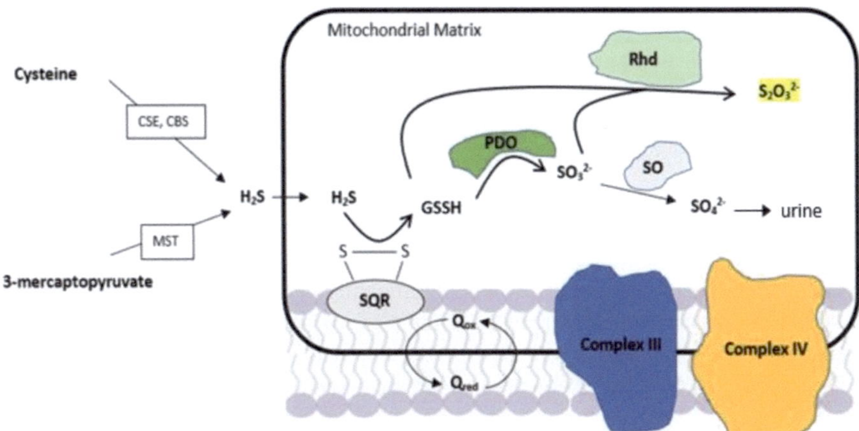

Fig. 10.1 Generation of thiosulfate from H_2S in the mitochondrial sulfide oxidation pathways. Hydrogen sulfide (H_2S) is produced by enzymes cystathionine γ-lyase (CSE) and cystathionine β-synthase (CBS) in the transsulfuration pathway. A third enzyme, 3-mercaptopyruvate sulfurtransferase (MST), also produces endogenous H_2S in the presence of the substrate 3-mercaptopyruvate. A membrane-bound sulfide, quinone oxidoreductase (SQR), oxidizes H_2S to persulfide, which is transferred to a glutathione (GSH). A persulfide dioxygenase (PDO) in the mitochondrial matrix oxides one glutathione persulfide (GSSH) to sulfite (H_2SO_3), which is then used in a sulfurtransferase reaction catalyzed by the enzyme rhodanese (Rhd) to form thiosulfate ($S_2O_3^{2-}$) by transferring a second glutathione persulfide from SQR to sulfite. Sulfite can be further oxidized by sulfite oxidase (SO) to form sulfate (SO_4^{2-}) and is subsequently excreted in urine. PDO and SO are oxygen-dependent enzymes

sulfur transferase (Fig. 10.1). Using an isolated mitochondria rat model, Hildebrandt et al. [30] proposed a method into the biochemical pathway of H_2S oxidation to thiosulfate. Firstly, as illustrated in Fig. 10.1, H_2S can react with a membrane-bound disulfide on quinone oxidoreductase (SQR) to generate a membrane-bound persulfide group (SQR-SSH). A persulfide dioxygenase in the mitochondrial matrix oxidizes one persulfide molecule to sulfite (H_2SO_3), which is then used in a sulfurtransferase reaction catalyzed by the enzyme rhodanese to form thiosulfate [30]. Rhodanese is a mitochondrial enzyme that transfers a sulfur atom from sulfane-containing donor to the thiophilic acceptor substrate [31]. The catalytic activity of rhodanese occurs via a double-displacement mechanism, where the active site, a cysteine residue (Cys247), accepts a sulfur atom from the persulfide intermediate state, followed by the transfer of sulfide sulfur from the enzyme to the nucleophilic acceptor sulfite, which produces thiosulfate (Fig. 10.1) [32]. Although human mitochondria also utilize this sulfide oxidation pathway, recent evidence suggests that glutathione (GSH) functions as a persulfide acceptor for human SQR to produce the persulfide intermediate [33, 34]. Most recently, Libiad et al. [35] found that the kinetic behavior of these enzymes favors SQR by using GSH as an acceptor to form glutathione persulfide (GSSH), which is then converted to thiosulfate by human rhodanese (Fig. 10.1). This is further confirmed by kinetic simulations in previous rat liver mitochondria studies with or without GSH, which supports GSSH as the first intermediate formed in the flow of the sulfide oxidation pathway [34].

After learning that H_2S can generate thiosulfate via the sulfide oxidation pathway, it is important to understand that the reverse reaction also occurs at a physiological level in tissue. In a study using recombinant human SQR in *Escherichia coli*, Jackson et al. [33] showed that the metabolism of thiosulfate is catalyzed by thiosulfate reductase, as it consumes two GSH molecules and results in the generation of sulfite, oxidized glutathione, and H_2S. Further evidence of the ability of thiosulfate to produce H_2S via a glutathione-dependent reduction was confirmed by a study in which exogenous thiosulfate treatment significantly decreased GSH/GSSG ratio to total sulfide ratio in a dose-dependent manner [36]. In addition, Olson et al. [37] found that H_2S generation from thiosulfate can also occur under the presence of 1,2-dithiole-3-thiones, an exogenous reducing agent. However, regardless of the exact mechanism of how sulfur is transferred, thiosulfate appears to be a key intermediate. Thus, thiosulfate (in the form of STS) is a major oxidation product of H_2S.

Biological Properties of Thiosulfate

In addition to thiosulfate being a stable, nontoxic metabolite of H_2S [38], it is also a sulfane sulfur, which is defined as sulfur atoms covalently bonded to other sulfur atoms, making it unstable and readily oxidizing in air and reducing with thiols [39,

40]. Compounds containing sulfane sulfur are known to possess cell regulatory effects through the activation or inactivation of enzymes and changing protein activities [41, 42]. The functions of sulfane sulfur include antioxidant regulation, tRNA sulfuration, and iron-sulfur protein formation [41, 43, 44]. The ability of mitochondrial enzymes to generate thiosulfate from H_2S and vice versa could have misinterpretations on which sulfur molecule conducts the biological signaling. In a mouse model of heart failure, Sen et al. [12] demonstrated that 3 mg/mL of oral thiosulfate can increase depleted H_2S levels. In addition, Tokuda et al. [45] observed the impact of H_2S gas on lipopolysaccharide (LPS)-induced inflammation in mice. They found that H_2S inhalation after LPS challenge increased plasma thiosulfate level and rhodanese activity, which prevented LPS-induced inflammation. The authors' opinion that thiosulfate may contribute to beneficial effects of H_2S inhalation was verified after they found that administering thiosulfate improved survival after LPS challenge in a dose-dependent manner. This suggests that it is thiosulfate, not H_2S, that participates as a signaling molecule in cellular regulatory processes [46].

Clinical Usefulness of STS

STS in the Treatment of Calcific Uremic Arteriolopathy in Dialysis Patients

The clinical usefulness of STS has grown over the years to include treatment of calcific uremic arteriolopathy (formerly known as calciphylaxis), which is a severe complication in patients with advanced chronic kidney disease in which calcium accumulates in blood vessels [47–49]. Predominantly seen in people with end-stage kidney disease, calcific uremic arteriolopathy is a predictor of cardiovascular death in long-term hemodialysis patients [50]. It is characterized by systemic medial calcification of the arterioles, leading to ischemia and subcutaneous necrosis. Promising results have been obtained through the use of intralesional STS. Areas of clinically active disease were treated with 250 mg/mL STS, resulting in the resolution of calciphylaxis lesions over a period of weeks with no recurrence of the disease [9]. Most recently, Peng et al. [11] conducted a systematic review of several cases on the use of STS for calcific uremic arteriolopathy and found that STS has a promising role as an effective therapy for calcific uremic arteriolopathy by acting as a calcium-chelating agent, binding to Ca^{2+}, and increasing its solubility. The authors also reported that STS possesses vasodilatory and antioxidant properties. Their findings were in agreement with previous reports that suggested that STS could combine with insoluble tissue calcium salts to form calcium thiosulfate, a salt that can later be dialyzed [11, 51–53]. Thus, treatment of calcific uremic arteriolopathy with STS is partly due to its antioxidant and calcium-chelating and vasodilatory properties.

Potential Clinical Applications of STS

STS in the Treatment of Renovascular Hypertension

As an H_2S donor molecule, STS is thought to have unexplored therapeutic potential in the context of many diseases. Over the past few years, a number of independent groups have discovered the beneficial effects of STS in animal models of disease (Table 10.1). For example, a recent study examined the protective properties of STS in angiotensin II-induced renovascular hypertension in rats [4]. The authors observed that 1 g/kg dose of STS treatment per day induced a lower plasma urea, and proteinuria, and improved creatinine clearance through its antioxidant property. They also attributed the protective effect of STS partly to its anti-inflammatory property, preventing angiotensin II-induced influx of macrophages [4]. This finding supports several previous reports that highlighted anti-inflammatory property of STS in downregulating pro-inflammatory genes such as IL-1β, TNF-α, and MAP-1 and reduced macrophage recruitment [5, 56, 57]. In a recent experimental rat model of hyperoxaluria and renal injury, 0.4 g/kg dose of STS treatment scavenged reactive oxygen species (ROS) in a dose-dependent manner, mitigated cellular hydrogen peroxide levels, and maintained superoxide dismutase activity [6]. It is important to

Table 10.1 Summary of mechanisms of action of STS in animal models of kidney diseases

Experimental model	STS concentration	Effect of STS	References
Hyperoxaluria in rats	0.4 g/kg/b.w.t.	– Preserved superoxide dismutase activity	[6]
Ethylene glycol-induced nephrolithiasis in rats	400 mg/kg b.w.t.	– Increased renal protection by modulating the mitochondrial K_{ATP} channel – Showed normal serum creatinine and renal tissue architecture	[54]
Angiotensin II-induced hypertension, proteinuria, and renal damage in rats	1 g/kg/day	– Increased GSH levels – Reduced influx of macrophages to near-control levels – Improved creatinine clearance	[4]
L-NNA-induced hypertensive nephropathy in rats	2 g/kg/day	– Enhanced GFR and ERPF – Protected against glomerulosclerosis – Lowered plasma urea and renal vascular resistance	[55]
Renal mitochondrial IRI in rats	400 mg/kg	– Maintained mitochondrial function – Increased NADH hydrogenase activity	[14]

ERPF effective renal plasma flow, *GFR* glomerular filtration rate, *GSH* glutathione, *IRI* ischemia-reperfusion injury, K_{ATP} *channel* adenosine triphosphate-sensitive potassium channel, *L-NNA* N-u-nitro-L-arginine, *NADH* nicotinamide adenine dinucleotide phosphate, *STS* sodium thiosulfate note that thiosulfate has two lone electron pairs: one at the single-bonded sulfur moiety of the disulfide bond and the other at the single-bonded oxygen [53]. This characteristic allows thiosulfate to act as an effective antioxidant by donating electrons to unpaired damaging electrons associated with mitochondrial ROS [37, 58, 59]. Further evidence of the antioxidant property of thiosulfate was confirmed in a mouse model of congestive heart failure by Sen et al. [12], where they reported that thiosulfate scavenged superoxide in myocardial tissue. In addition, thiosulfate can react with superoxide to form glutathione, a thiol-dependent antioxidant system in mammalian cells [3]. In conclusion, STS possesses potent antioxidant and anti-inflammatory properties, which protect against renovascular hypertension and other models of renal injury.

STS Against Renal Ischemia-Reperfusion Injury

An additional area in which STS has been reported to show protective effects is in animal models of ischemia-reperfusion injury (IRI) (Table 10.1). IRI is defined as tissue injury due to temporary cessation of blood flow (ischemia) and subsequent restoration of blood flow (reperfusion) to the ischemic tissue [60]. Chronic inflammation, excessive ROS production, ATP depletion, accumulation of succinate, and induction of cellular apoptotic pathways are major molecular events associated with IRI [61–63]. The first major molecular event of IRI occurs when cells are deprived of adequate oxygen due to cessation of blood flow. Lack of oxygen results in energy depletion since the cells are unable to synthesize ATP [64]. The depletion of ATP causes a rise in inorganic phosphate and inhibition of Na^+/K^+ pumps, resulting in increased intracellular Ca^{2+} concentration and mitochondrial inner membrane permeability [65]. Additionally, prolonged ischemic time can damage multiple complexes in the electron transport chain (ETC), causing it to be more prone to electron leakage [66]. The second molecular event in IRI occurs when blood flow is restored to the ischemic tissue. Reperfusion is often characterized by increased formation of ROS, decreased ATP production, and cell death [67]. Previous studies have shown that overproduction of ROS occurs from the mitochondrial ETC when oxygen is reintroduced to the cell, with the oxygenation of succinate as a main superoxide-generating species via reverse electron transport [62, 63, 67]. ROS can damage proteins of the ETC complexes, which further inhibits ATP production and increases electron leakage [68]. Cellular ATP depletion initiates translocation of pro-apoptotic proteins such as BAX, which causes mitochondrial swelling and induces efflux of cytochrome c and apoptosis-inducing factor [69]. These factors in turn activate caspase-3 apoptotic signaling cascade, initiating cellular apoptosis.

In an experimental model of renal IRI, in which isolated rat mitochondria were subjected to physiological oxidative stress by nitrogen gas purging, treatment with STS induced renal protection and maintained mitochondrial functional integrity by markedly reducing oxidative stress and deteriorated mitochondrial enzyme activities compared to untreated groups [14]. Apart from the kidney, Marutani et al. [70]

also reported that 10 mg/kg dose of STS inhibits caspase-3 activity via persulfidation of the same active site, Cys-163, and protects against neuronal IRI in mice. Additionally, STS was shown to activate Erk 1/2 and block the c-Jun N-terminal kinase (JNK), which led to inhibition of apoptosis by preventing dephosphorylation of the pro-apoptotic protein, Bad, and downregulation of anti-apoptotic protein, Bcl-2 [71–73].

The protective effect of STS observed in different experimental models of IRI is partly attributable to its ability to activate mitochondrial adenosine triphosphate (ATP)-sensitive potassium (K_{ATP}) channels, suggesting that the opening of these channels may have inhibited mitochondrial permeability transition [12, 13]. This observation confirms previous studies in which H_2S stimulated the opening of K_{ATP} channels by blocking phosphorylation of the transcription factors forkhead box O (FOXO1 and FOXO3a) in rat vascular smooth muscle cells, leading to reduced Ca^{2+} influx and preventing the opening of mitochondrial permeability transition pores [74, 75]. Further evidence of STS maintaining mitochondrial integrity was confirmed in a study by Mohan et al. [14], where isolated rat mitochondria were subjected to physiological oxidative stress. The results showed that the pretreated STS group had higher renal mitochondrial enzyme activity due to its increased NADH dehydrogenase activity compared to the nontreated group [14]. In summary, STS modulates several molecular pathways in the mitochondria, leading to protection against IRI.

Use of STS as an H_2S Donor Drug

Considering that STS is already a clinically viable H_2S donor drug approved by the FDA and is also in clinical trials along with other H_2S donor drugs such as GIG-1001, SG1002, ATB-436, and zofenopril for cardiovascular diseases, intestinal disorders, and other conditions [76], it is important to translate these promising experimental findings about STS to clinical practice. As such, STS-related therapeutic research is a rapidly emerging field, with many studies done on H_2S-related cytoprotective effects. One example is signaling mechanism of the antioxidant and transcription factor nuclear factor erythroid-related factor 2 (Nrf2), which is partly attributable to H_2S effects [77] (Fig. 10.2). Previous studies have shown that H_2S activates Nrf2-dependent signaling, which produces antioxidant proteins to mitigate animal models of inflammatory acute liver failure and cardiovascular disease [78–81]. Under normal conditions, Nrf2 is captured by Keap1 proteins in the cytoplasm [82]. However, when exposed to oxidative stress, Nrf2 avoids Keap1 and is translocated into the nucleus in order to bind to antioxidant response elements (AREs) to induce the expression of various antioxidant gene clusters [77, 81, 83]. In a recent study by Koike et al. [84, 85], they discovered that addition of sulfane sulfurs increased Nrf2 accumulation in the nucleus of neuroblastoma cells through the structural change of Keap1 protein. Specifically, the sulfane sulfurs triggered a persulfidation reaction of

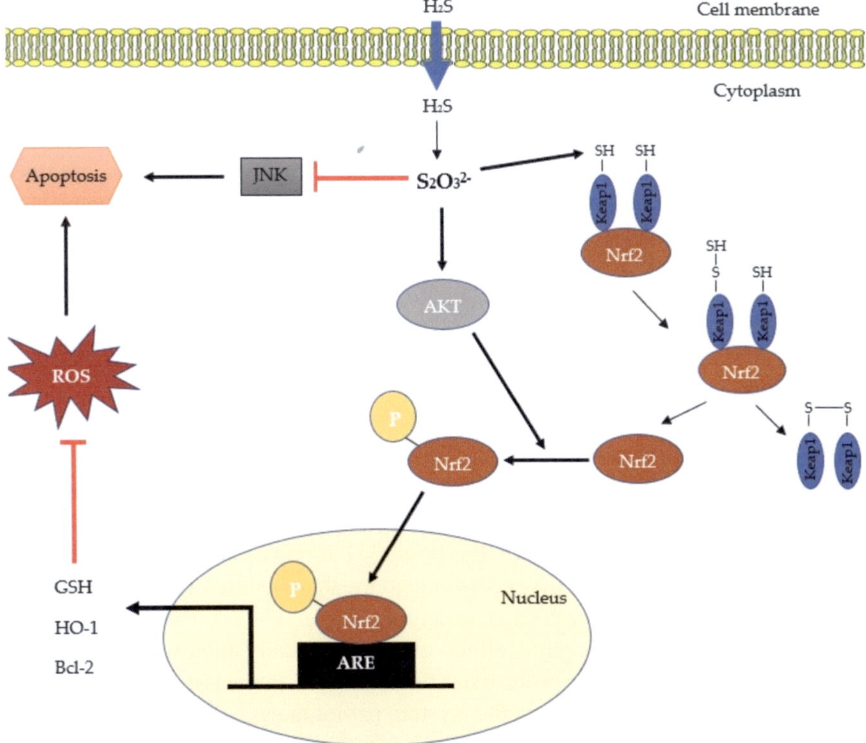

Fig. 10.2 Proposed overview of cytoprotective effects of thiosulfate against oxidative stress. Thiosulfate ($S_2O_3^{2-}$) is produced from hydrogen sulfide (H_2S) via sulfide oxidation pathway. The bound sulfur on thiosulfate activates the Nrf2 system through the structural change of Keap1 proteins and induction of phosphorylated AKT. The nuclear translocation of phosphorylated Nrf2 binds to ARE to promote the expression of various antioxidative gene clusters. Thiosulfate also contributes to anti-apoptotic signaling via inhibition of JNK phosphorylation. *ROS* reactive oxygen species, *GSH* glutathione, *HO-1* heme oxygenase-1, *Bcl-2* B-cell lymphoma-2, *ARE* antioxidant response element, *Nrf2* nuclear factor erythroid-related factor 2, *Keap1* Kelch-like ECH-associated protein 1, *AKT* protein kinase B, *JNK* c-Jun N-terminal kinases

the cysteine residue in Keap1, which led to Keap1-forming homodimers with another Keap1 protein or heterodimers with another protein (Fig. 10.2). It has also been reported that persulfidated proteins are protective against oxidative stress-induced damage and thereby preserve the function of the persulfidated cysteine residues [86]. The authors further reported that the polysulfide induced AKT phosphorylation, which triggered the phosphorylation of Nrf2, resulting in nuclear translocation. This suggests that sulfane sulfurs, such as thiosulfate, activate Nrf2 signaling pathway through the structural change of Keap1 protein and phosphorylation of AKT (Fig. 10.2). These findings support a recent study about a mice model of acute liver failure, where administration of 2 g/kg STS attenuated liver injury by enhancing AKT phosphorylation and inducing Nrf2-dependent antioxidant proteins

[21]. In addition, the authors showed that STS treatment also inhibited phosphorylation of JNK, a protein that is upregulated by inflammatory cytokines and extracellular stresses and plays a critical role in apoptotic signaling [87]. A proposed mechanism of how thiosulfate interacts with Nrf2 signaling pathway to induce cytoprotective effects against oxidative stress is shown in Fig. 10.2.

Many of the biochemical characteristics of H_2S signaling that provide cytoprotective effects, such as persulfidation of signaling proteins, can be accomplished with thiosulfate instead. For example, a study by Giovinazzo et al. [88] showed that H_2S donor molecule GYY4137 inhibits Tau hyperphosphorylation by persulfidation of kinase GSK3β, ultimately ameliorating cognitive and motor deficits in Alzheimer's disease. STS, as we previously mentioned, has been shown to trigger persulfidation reactions in the sulfur oxidation pathway [37] and in the Nrf2 signaling pathway [84]. Multiple studies on H_2S prodrugs reported to be beneficial in cardiovascular systems also involve similar biochemical mechanism to STS, such as persulfidation in SP1-mediated transcription to preserve endothelial function [89, 90], persulfidation in regulation of PYK2-mediated eNOS phosphorylation to mediate cardioprotection [91], and persulfidation in ERK/MEK1/PARP-mediated DNA damage repair and cell survival [92]. It is possible but remains to be studied whether modulation of STS pathways may contribute to the therapeutic actions of the experimental H_2S prodrugs. Since STS is widely available as a key metabolite of H_2S with similar biochemical signaling effects and as a clinically approved drug, further studies are warranted on the protective effects of STS in central nervous system, cardiovascular system, and many other system pathologies.

Use of STS in Kidney Transplantation

Following our compelling success in different animal models of kidney transplantation with the use of H_2S-supplemented University of Wisconsin (UW) solution for static cold storage, it is important to translate these promising experimental findings to clinical practice using STS. Hence, we decided to investigate whether STS-supplemented UW solution would be suitable for renal graft preservation. In our recent rat model of syngeneic orthotopic kidney transplantation, we found that kidneys stored in STS-supplemented UW solution prolonged transplant recipient survival, with improved acute tubular necrosis scores and graft function compared to UW-stored kidneys without STS treatment [93]. Serum creatinine levels also showed that while STS-treated rats exhibited significantly decreased serum creatinine at postoperative day 3 compared to UW-treated rats (without STS), serum creatinine levels in the former group were not statistically different from those of sham-operated rats [93]. Overall, supplementing organ preservation solutions with STS may be a promising approach, as it requires minimal modification of existing clinical protocols and is also cost-effective. However, mechanistic properties of STS on renal IRI need to be studied further.

STS in the Treatment of Chronic Kidney Disease

As discussed in Chap. 3, chronic kidney disease (CKD) is a major global health issue and is characterized by irreversible pathological processes that involve progressive loss of renal function, chronic inflammation, ROS-induced oxidative stress, and glomerular and tubular injury, all of which culminate in the development of end-stage renal disease (ESRD). At the molecular level, overproduction of ROS from damaged mitochondria of renal tubular cells is a major factor in CKD progression, as it overwhelms the cell's antioxidant defense system and induces apoptosis via activation of a cascade of pathological signaling pathways that involve DNA damage, increased expression of initiator and executioner caspases, and cleavage of poly-(ADP-ribose)-polymerase [94, 95]. Interestingly, excess ROS has also been identified recently as a mediator of ferroptosis (a type programmed cell death that is dependent on iron) by inhibiting the activity of glutathione peroxidase 4 (GPX4) and propagating lipid peroxidation chain reaction in animal models of CKD [96–98]. As current antioxidant therapy for CKD confers significant adverse side effects that limits their approval in clinical trials [99, 100], these pieces of empirical evidence suggest immediate development or identification of potent antioxidant agents with less adverse effects or the use of drug repositioning (or repurposing) as an off-label pharmacological tool to inhibit ROS-induced molecular events and prevent or retard CKD progression.

In a recent rat model of 5/6 nephrectomy, a common animal model of CKD with progressive albuminuria and loss of renal function, in which two-thirds of the left kidney was infarcted by ligation of left renal artery and subsequent right nephrectomy, Cheng et al. [101] reported renal dysfunction and impaired glomeruli and tubules, as seen in increased levels of urinary protein, blood urea nitrogen, and serum creatinine in untreated CKD rats, along with apoptosis, ferroptosis, fibrosis and inflammation, and systemic hypertension. The authors also observed high levels of renal and plasma reactive oxygen-derived free radicals such as hydrogen peroxide and hypochlorous acid, which are indicative of increased oxidative stress in this group of experimental animals. Remarkably, intraperitoneal administration of 0.1 g/kg STS three times/week for 4 weeks in CKD rats attenuated these pathological changes including amelioration of CKD-induced oxidative stress parameters, leading to preservation of renal structure and significant improvement in renal function [101]. This implies that STS exhibits antioxidant, anti-apoptotic, anti-ferroptotic, anti-fibrotic, and anti-inflammatory effects that confer renal protection and prevent CKD progression. In the same study, STS strongly downregulated renal expression of Drp-1 (a promotor of mitochondrial fission and mediator of cytochrome c release during apoptosis), while it markedly upregulated renal expression of OPA-1 (a promotor of mitochondrial fusion that preserves mitochondrial structure) to normal levels [101]. This finding suggests that STS plays a key role in preserving mitochondrial dynamics and integrity, which partly contributes to prevention of CKD progression. Interestingly, no adverse effect of STS administration was reported in this study. However, one clinical study reported metabolic acidosis in a patient with calcific uremic arteriolopathy following intravenous administration of STS [102]. Conversely, significant reduction in STS dose improved the patient's situation, highlighting the importance of starting and maintaining a low therapeutic dose to avoid any potential adverse effects. Although the preclinical report about the reno-protective effect of STS in CKD holds a clinical promise, it requires further studies by other research groups to accentuate and validate the finding. In summary, STS may be used as a drug-repositioning strategy to prevent or retard CKD progression.

STS in the Treatment of Uremic Pruritus

Uremic pruritus, also called CKD-associated pruritus (CKD-aP), is a frequent and compromising symptom of itchy skin in patients with advanced CKD and ESRD. Clinically, it is defined as daily or near-daily itching in the absence of comorbid conditions such as dermatological, hepatobiliary, hematological, endocrinological, neurological, and psychiatric disorders; drug intake; as well as solid tumors. CKD-aP may be localized or generalized and causes considerable discomfort, with a varying presentation ranging from intermittent discomfort to persistent and complete restlessness during day- and nighttime, thus significantly impairing the quality of life of patients, along with depressive symptoms [103, 104]. There are clinical reports showing that over 40% of dialysis patients have CKD-aP, with a higher mortality rate due to sleep disturbance and other associated causes than non-CKD-aP dialysis patients [105, 106]. The underlying pathogenic mechanism of CKD-aP is poorly understood. However, histamine, parathormone, albumin, inflammatory markers, and metabolism of minerals such as magnesium, calcium, and phosphorus have been associated with its pathogenesis and progression and may also be a consequence of a neuropathic mechanism via opioid-receptor derangements [104, 107, 108]. Although there is currently no universally effective therapy, treatments of CKD-aP include topical therapies with or without anti-inflammatory agents; systemic therapies with gabapentin, pregabalin, μ-opioid receptor antagonists and κ-agonists, and anti-inflammatory drugs; phototherapy; and complementary alternative therapies such as acupuncture [104]. However, therapeutic success is limited due to severe adverse effects and low number of randomized, placebo-controlled trials [109, 110]. Also, there are contradictory results on putative effective novel therapeutic options [111–114]. Therefore, there is urgent need to identify safe and effective complementary therapies.

In a recent retrospective study involving 24 hemodialysis patients with CKD-aP, who received intravenous administration of 3.2 g STS in 20 mL of normal saline three times/week for 8 weeks, Song et al. [115] observed significantly lower visual analog scale (VAS, a pain rating scale) and detailed pruritus score (DPS) following 8 weeks of STS therapy compared to 20 CKD-aP hemodialysis patients who received 10 mg/day of loratadine (an antihistamine). All biological parameters were not affected, and no adverse effects or mortalities were recorded after treatment

[115]. Mechanistically, the antipruritic action of STS has been attributed to its vasodilation property, which increases the synthesis of nitric oxide (a vasodilator), thereby reducing local inflammation and pruritogen production [104, 115]. The positive clinical outcome with STS administration in CKD-aP patients was supported by a later systematic review and meta-analysis of randomized controlled trials in which STS group of CKD-aP patients exhibited markedly decreased DPS without remarkable adverse effects compared to control group [116], indicating that STS could represent a safe and effective complementary therapy for hemodialysis patients with CKD-aP. However, these studies used only a small patient population and short duration of treatment. Therefore, a larger sample size with further studies focused on different doses of STS, frequency of its administration, and close monitoring for long-term effects will provide more insights on the pharmacological and therapeutic implications of STS in CKD-aP.

Conclusion

Although H_2S is a major contributor to altering cellular physiology in various ways, STS appears to play a significant role in biological signaling as well. Several studies have elucidated the ability of mitochondrial enzymes to generate thiosulfate from H_2S through a sulfide oxidation pathway. Emerging data on the biological effects of STS and its close chemical relationship with H_2S support the development of STS-based therapeutics. Besides its clinical usefulness, STS has also been shown experimentally to effectively protect against renovascular hypertension and other renal pathologies such as renal IRI, chronic kidney disease, and uremic pruritus. In the context of kidney transplantation, modification of the preservation solutions with STS may be a simple, inexpensive, and nontoxic novel therapeutic strategy to mitigate cold IRI in donor kidneys to ultimately improve renal graft outcomes and minimize posttransplant complications. However, the underlying protective molecular mechanisms of this novel approach will need further investigation.

Conflict of Interest None.

References

1. Ma X, Yu J, Yan R, Yan M, Xu Q. Promoting effect of crystal water leading to catalyst-free synthesis of heteroaryl thioether from heteroaryl chloride, sodium thiosulfate pentahydrate, and alcohol. J Org Chem. 2019;84:11294–300. https://doi.org/10.1021/acs.joc.9b01670.
2. World Health Organization. World Health Organization model list of essential medicines: 21st list 2019. Geneva: World Health Organization; 2019.
3. Mishanina TV, Libiad M, Banerjee R. Biogenesis of reactive sulfur species for signaling by hydrogen sulfide oxidation pathways. Nat Chem Biol. 2015;11:457–64. https://doi.org/10.1038/nchembio.1834.

4. Snijder PM, Frenay A-RS, Koning AM, Bachtler M, Pasch A, Kwakernaak AJ, Berg EVD, Bos EM, Hillebrands J-L, Navis G, et al. Sodium thiosulfate attenuates angiotensin II-induced hypertension, proteinuria and renal damage. Nitric Oxide. 2014;42:87–98. https://doi.org/10.1016/j.niox.2014.10.002.

5. Song K, Wang F, Li Q, Shi Y-B, Zheng H-F, Peng H, Shen H-Y, Liu C-F, Hu L-F. Hydrogen sulfide inhibits the renal fibrosis of obstructive nephropathy. Kidney Int. 2014;85:1318–29. https://doi.org/10.1038/ki.2013.449.

6. Bijarnia RK, Bachtler M, Chandak PG, van Goor H, Pasch A. Sodium thiosulfate ameliorates oxidative stress and pre-serves renal function in hyperoxaluric rats. PLoS One. 2015;10:e0124881.

7. Roorda M, Miljkovic JL, van Goor H, Henning RH, Bouma HR. Spatiotemporal regulation of hydrogen sulfide signaling in the kidney. Redox Biol. 2021;43:101961. https://doi.org/10.1016/j.redox.2021.101961.

8. Bebarta VS, Brittain M, Chan A. Sodium nitrite and sodium thiosulfate are effective against acute cyanide poisoning when administered by intramuscular injection. Ann Emerg Med. 2017;69:718–25.

9. Tsang RY, Al-Fayea T, Au HJ. Cisplatin overdose: toxicities and management. Drug Saf. 2009;32:1109–22.

10. Strazzula L, Nigwekar SU, Steele D, Tsiaras W, Sise M, Bis S, Smith GP, Kroshinsky D. Intralesional sodium thiosulfate for the treatment of calciphylaxis. JAMA Dermatol. 2013;149:946–9. https://doi.org/10.1001/jamadermatol.2013.4565.

11. Peng T, Zhuo L, Wang Y, Jun M, Li G, Wang L, Hong D. Systematic review of sodium thiosulfate in treating calciphylaxis in chronic kidney disease patients. Nephrology (Carlton). 2017;23:669–75. https://doi.org/10.1111/nep.13081.

12. Sen U, Vacek TP, Hughes WM, Kumar MS, Moshal KS, Tyagi N, Metreveli NS, Hayden MR, Tyagi SC. Cardioprotective role of sodium thiosulfate on chronic heart failure by modulating endogenous H_2S generation. Pharmacology. 2008;82:201–13. https://doi.org/10.1159/000156486.

13. Cancherini DV, Trabuco LG, Rebouças NA, Kowaltowski AJ. ATP-sensitive K^+ channels in renal mitochondria. Am J Physiol Physiol. 2003;285:F1291–6. https://doi.org/10.1152/ajprenal.00103.2003.

14. Kurian GA, Mohan D, Balasubramanian ED, Ravindran S. Renal mitochondria can withstand hypoxic/ischemic injury secondary to renal failure in uremic rats pretreated with sodium thiosulfate. Indian J Pharmacol. 2017;49:317–21. https://doi.org/10.4103/ijp.IJP_751_16.

15. Abe K, Kimura H. The possible role of hydrogen sulfide as an endogenous neuromodulator. J Neurosci. 1996;16:1066–71. https://doi.org/10.1523/jneurosci.16-03-01066.1996.

16. Polhemus DJ, Lefer DJ. Emergence of hydrogen sulfide as an endogenous gaseous signaling molecule in cardiovascular disease. Circ Res. 2014;114:730–7. https://doi.org/10.1161/circresaha.114.300505.

17. Blackstone E, Morrison M, Roth MB. H_2S induces a suspended animation-like state in mice. Science. 2005;308:518. https://doi.org/10.1126/science.1108581.

18. Yamamoto J, Sato W, Kosugi T, Yamamoto T, Kimura T, Taniguchi S, Kojima H, Maruyama S, Imai E, Matsuo S, et al. Distribution of hydrogen sulfide (H_2S)-producing enzymes and the roles of the H_2S donor sodium hydrosulfide in diabetic nephropathy. Clin Exp Nephrol. 2012;17:32–40. https://doi.org/10.1007/s10157-012-0670-y.

19. Dugbartey GJ. Diabetic nephropathy: a potential savior with 'rotten-egg' smell. Pharmacol Rep. 2017;69:331–9.

20. Dugbartey GJ. H_2S as a possible therapeutic alternative for the treatment of hypertensive kidney injury. Nitric Oxide. 2017;64:52–60. https://doi.org/10.1016/j.niox.2017.01.002.

21. Shirozu K, Tokuda K, Marutani E, Lefer D, Wang R, Ichinose F. Cystathionine γ-lyase deficiency protects mice from galactosamine/lipopolysaccharide-induced acute liver failure. Antioxid Redox Signal. 2014;20:204–16. https://doi.org/10.1089/ars.2013.5354.

22. Dugbartey GJ, Bouma HR, Lobb I, Sener A. Hydrogen sulfide: a novel nephroprotectant against cisplatin-induced renal toxicity. Nitric Oxide. 2016;57:15–20. https://doi.org/10.1016/j.niox.2016.04.005.
23. Kimura Y, Goto Y-I, Kimura H. Hydrogen sulfide increases glutathione production and suppresses oxidative stress in mitochondria. Antioxid Redox Signal. 2010;12:1–13. https://doi.org/10.1089/ars.2008.2282.
24. Whiteman M, Armstrong JS, Chu SH, Jia-Ling S, Wong B-S, Cheung NS, Halliwell B, Moore PK. The novel neuromodulator hydrogen sulfide: an endogenous peroxynitrite 'scavenger'? J Neurochem. 2004;90:765–8. https://doi.org/10.1111/j.1471-4159.2004.02617.x.
25. Filipovic MR, Miljkovic J, Allgäuer A, Chaurio R, Shubina T, Herrmann M, Ivanovic-Burmazovic I. Biochemical insight into physiological effects of H$_2$S: reaction with peroxynitrite and formation of a new nitric oxide donor, sulfinyl nitrite. Biochem J. 2012;441:609–21.
26. Shibuya N, Koike S, Tanaka M, Ishigami-Yuasa M, Kimura Y, Ogasawara Y, Fukui K, Nagahara N, Kimura H. A novel pathway for the production of hydrogen sulfide from D-cysteine in mammalian cells. Nat Commun. 2013;4:1366. https://doi.org/10.1038/ncomms2371.
27. Burnie R, Smail S, Javaid MM. Calciphylaxis and sodium thiosulphate: a glimmer of hope in desperate situation. J Ren Care. 2013;39:71–6. https://doi.org/10.1111/j.1755-6686.2013.12008.x.
28. Nigwekar SU, Brunelli SM, Meade D, Wang W, Hymes J, Lacson E Jr. Sodium thiosulfate therapy for calcific uremic arteriolopathy. Clin J Am Soc Nephrol. 2013;8:1162–70.
29. Li L, Whiteman M, Guan YY, Neo KL, Cheng Y, Lee SW. Characterization of a novel, water-soluble hydrogen sulfide-releasing molecule (GYY4137): new insights into the biology of hydrogen sulfide. Circulation. 2008;117:2351–60.
30. Hildebrandt TM, Grieshaber MK. Three enzymatic activities catalyze the oxidation of sulfide to thiosulfate in mammalian and invertebrate mitochondria. FEBS J. 2008;275:3352–61. https://doi.org/10.1111/j.1742-4658.2008.06482.x.
31. Westley J, Adler H, Westley L, Nishida C. The sulfurtransferases. Fundam Appl Toxicol. 1983;3:377–82.
32. Kruithof PD, Lunev S, Lozano SPA, Batista FDA, Al-Dahmani ZM, Joles JA, Dolga AM, Groves MR, van Goor H. Unraveling the role of thiosulfate sulfurtransferase in metabolic diseases. Biochim Biophys Acta (BBA) Mol Basis Dis. 2020;1866:165716. https://doi.org/10.1016/j.bbadis.2020.165716.
33. Jackson MR, Melideo SL, Jorns MS. Human sulfide: quinone oxidoreductase catalyzes the first step in hydrogen sulfide metabolism and produces a sulfane sulfur metabolite. Biochemistry. 2012;51:6804–15. https://doi.org/10.1021/bi300778t.
34. Bartholomew TC, Powell GM, Dodgson KS, Curtis CG. Oxidation of sodium sulphide by rat liver, lungs and kidney. Biochem Pharmacol. 1980;29:2431–7. https://doi.org/10.1016/0006-2952(80)90346-9.
35. Libiad M, Yadav PK, Vitvitsky V, Martinov M, Banerjee R. Organization of the human mitochondrial hydrogen sulfide oxidation pathway. J Biol Chem. 2014;289:30901–10. https://doi.org/10.1074/jbc.m114.602664.
36. Leskova A, Pardue S, Glawe JD, Kevil CG, Shen X. Role of thiosulfate in hydrogen sulfide-dependent redox signaling in endothelial cells. Am J Physiol Circ Physiol. 2017;313:H256–64. https://doi.org/10.1152/ajpheart.00723.2016.
37. Olson KR, DeLeon ER, Gao Y, Hurley K, Sadauskas V, Batz C, Stoy GF. Thiosulfate: a readily accessible source of hydrogen sulfide in oxygen sensing. Am J Physiol Regul Integr Comp Physiol. 2013;305:R592–603. https://doi.org/10.1152/ajpregu.00421.2012.
38. Bilska-Wilkosz A, Iciek M, Górny M, Kowalczyk-Pachel D. The role of hemoproteins: hemoglobin, myoglobin and neuroglobin in endogenous thiosulfate production processes. Int J Mol Sci. 2017;18:1315. https://doi.org/10.3390/ijms18061315.
39. Koike S, Ogasawara Y. Sulfur atom in its bound state is a unique element involved in physiological functions in mammals. Molecules. 2016;21:1753. https://doi.org/10.3390/molecules21121753.

40. Wood JL. Sulfane sulfur. Methods Enzymol. 1987;143:25–9.
41. Iciek M, Włodek L. Biosynthesis and biological properties of compounds containing highly reactive, reduced sulfane sulfur. Pol J Pharmacol. 2002;53:215–25.
42. Mustafa AK, Gadalla MM, Sen N, Kim S, Mu W, Gazi SK, Barrow RK, Yang G, Wang R, Snyder SH. HS signals through protein S-sulfhydration. Sci Signal. 2009;2:ra72.
43. Umbreit J. Methemoglobin—it's not just blue: a concise review. Am J Hematol. 2007;82:134–44.
44. Sakaguchi M, Marutani E, Shin H, Chen W, Hanaoka K, Xian M, Ichinose F. Sodium thiosulfate attenuates acute lung injury in mice. Anesthesiology. 2014;121:1248–57.
45. Tokuda K, Kida K, Marutani E, Crimi E, Bougaki M, Khatri A, Kimura H, Ichinose F. Inhaled hydrogen sulfide prevents endotoxin-induced systemic inflammation and improves survival by altering sulfide metabolism in mice. Antioxid Redox Signal. 2012;17:11–21. https://doi.org/10.1089/ars.2011.4363.
46. Toohey JI. Sulfur signaling: is the agent sulfide or sulfane? Anal Biochem. 2011;413:1–7.
47. Burnie R, Smail S, Javaid MM. Calciphylaxis and sodium thiosulfate: a glimmer of hope in desperate situation. J Ren Care. 2013;39:71–6.
48. Meillier A, Heller C. Acute cyanide poisoning: hydroxocobalamin and sodium thiosulfate treatments with two outcomes following one exposure event. Case Rep Med. 2015;2015:1–4. https://doi.org/10.1155/2015/217951.
49. Yu Z, Gu L, Pang H, Fang Y, Yan H, Fang W. Sodium thiosulfate: an emerging treatment for calciphylaxis in dialysis patients. Case Rep Nephrol Dial. 2015;5:77–82. https://doi.org/10.1159/000380945.
50. Goel SK, Bellovich K, McCullough PA. Treatment of severe metastatic calcification and calciphylaxis in dialysis patients. Int J Nephrol. 2011;2011:1–5. https://doi.org/10.4061/2011/701603.
51. Yatzidis H. Successful sodium thiosulphate treatment for recurrent calcium urolithiasis. Clin Nephrol. 1985;23:63–7.
52. Hayden MR, Goldsmith DJA. Sodium thiosulfate: new hope for the treatment of calciphylaxis. Semin Dial. 2010;23:258–62. https://doi.org/10.1111/j.1525-139x.2010.00738.x.
53. Olaoye OA, Koratala A. Calcific uremic arteriolopathy. Oxf Med Case Rep. 2017;2017:omx055. https://doi.org/10.1093/omcr/omx055.
54. Baldev N, Sriram R, Prabu P, Gino AK. Effect of mitochondrial potassium channel on the renal protection mediated by sodium thiosulfate against ethylene glycol induced nephrolithiasis in rat model. Int Braz J Urol. 2015;41:1116–25. https://doi.org/10.1590/s1677-5538.ibju.2014.0585.
55. Nguyen IT, Klooster A, Minnion M, Feelisch M, Verhaar MC, van Goor H, Joles JA. Sodium thiosulfate improves renal function and oxygenation in L-NNA—induced hypertension in rats. Kidney Int. 2020;98:366–77. https://doi.org/10.1016/j.kint.2020.02.020.
56. Lobb I, Davison M, Carter D, Liu W, Haig A, Gunaratnam L, Sener A. Hydrogen sulfide treatment mitigates renal allograft ischemia-reperfusion injury during cold storage and improves early transplant kidney function and survival following allogeneic renal transplantation. J Urol. 2015;194:1806–15.
57. Grewal J, Lobb I, Saha M, Haig A, Jiang J, Sener A. MP29-16 hydrogen sulfide supplementation mitigates effects of ischemia reperfusion injury in a murine model of donation after cardiac death renal transplantation. J Urol. 2016;195:1100. https://doi.org/10.1016/j.juro.2016.02.1100.
58. Hayden MR, Tyagi SC, Kolb L, Sowers JR, Khanna R. Vascular ossification–calcification in metabolic syndrome, type 2 diabetes mellitus, chronic kidney disease, and calciphylaxis-calcific uremic arteriolopathy: the emerging role of sodium thio-sulfate. Cardiovasc Diabetol. 2005;4:4.
59. Szabó C. Hydrogen sulphide and its therapeutic potential. Nat Rev Drug Discov. 2007;6:917–35. https://doi.org/10.1038/nrd2425.
60. Dorweiler B, Pruefer D, Andrasi TB, Maksan SM, Schmiedt W, Neufang A, Vahl CF. Ischemia-reperfusion injury. Eur J Trauma Emerg Surg. 2007;33:600–12.

61. Summers DM, Watson CJ, Pettigrew GJ, Johnson RJ, Collett D, Neuberger JM, Bradley JA. Kidney donation after circulatory death (DCD): state of the art. Kidney Int. 2015;88:241–9. https://doi.org/10.1038/ki.2015.88.
62. Chouchani ET, Pell VR, Gaude E, Aksentijević D, Sundier SY, Robb EL, Logan A, Nadtochiy SM, Ord ENJ, Smith AC, et al. Ischaemic accumulation of succinate controls reperfusion injury through mitochondrial ROS. Nature. 2014;515:431–5. https://doi.org/10.1038/nature13909.
63. Chouchani ET, Pell VR, James AM, Work L, Saeb-Parsy K, Frezza C, Krieg T, Murphy MP. A unifying mechanism for mitochondrial superoxide production during ischemia-reperfusion injury. Cell Metab. 2016;23:254–63. https://doi.org/10.1016/j.cmet.2015.12.009.
64. Kezic A, Spasojevic I, Lezaic V, Bajcetic M. Mitochondria-targeted antioxidants: future perspectives in kidney ischemia reperfusion injury. Oxid Med Cell Longev. 2016;2016:2950503.
65. Kowaltowski AJ, Castilho RF, Grijalba MT, Bechara EJ, Vercesi AE. Effect of inorganic phosphate concentration on the nature of inner mitochondrial membrane alterations mediated by Ca^{2+} ions. J Biol Chem. 1996;271:2929–34. https://doi.org/10.1074/jbc.271.6.2929.
66. Thomas DD, Heinecke JL, Ridnour LA, Cheng RY, Kesarwala AH, Switzer CH, McVicar DW, Roberts DD, Glynn S, Fukuto JM, et al. Signaling and stress: the redox landscape in NOS_2 biology. Free Radic Biol Med. 2015;87:204–25. https://doi.org/10.1016/j.freeradbiomed.2015.06.002.
67. Martinou JC, Green DR. Breaking the mitochondrial barrier. Nat Rev Mol Cell Biol. 2001;2:63–7.
68. Becker LB. New concepts in reactive oxygen species and cardiovascular reperfusion physiology. Cardiovasc Res. 2004;61:461–70. https://doi.org/10.1016/j.cardiores.2003.10.025.
69. McCully JD, Wakiyama H, Hsieh Y-J, Jones M, Levitsky S. Differential contribution of necrosis and apoptosis in myocardial ischemia-reperfusion injury. Am J Physiol Circ Physiol. 2004;286:H1923–35. https://doi.org/10.1152/ajpheart.00935.2003.
70. Marutani E, Yamada M, Ida T, Tokuda K, Ikeda K, Kai S, Shirozu K, Hayashida K, Kosugi S, Hanaoka K, et al. Thiosulfate mediates cytoprotective effects of hydrogen sulfide against neuronal ischemia. J Am Hear Assoc. 2015;4:2125. https://doi.org/10.1161/jaha.115.002125.
71. Ohtaki H, Nakamachi T, Dohi K, Aizawa Y, Takaki A, Hodoyama K, Yofu S, Hashimoto H, Shintani N, Baba A, et al. Pituitary adenylate cyclase-activating polypeptide (PACAP) decreases ischemic neuronal cell death in association with IL-6. Proc Natl Acad Sci U S A. 2006;103:7488–93. https://doi.org/10.1073/pnas.0600375103.
72. Benakis C, Bonny C, Hirt L. JNK inhibition and inflammation after cerebral ischemia. Brain Behav Immun. 2010;24:800–11. https://doi.org/10.1016/j.bbi.2009.11.001.
73. Nijboer CH, Bonestroo HJ, Zijlstra J, Kavelaars A, Heijnen CJ. Mitochondrial JNK phosphorylation as a novel therapeutic target to inhibit neuroinflammation and apoptosis after neonatal ischemic brain damage. Neurobiol Dis. 2013;54:432–44. https://doi.org/10.1016/j.nbd.2013.01.017.
74. Zhao W, Zhang J, Lu Y, Wang R. The vasorelaxant effect of H_2S as a novel endogenous gaseous KATP channel opener. EMBO J. 2001;20:6008–16.
75. Sun Y, Huang Y, Zhang R, Chen Q, Chen J, Zong Y, Liu J, Feng S, Liu AD, Holmberg L, et al. Hydrogen sulfide upregulates KATP channel expression in vascular smooth muscle cells of spontaneously hypertensive rats. J Mol Med. 2014;93:439–55. https://doi.org/10.1007/s00109-014-1227-1.
76. Wallace JL, Vaughan D, Dicay M, Macnaughton WK, De Nucci G. Hydrogen sulfide-releasing therapeutics: translation to the clinic. Antioxid Redox Signal. 2018;28:1533–40. https://doi.org/10.1089/ars.2017.7068.
77. Calvert J, Jha S, Gundewar S, Elrod J, Ramachandran A, Pattillo CB, Kevil C, Lefer DJ. Hydrogen sulfide mediates cardioprotection through Nrf2 signaling. Circ Res. 2009;105:365–74. https://doi.org/10.1161/circresaha.109.199919.
78. Das J, Ghosh J, Roy A, Sil PC. Mangiferin exerts hepatoprotective activity against D-galactosamine induced acute toxicity and oxidative/nitrosative stress via Nrf2–NFκB pathways. Toxicol Appl Pharmacol. 2012;260:35–47. https://doi.org/10.1016/j.taap.2012.01.015.

79. MacGarvey NC, Suliman HB, Bartz RR. Activation of mitochondrial biogenesis by heme oxygenase-1-mediated NF-E2-related factor-2 induction rescues mice from lethal *Staphylococcus aureus* sepsis. Am J Respir Crit Care Med. 2012;185:851–61.

80. Calvert JW, Elston M, Nicholson CK. Genetic and pharmacologic hydrogen sulfide therapy attenuates ischemia-induced heart failure in mice. Circulation. 2010;122:11–9.

81. Peake BF, Nicholson CK, Lambert JP. Hydrogen sulfide preconditions the db/db diabetic mouse heart against ischemia-reperfusion injury by activating Nrf2 signaling in an Erk-dependent manner. Am J Physiol Heart Circ Physiol. 2013;304:H1215–24.

82. Itoh K, Chiba T, Takahashi S. An Nrf2/small Maf heterodimer mediates the induction of phase II detoxifying enzyme genes through antioxidant response elements. Biochem Biophys Res Commun. 1997;236:313–22.

83. Hourihan JM, Kenna JG, Hayes JD. The gasotransmitter hydrogen sulfide induces Nrf2-target genes by inactivating the Keap1 ubiquitin ligase substrate adaptor through formation of a disulfide bond between Cys-226 and Cys-613. Antioxid Redox Signal. 2013;19:465–81. https://doi.org/10.1089/ars.2012.4944.

84. Koike S, Ogasawara Y, Shibuya N, Kimura H, Ishii K. 77 Polysulfide exerts a protective effect against cytotoxicity caused by *t*-butylhydroperoxide through Nrf2 signaling in neuroblastoma cells. FEBS Lett. 2013;587:3548–55.

85. Zivanovic J, Kouroussis E, Kohl JB, Adhikari B, Bursac B, Schott-Roux S, Petrovic D, Miljkovic JL, Thomas-Lopez D, Jung Y, et al. Selective persulfide detection reveals evolutionarily conserved antiaging effects of S-sulfhydration. Cell Metab. 2019;30:1152–1170. e13. https://doi.org/10.1016/j.cmet.2019.10.007.

86. Miller DL, Roth MB. Hydrogen sulfide increases thermotolerance and lifespan in *Caenorhabditis elegans*. Proc Natl Acad Sci U S A. 2007;104:20618–22. https://doi.org/10.1073/pnas.0710191104.

87. Takekawa M, Tatebayashi K, Saito H. Conserved docking site is essential for activation of mammalian MAP kinase kinases by specific MAP kinase kinase kinases. Mol Cell. 2005;18:295–306. https://doi.org/10.1016/j.molcel.2005.04.001.

88. Giovinazzo D, Bursac B, Sbodio JI, Nalluru S, Vignane T, Snowman AM, Albacarys LM, Sedlak TW, Torregrossa R, Whiteman M, et al. Hydrogen sulfide is neuroprotective in Alzheimer's disease by sulfhydrating GSK3β and inhibiting tau hyperphosphorylation. Proc Natl Acad Sci U S A. 2021;118:e2017225118. https://doi.org/10.1073/pnas.2017225118.

89. Yang P, Zhang Y, Pang J. Loss of Jak2 impairs endothelial function by attenuating Raf-1/MEK1/Sp-1 signaling along with altered eNOS activities. Am J Pathol. 2013;183:617–25.

90. Saha S, Chakraborty PK, Xiong X. Cystathionine β-synthase regulates endothelial function via protein S-sulfhydration. FASEB J. 2016;30:441–56.

91. Bibli SI, Szabo C, Chatzianastasiou A. Hydrogen sulfide preserves endothelial nitric oxide synthase function by inhibiting proline-rich kinase 2: implications for cardiomyocyte survival and cardioprotection. Mol Pharmacol. 2017;92:718–30.

92. Zhao K, Ju Y, Li S, Altaany Z, Wang R, Yang G. S-Sulfhydration of MEK1 leads to PARP-1 activation and DNA damage repair. EMBO Rep. 2014;15:792–800.

93. Zhang MY, Dugbartey GJ, Juriasingani S, Akbari M, Liu W, Haig A, McLeod P, Arp J, Sener A. Sodium thiosulfate-supplemented UW solution protects renal grafts against prolonged cold ischemia-reperfusion injury in a murine model of syngeneic kidney transplantation. Biomed Pharmacother. 2022;145:112435. https://doi.org/10.1016/j.biopha.2021.112435.

94. Chien CT, Lee PH, Chen CF, Ma MC, Lai MK, Hsu SM. de Novo demonstration and co-localization of free-radical production and apoptosis formation in rat kidney subjected to ischemia/reperfusion. J Am Soc Nephrol. 2001;12(5):973–82.

95. Yang CC, Yao CA, Yang JC, Chien CT. Sialic acid rescues repurified lipopolysaccharide-induced acute renal failure via inhibiting TLR4/PKC/gp91-mediated endoplasmic reticulum stress, apoptosis, autophagy, and pyroptosis signaling. Toxicol Sci. 2014;141(1):155–65.

 96. Su LJ, Zhang JH, Gomez H, Murugan R, Hong X, Xu D, Jiang F, Peng ZY. Reactive oxygen species-induced lipid peroxidation in apoptosis, autophagy, and ferroptosis. Oxid Med Cell Longev. 2019;2019:5080843.
 97. Zhuo WQ, Wen Y, Luo HJ, Luo ZL, Wang L. Mechanisms of ferroptosis in chronic kidney disease. Front Mol Biosci. 2022;9:975582.
 98. Zhou Y, Zhang J, Guan Q, Tao X, Wang J, Li W. The role of ferroptosis in the development of acute and chronic kidney diseases. J Cell Physiol. 2022;237(12):4412–27.
 99. Jialal I, Fuller CJ, Huet BA. The effect of alpha-tocopherol supplementation on LDL oxidation. A dose-response study. Arterioscler Thromb Vasc Biol. 1995;15(2):190–8.
100. Huang KC, Yang CC, Lee KT, Chien CT. Reduced hemodialysis-induced oxidative stress in end-stage renal disease patients by electrolyzed reduced water. Kidney Int. 2003;64(2):704–14.
101. Cheng YH, Yao CA, Yang CC, Hsu SP, Chien CT. Sodium thiosulfate through preserving mitochondrial dynamics ameliorates oxidative stress induced renal apoptosis and ferroptosis in 5/6 nephrectomized rats with chronic kidney diseases. PLoS One. 2023;18(2):e0277652.
102. Selk N, Rodby RA. Unexpectedly severe metabolic acidosis associated with sodium thiosulfate therapy in a patient with calcific uremic arteriolopathy. Semin Dial. 2011;24(1):85–8.
103. Shirazian S, Aina O, Park Y, Chowdhury N, Leger K, Hou L, Miyawaki N, Mathur VS. Chronic kidney disease-associated pruritus: impact on quality of life and current management challenges. Int J Nephrol Renovasc Dis. 2017;10:11–26.
104. Verduzco HA, Shirazian S. CKD-associated pruritus: new insights into diagnosis, pathogenesis, and management. Kidney Int Rep. 2020;5:1387–402.
105. Mathur VS, Lindberg J, Germain M, et al. A longitudinal study of uremic pruritus in hemodialysis patients. Clin J Am Soc Nephrol. 2010;5(8):1410–9.
106. Ozen N, Cinar FI, Askin D, Mut D. Uremic pruritus and associated factors in hemodialysis patients: a multi-center study. Kidney Res Clin Pract. 2018;37:138–47.
107. Kimmel M, Alscher DM, Dunst R, Braun N, Machleidt C, Kiefer T, Stülten C, van der Kuip H, Pauli-Magnus C, Raub U, Kuhlmann U, Mettang T. The role of micro-inflammation in the pathogenesis of uraemic pruritus in haemodialysis patients. Nephrol Dial Transplant. 2006;21(3):749–55.
108. Rayner HC, Larkina M, Wang M, et al. International comparisons of prevalence, awareness, and treatment of pruritus in people on hemodialysis. Clin J Am Soc Nephrol. 2017;12:2000–7.
109. Wikström B, Gellert R, Ladefoged SD, et al. Kappa-opioid system in uremic pruritus: multicenter, randomized, double-blind, placebo-controlled clinical studies. J Am Soc Nephrol. 2005;16:3742–7.
110. Eusebio-Alpapara KMV, Castillo RL, Dofitas BL. Gabapentin for uremic pruritus: a systematic review of randomized controlled trials. Int J Dermatol. 2020;59:412–22.
111. De Marchi S, Cecchin E, Villalta D, Sepiacci G, Santini G, Bartoli E. Relief of pruritus and decreases in plasma histamine concentrations during erythropoietin therapy in patients with uremia. N Engl J Med. 1992;326(15):969–74.
112. Balaskas EV, Uldall RP. Erythropoietin treatment does not improve uremic pruritus. Perit Dial Int. 1992;12(3):330–1.
113. Peer G, Kivity S, Agami O, Fireman E, Silverberg D, Blum M, Laina A. Randomised crossover trial of naltrexone in uraemic pruritus. Lancet. 1996;348(9041):1552–4.
114. Pauli-Magnus C, Mikus G, Alscher DM, et al. Naltrexone does not relieve uremic pruritus: results of a randomized, placebo-controlled crossover-study. J Am Soc Nephrol. 2000;11(3):514–9.
115. Song YH, Wang SY, Lang JH, Xiao YF, Cai GY, Chen XM. Therapeutic effect of intravenous sodium thiosulfate for uremic pruritus in hemodialysis patients. Ren Fail. 2020;42:987–93.
116. Lu PH, Chuo HE, Kuo KL, Liao JF, Lu PH. Clinical efficacy and safety of sodium thiosulfate in the treatment of uremic pruritus: a meta-analysis of randomized controlled trials. Toxins (Basel). 2021;13(11):769.

Index

A

Acute coronary syndrome, 194
Acute kidney injury (AKI), 121–123, 126, 127, 144, 149
Adenosine triphosphate (ATP), 160
Adenosine triphosphate (ATP)-sensitive potassium (K_{ATP}) channels, 3, 96, 97, 151
Adipocyte-derived relaxing factor, 97
AKT phosphorylation, 211
Albuminuria, 149
Allogeneic transplantation, 187
Allyl disulfide, 153
Alpha-blockers, 150
Alpha-lipoic acid (ALA), 14
Alzheimer's disease, 212
Ameliorates
    anti-inflammatory property, 27, 28
    antioxidant action, 25–27
    apoptotic machinery and proximal tubular cells, 28
    endogenous and exogenous H_2S, 25
    nephrotoxic metabolites, 26
Aminooxycetic acid (AOAA), 7, 164, 167, 168
Aminopeptidase N (APN), 26
Anemia, 45, 46
Anemia of inflammation (AI), 45
Anemia-relieving effect, 45, 46
Angiotensin II (Ang II), 48, 147
Ang II-induced hypertension, 51, 103–105
Angiotensin-converting enzyme (ACE) inhibitor, 147
Angiotensin-converting enzyme 2 (ACE2), 120, 121, 123, 124, 129–132, 135
Anti-inflammatory cytokines, 133, 190
Anti-inflammatory effects, 173
Antioxidants, 210
    effect, 168, 190
    therapy, 213
AP123, 128
AP39, 128, 187
Apolipoprotein L1 (APOL1), 126, 127
Apoptosis, 28, 131, 132, 145, 188
Apoptotic index, 192
AQP-2 protein expression, 9
Aquaporins (AQPs), 4, 12–14
Artificial intelligence-based binding affinity, 129
ATB-346, 129, 154
Atherosclerosis, 94
Autopsy, 122
Autosomal dominant polycystic kidney disease (ADPKD)
    definition, 53
    development, 53
    pharmacological agent, 55, 56
    vascular endothelial dysfunction
        inflammation, 54
        oxidative stress, 54, 55

B

Benign prostatic hyperplasia, 144
β-lactam antibiotics, 29
Blood pressure (BP), 93, 94
Blood urea nitrogen (BUN), 122

© The Editor(s) (if applicable) and The Author(s), under exclusive license to Springer Nature Switzerland AG 2023
G. J. Dugbartey, A. Sener, *Hydrogen Sulfide in Kidney Diseases*,
https://doi.org/10.1007/978-3-031-44041-0

C
Calcific uremic arteriolopathy, 207
Calcium-Based nephrolithiasis
    clinical application, 109, 110
    genetic factor, 107
    H_2S attenuates, 108, 109
    hypercalciuria, 107
    oxalate, 107, 108
    prevalence, 106, 107
Calcium oxalate (CaOx), 107, 108
CaOx dihydrate (COD), 108
CaOx monohydrate (COM), 108
Carbon monoxide (CO), 151
Cardiac fibrosis, 188
Cardiomyocytes, 188
Cardioprotection, 188, 189
Cardiopulmonary arrest, 2
Cardiovascular system, 212
    blood pressure-lowering effect, 95, 97, 98
    K_{ATP} channels, 97
    malfunction, 98–100
Caspase-mediated apoptotic pathway, 145
Cellular ATP depletion, 209
Cellular oxidative metabolism, 186
Cellular processes, 154
Cellular signaling pathways, 204
Chemotherapy, 124
Chronic hypoxia hypothesis, 40
Chronic kidney disease (CKD), 123, 144,
        213, 214
    characteristics, 41
    classification, 40
    clinical trials, 41
    cytoplasm and mitochondria, 41
    definition, 40
    EPO production and anemia, 45, 46
    gasotransmitters, 51
    HIF and progression, 42–44
    medullary oxygenation and hypoxia, 42
    mortality, 39
    oxidative and endoplasmic reticulum
        stress, 49–51
    pathophysiology, 40, 41
    renal fibrosis and inflammatory
        response, 46–48
Chronic renal injury, 149
Cisplatin- and gentamicin-induced acute
        kidney injury (AKI)
    ameliorates
        anti-inflammatory property, 27, 28
        antioxidant action, 25–27
        apoptotic machinery and proximal
            tubular cells, 28
        endogenous and exogenous H_2S, 25
        nephrotoxic metabolites, 26
    clinical reports, 24
    definition, 23
    gentamicin
        β-lactam antibiotics, 29
        clinical manifestations, 29
        complication, 29
        hydrogen sulfide attenuates, 30–32
        mechanisms, 30, 31
    high-dose cisplatin therapy, 24
    history, 23
    limitations, 32, 33
    RBF and GFR, 29
    tubular injury pathway, 24
c-Jun N-terminal kinase (JNK), 210
CKD-associated pruritus (CKD-aP), 214
Cl^-/HCO_3^- exchanger, 9
Cold ischemia/reperfusion injury (IRI)
    effects and mechanisms, 172
    heart transplantation, 187
        antioxidant defense system, 189
        antioxidant effect, 189
        apoptotic machinery, 188
        cyclophilin D-independent
            mechanism, 188
        DATS-MSN treatment, 188
        graft performance, 188
        in vitro and in vivo murine model, 187
    H2S suppresses renal inflammation,
        172, 173
    induces renal vasodilation, 171
    inhibits apoptosis, 170
    intestinal transplantation, 192, 193
    kidney transplantation, 185–187
    limitations, 194, 195
    liver transplantation, 191
    lung transplantation, 189, 190
    mitochondrial homeostasis, 170
    pancreas transplantation, 191, 192
    preservation, 160, 161
    protects and prolongs renal graft
        function, 167
    scavenges ROS and preserves renal
        function, 167, 168
    sources of production
        endogenous source, 183
        enzymatic production, 183, 184
        exogenous sources, 184, 185
        non-enzymatic production, 184
    translation from bench to bedside, 193, 194
Cold-stored porcine kidneys, 7
Collagen, 70

Congenital obstructive nephropathy, 144
Congestive heart failure (CHF), 154
COVID-19-related kidney injury
    ACE2, 120
    AKI, 121–123
    antiviral action of H2S and
            mechanisms, 129–133
    antiviral agents, 127
    APOL1, 126, 127
    CKD, 123
    diabetic nephropathy, 123, 124
    endogenous and exogenous sources of
            H2S, 128, 129
    ESRD, 125, 126
    kidney infarction, 124, 125
    kidney transplantation, 126
    potential biomarker, final outcome,
            133, 134
    renal cancer, 124
    treatment, 127, 128
Cyclosporine, 171
Cystathionine beta-synthase (CBS), 3, 5–9, 11,
        128, 151, 205
Cystathionine gamma-lyase (CSE), 3, 5, 7–9,
        128, 151, 205
Cyclosporine-induced vasoconstriction, 7, 171
Cysteine, 188
Cytochrome c oxidase, 4
Cytokine-storm syndrome, 120, 133
Cytoprotective effects, 211, 212
Cytoprotective pathways, 164

D
Damage-associated molecular patterns
        (DAMPs), 146
D-amino acid oxidase (DAO), 95, 128, 161,
        183, 184
D-cysteine, 4, 95, 128, 205
Delayed graft function (DGF), 160
Detrimental effects, 164
Diabetic kidney disease (DKD)
    clinical application, 82, 83
    clinical manifestations, 71
    cytosolic enzymes, 71, 72
    definition, 69
    ECM, 70
    FSGS, 80–82
    future perspectives, 82, 83
    gasotransmitters, 71
    glomeruli, 72
    glycation end-products and
            dyslipidemia, 70
    history, 70

    hyperglycemia
        inflammation, 76, 77
        renal fibrosis, 73, 75, 76
        ROS production, 73, 74
    hypertension, 70
    in vitro and in vivo studies, 71
    limitations, 80
    RAAS, 77–79
    renal functional changes, 79
    therapeutic agents, 70
    vascular complications, 72
Diabetic nephropathy, 123, 124
Diallyl disulfide (DADS), 26, 30–32
Diallyl sulfide (DAS), 26, 31, 32
Disseminated intravascular coagulopathy
        (DIC), 125
Diuretics, 149
Donation-after-cardiac-death (DCD), 171
Dopamine, 132, 164
D-penicillamine, 150

E
Electron donor, 166
Electron microscopy, 122
Electron transport chain (ETC), 166, 169, 183,
        187, 204, 209
Enalapril, 147
Endoplasmic reticulum stress, 49–51
End-organ dysfunction, 182
Endothelial NOS (eNOS), 154
Endothelium-derived hyperpolarizing
        factor, 97
Endothelium-derived relaxing factor, 97
End-stage renal disease (ESRD), 40, 43–46,
        125, 126, 144
Epithelial-mesenchymal transition (EMT),
        147, 148, 153
Epithelial sodium channels (ENac), 100
Erythropoietin (EPO), 45, 46
Expanded criteria donors (ECD), 174
Extracellular matrix (ECM), 70, 146, 151, 154
Ex vivo reperfusion, 191

F
Fibroblasts, 147
Fibrosis, 146
Fibrotic pathway, 147
Flank pain, 150
Focal segmental glomerulosclerosis
        (FSGS), 80–82
Food and Drugs Administration
        (FDA), 204

G
Gamma-glutamyl transpeptidase (GGT), 26
Gaseous signaling molecules, 120
Gasotransmitters, 97, 150, 154, 161, 182, 189,
        195, 204
Gene expression, 131
Gene transcription, 130, 132
Gentamicin
        β-lactam antibiotics, 29
        clinical manifestations, 29
        complication, 29
        hydrogen sulfide attenuates, 30–32
        mechanisms, 30, 31
Glomerular atrophy, 171
Glomerular basement membrane (GBM), 70
Glomerular filtration rate (GFR), 29, 100, 101,
        145, 187
Glomerulopathy, 127
Glucose-induced kidney injury, 154, 155
Glucose-lowering effect, 76
Glutathione (GSH), 74, 129, 188, 205, 206
Glutathione peroxidase 4 (GPX4), 213
Glutathione persulfide (GSSH), 206
Glutathione-S-transferase (GST), 26
Graft function, 167, 170, 171
GYY4137, 153, 161, 184, 193, 212

H
Heart transplantation, 187–189
Hematuria, 122
Hemodialysis, 214
Hemodynamics, 144
Hepcidin, 45
Hibernation, 161
High-salt-induced hypertension, 10, 98, 105
Homocysteine, 168
Human metapneumovirus, 133
Hydrogen gas, 192
Hydrogen sulfide (H2S)
        cold ischemia/reperfusion injury (*see* Cold
                ischemia/reperfusion injury (IRI))
        donor, 128, 130–133, 152
                molecules, 182, 185, 187–195
        endogenous source, 183
        enzymatic production, 183, 184
        exogenous sources, 184, 185
        non-enzymatic production, 184
        renal graft preservation (*see* Renal graft
                preservation)
Hydroxychloroquine, 134
Hyperglycemia
        inflammation, 76, 77
        renal fibrosis, 73, 75, 76

ROS production, 73, 74
Hyperhomocysteinemia (HHcy), 7, 51–53, 81
Hyperhomocysteinemia-induced
        cardiomyocyte injury, 132
Hyperkalemia, 150
Hyperoxaluria, 208
Hypertensive nephropathy
        atherosclerosis, 94
        blood pressure, 93, 94
        cardiovascular system
                blood pressure-lowering effect,
                        95, 97, 98
                K_{ATP} channels, 96, 97
                malfunction, 98–100
        clinical application, 109, 110
        endogenous and exogenous
                sources, 94–96
        fibrosis, 104, 105
        fluid and electrolyte balance, 93
        gasotransmitter, 106
        nitric oxide and carbon monoxide, 94
        RAAS, 101, 102
        RBF and GFR, 100, 101
        renal dysfunction, 93
        renal inflammation, 103, 104
        renal tubular function, 100
        ROS-induced oxidative stress, 102, 103
        vascular and antihypertensive effects, 94
Hypometabolism, 185
Hypothermia, 185
Hypoxia-inducible factor (HIF), 40, 42–44

I
Inducible NOS (iNOS), 154, 155
Inflammation, 152
Integrity, 213
Interleukin-6 (IL-6), 133
Intestinal transplantation, 192, 193
Intracellular messenger molecule, 128
Intravenous sodium sulfide (IK-1001),
        153, 154
Isatis indigotica, 129
Ischemia, 165, 166, 169
Ischemia-reperfusion injury (IRI), 51, 151,
        160, 161, 209, 210
        See also Cold ischemia/reperfusion
                injury (IRI)
Ischemic injury, 160

K
Kaliuresis, 7, 8
Kidney infarction, 124, 125

Kidney injury molecule (KIM-1), 132
Kidney transplantation, 126, 185–187, 212

L
L-arginine, 151
L-cysteine, 3, 4, 71, 94, 95, 128, 151
Lethal effect, 2
Leukocyte adhesion molecules, 104
Liver transplantation, 191
Loratadine, 214
Lorsartan, 147
Lung transplantation, 189, 190

M
Macrophages, 146
Macula densa cells, 10
Malondialdehyde (MDA), 152
Mammalian hibernation, 161–164
Matrix metalloproteinase (MMP), 105
Matrix metalloproteinase (MMP-9), 81
Mediators, 173
Mesenteric perfusion, 193
Mesoporous silica nanoparticles (MSN), 188
Metabolic rate, 163, 166
Middle East Respiratory Syndrome (MERS-CoV), 120
Mitochondrial adenosine triphosphate (ATP)-sensitive potassium (KATP) channel, 210
Mitochondrial dynamics, 213
Mitochondrial integrity, 170
Mitochondrial permeability transition pore (MPTP), 28, 169, 170
Mitochondrial respiratory chain, 166
Mitochondrial-targeting molecule, 168
Mitogen-activated protein kinases (MAPK), 27
Molecular pathways, 194
Monocyte chemoattractant protein-1 (MCP-1), 54, 146
Mortality, 123
mRNA expression, 187
Multisystem organ dysfunction, 133–134

N
Na$^+$/K$^+$-ATPase activity, 8, 9, 100
N-acetylcysteine (NAC), 130, 131, 134, 168
Natriuresis, 7, 8
Nephrectomy, 213
Nephrotic syndrome, 80

Neurotransmitters, 163
NF-κB expression, 152
Nipah virus, 133
Nitric oxide (NO), 3, 150, 154
Nitric oxide synthases (NOS), 150
NO/cGMP/sGC/PKG pathway, 8
Non-steroidal anti-inflammatory drugs (NSAID), 150, 154
Normoglycemia, 191
Nuclear factor erythroid-related factor 2 (Nrf2), 210

O
Obesity, 126
Obstructive nephropathy
  animal models, 149
  endogenous gasotransmitters, 150, 151
    GYY4137, H2S donor, 153
    H2S in, 151–153
  pathogenesis of, 144, 148
    hemodynamics and functional changes, 144, 145
    renal interstitial inflammation, 146
    renal tubular cell death, 145
    tubulointerstitial fibrosis, 146, 147
  pharmacological treatments, 149, 150
  recovery of renal function, 148, 149
  research and development, clinically viable H2S donors, 153, 154
Odds ratio (OR), 122
Olfactory paralysis, 2
Osteopontin, 54
Oxidative and endoplasmic reticulum stress, 49–51
Oxygen consumption, 147

P
Pancreas transplantation, 191, 192
Pattern recognition receptors (PRRs), 131
Perfusion, 165, 171
Persulfide dioxygenase, 206
Phenylephrine-induced vasoconstriction, 97
Platelet–leukocyte aggregates, 134
Porcine model, 7
Post-obstructive renal function, 149
Post-transplant outcome, 194
Potassium citrate, 149–150
Pro-inflammatory cytokines, 150, 151
Pro-inflammatory elements, 192
Pro-inflammatory genes, 208
Pro-inflammatory mediators, 133, 146

Pro-inflammatory pathway, 133
Propargylglycine (PAG), 7
Prostacyclin, 144
Prostaglandin, 144
Prostate cancer, 144
Proteinuria, 122
Proximal tubular epithelial cell (PTEC)
          gene, 124

Q
Quiescent proximal tubular cells, 24
Quinone oxidoreductase, 205

R
Rapamycin, 167
Reactive oxygen species (ROS), 129, 145,
          152, 161, 185, 208, 213
Renal blood flow (RBF), 4, 7, 29, 100,
          101, 167
Renal cancer, 124
Renal cell carcinoma (RCC), 124
Renal damage, 144
Renal fibrosis, 46–48, 73, 75, 76, 104, 105,
          152, 154, 155
Renal graft, 160, 170–172
     preservation
          ATP stimulation, low
               concentrations, 166
          cold preservation, 160, 161
          enzymatic pathways, 161
          induces renal vasodilation, 171, 172
          inhibits apoptosis, 170
          ischemia, 165, 166
          lower metabolic rate, at high
               concentrations, 166
          mammalian hibernation, 161–164
          mitochondrial homeostasis, 170
          protects and prolongs renal graft
               function, 167
          scavenges ROS and preserves renal
               function, 167, 168
          suppresses renal inflammation, cold
               IRI, 172, 173
     quality, 182
Renal injury, 167, 208
Renal ischemia-reperfusion injury, 8, 182
Renal system
     cellular physiology, 7
     endogenous biological signaling
          molecule, 3, 4

excretory function, 7–9
functional anatomy, 4, 5
history, 1–3
oxygen sensor, 9, 10
production, 5–7
RAAS, 10, 11
renal water handling, 12–14
Renal tubular function, 100
Renin-angiotensin-aldosterone system
          (RAAS), 10, 11, 48, 77–79, 101,
          102, 121, 145
Renoprotective effect, 164, 214
Renovascular hypertension, 208, 209
Reperfusion, 188
Reverse reaction, 206
Rhodanase, 206
ROS-scavenging property, 190

S
Sepsis-induced myocardial dysfunction
          (SIMD), 131
Serum concentration, 131
Severe acute respiratory syndrome corona
          virus-2 (SARS-CoV-2), 120–124,
          126, 128–132, 135
Significant activation of sirtuin1 (SIRT1)
          signaling, 190
Sodium citrate, 150
Sodium hydrosulfide (NaHS), 96–98,
          100–103, 105, 108
Sodium polysulthionate (SG-1002), 153, 154
Sodium thiosulfate (STS), 129
     biological properties, 206, 207
     clinical applications
          CKD, 213, 214
          H2S donor drugs, 210–212
          IRI, 209, 210
          kidney transplantation, 212
          renovascular hypertension, 208, 209
          uremic pruritus, 214, 215
     clinical usefulness of, 207
     FDA, 204
     gasotransmitter, 204
     H2S generation, thiosulfate, 205, 206
     mechanisms of action, 208
     metabolic pathways, 205
     mitochondrial sulfide oxidation pathway,
          205, 206
     toxic effect, H2S, 204
Spontaneously hypertensive rats (SHR), 94,
          97–100, 103–105

Static cold storage (SCS), 185, 187, 192, 193
Streptozotocin (STZ), 76–80, 191
Sulfane sulfur, 206
Sulfide oxidation pathway, 205, 206, 211, 215
Sulfur dioxygenase, 205
Sulfur oxidation pathway, 212
Sulfur transferase, 206
Superoxide dismutase (SOD), 74, 152
Suppression, 163
Sympathetic nervous system, 131

T
TGF-β1, 146–148, 154
Therapeutic hypothermia, 132
Thiosulfate, 185, 205–207, 209
3-chymotrypsin-like protease, 129
3-mercaptopyruvate sulfurtransferase
    (3-MST), 128, 151, 161, 205
Thrombolytic/anti-thrombotic property, 134
Tiopronin, 150
Tissue hypoxia, 166
Toll-like receptors (TLRs), 131
Torpor, 165
Torpor-arousal cycle, 161–163
Toxicity, 183
Transcription factor, 210
Transmembrane protease serine 2
    (TMPRSS2), 120
Trans-sulfuration pathway, 183
Trypanosomiasis, 126
Tubular system, 4
Tubulointerstitial fibrosis, 46, 151
Tubulointerstitial hypoxia, 40
Tumour necrosis factor α (TNF-α), 145, 147
Two-kidney-one-clip (2K1C) model, 10
Type 1 diabetes mellitus, 191
Type 2 diabetes mellitus, 154, 155, 194

U
Ulcerative colitis, 44
Unilateral ureteral obstruction and
    reimplantation (UUO-R)
    model, 149
Unilateral ureteral/urinary obstruction (UUO),
    47, 48, 50, 144, 145, 148, 149,
    151, 155
    see also Obstructive nephropathy
United States Food and Drug Administration
    (FDA), 127, 193
University of Wisconsin (UW) solution, 160, 212
Uremic pruritus, 214, 215
Urinary obstruction, 144, 145, 151, 155

V
Vascular endothelial dysfunction
    inflammation, 54
    oxidative stress, 54, 55
Vascular smooth muscle cells
    (VSMCs), 96, 97
Vasoconstriction, 145, 147, 171
Vasodilation, 171, 186, 215
Vasodilatory effect, 8, 171
Vasorelaxant effect, 154
Vimentin, 147, 148
Vitamin deficiency, 49
von Willebrand factor antigen, 125

X
Xanthine oxidase inhibitors, 150

Z
Zofenopril, 129, 154, 210
Zucker diabetic fatty (ZDF), 80

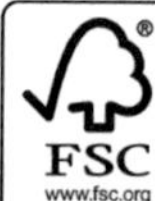

MIX
Papier aus verantwortungsvollen Quellen
Paper from responsible sources
FSC® C105338

If you have any concerns about our products,
you can contact us on
ProductSafety@springernature.com

In case Publisher is established outside the EU,
the EU authorized representative is:
**Springer Nature Customer Service Center GmbH
Europaplatz 3, 69115 Heidelberg, Germany**

Printed by Libri Plureos GmbH
in Hamburg, Germany